•

HEALTH CARE AND
THE ETHICS OF ENCOUNTER

•

STUDIES IN SOCIAL MEDICINE

Allan M. Brandt and Larry R. Churchill, editors

LAURIE ZOLOTH

HEALTH CARE
AND THE ETHICS
OF ENCOUNTER

A Jewish Discussion
of Social Justice

THE UNIVERSITY OF NORTH CAROLINA PRESS

Chapel Hill and London

Set in Electra with MetaPlus by Keystone Typesetting, Inc.

Manufactured in the United States of America

The paper in this book meets the guidelines for permanence and
durability of the Committee on Production Guidelines for
Book Longevity of the Council on Library Resources.

Library of Congress Cataloging-in-Publication Data

Zoloth, Laurie.
Health care and the ethics of encounter :
a Jewish discussion of social justice / by Laurie Zoloth.
p. cm. — (Studies in social medicine)

Based on the author's dissertation (doctoral)—Graduate Theological
Union in California, 1993. Includes bibliographical references and index.
ISBN 0-8078-2418-6 (cloth: alk. paper)
ISBN 0-8078-4828-X (pbk.: alk. paper)
1. Health care rationing—Religious aspects—Judaism.
2. Right to health care—Religious aspects—Judaism.
3. Distributive justice—Religious aspects—Judaism.
I. Title.   II. Series.
RA410.5.Z65 1998
296.3'642—dc21   97-45978
                                                      CIP

03 02 01 00 99   5 4 3 2 1

CONTENTS

•

FOREWORD

•

A scholarly series is typically begun in order to define a field, to set forth standards for research in that field, or to call attention to an area of growing social importance. All three aims are appropriate to Studies in Social Medicine.

The term "social medicine" dates from the work of Jules Guerin, Rudolf Virchow, and other nineteenth-century physicians and served to underscore their conviction that medicine should address the human misery resulting from industrialization. Donald Madison, a contemporary social medicine faculty member at the University of North Carolina, has traced the various movements and ambitions of those who espouse social medicine from Guerin and Virchow to the present. He identifies several common themes. Among these are investigations of the causes and distribution of diseases, an emphasis on prevention, concern for the organization and delivery of health services, a focus on "community," and the importance of political action and public policy in matters of health. These themes are not confined to specific disciplines, but name areas of focus associated with deeply held convictions that motivate both scholarly studies and practical action.

Contemporary scholars who claim this agenda for their work come from a wide variety of disciplines, including medical history, health care ethics, medical sociology and anthropology, the politics and economics of health care, and literary studies of health and disease, as well as the more traditional fields of social epidemiology, prevention, and public health. This broad array of disciplines is appropriate, as medicine has enlarged its realm of influence by measure of both dollars and cultural impact, and as American society itself has become increasingly and more self-consciously concerned with health.

In inaugurating Studies in Social Medicine we intentionally cast a large and indeterminate net. We hope to publish volumes by scholars in each of the areas mentioned above, but with the essential prerequisite that all such work must enhance our understanding of the interaction between medicine, health care, and the larger society. We seek new ways to understand the shifts in the social environment that affect medicine and health care, as well as changes in medical practices and with medical professionals and their patients that alter the social, ethical, or political ecology.

Health Care and the Ethics of Encounter, one of the first books in this social medicine series, is an emblematic volume for these aims. This book emerged from Zoloth's academic research in a religious studies doctoral program, but it is marked throughout by her practical work as a consulting bioethicist, a mother, a feminist, and most recently, the director of a university academic program in Jewish studies that is oriented to engagement with community. She is a practitioner in each of these realms, but one who refuses to treat these realms as separated. As she notes in the Introduction, this book was born of her efforts to put the voices from these many spheres of activity into conversation.

This book is broad and ambitious in its scope. It deals with the larger social meanings to be discerned from the Oregon Health Care Plan and contains the best explication yet available of this effort. Zoloth defines what is important about the Oregon experiment as an example of how people can learn to talk to one another, as a breakthrough in conversation. She demonstrates how the language of communal responsibility can transcend the usual idioms of reform and present a paradigm for thinking and talking that values both individual and communal life. The question for Zoloth is not "What are my rights?" but "How can we live together?" probing past possessive individualism to embrace individuals in a social context. Part of the originality of Zoloth's work is that she finds a compelling way to argue her thesis through a fresh reading of the scriptural account of Ruth and Naomi, drawing upon the work of Emmanuel Levinas, among others. The result is a volume offering many insights into the social meaning of health care in American society—a place to begin the next national conversation about reforming our health care system.

Allan M. Brandt
Larry R. Churchill

PREFACE

•

The social world around us is tempted by new yearning and shaken with crisis—a crisis of scarce resources, increasing demands for services, and increasingly contentious arguments about the just allocation of contested public goods. In these arguments, the politics of personal identity, the ethical principle of autonomy and its association with individual rights, and the philosophic claim of entitlement have become central. But the vision that a claim of entitlement projects is increasingly problematic in the face of profound social trouble and a flight from the shared goods of the public square. A rift grows between global wealth and global scarcity. Our arguments seem to be increasingly circular, a competition won by power rather than justice. What is amiss? Why has a theory of justice failed to give workable solutions to a practical public yearning for justice?

Many theorists, both secular and religious—among them, Larry R. Churchill, Robert Bellah, and Carol Gilligan—have suggested that in moral philosophy the very concepts of individualism and entitlement must be challenged; they claim that addressing the problem of justice in a crisis of allocation requires different language—the language of communal responsibility—rather than the language of individual entitlement. These theorists suggest that there are two crises, the crisis of scarce resources and the crisis of language within the discourse of ethics adequate to frame a response. Many arguments have been advanced, in popular culture and in academic theory, for the necessity of a new language of morality. This book is an agreement with and a continuation of those arguments. So why another book about the discourse of justice and public policy?

I believe another book is warranted because I intend to add another voice. The debate has been far-reaching yet incomplete: as a rule it has been largely marked by the silence of the moral voice of the Jewish textual tradition.

Why should we introduce, and value, a distinctive Jewish moral voice? This is a question that I will ask insistently. It is a question about the use of the particular in the work of the public, and about the role of the religious in the conversation on policy. In large part we should heed this voice because the Jewish tradition normatively envisions an ethics of conversational encounter that is deeply social and deeply public. The Jewish tradition offers resources of method, text, and history for the recovery of a language of public values of *community* that addresses the conceptual and framing issues raised by the critical allocation debate. It is precisely such a language that ethicists in the feminist, Christian, and secular traditions have called for. Reclaiming this language means giving serious attention to an ethical decision-making model that is contextual and narrative—and conversational. This model entails an ethics organized around an encounter rooted in a moral community of meaning—an ethics of encounter—and it changes the way ethics can enter the actual public arena. Additionally, a recovered Jewish moral voice is critical because the debate so far has failed: all the exhortations, the careful drafting of theory, the ordinary conversation at the clinical level and at the policy level have not been able to answer the basic questions of who gets what and why, the question of social justice.

This Jewish ethical position insists on three methodological necessities. First, there is an inherent link between private desire and decision and public acts of moral choice. Conscience (the individual, interior discernment of the morally appropriate choice) and human community (the interdependent relationships between the self and the other) are mutually shaped and shaping, constructed by and constructing any social order. Second, not only are public and private acts inherently linked, but the focus on community means we must make a shift in the paradigm of analysis from the agent of moral action (defined as an individual actor) to the nature of moral agency itself. Ethics is a collective gesture that needs a language of mutuality and interdependence. Third, the focus on community needs a full, multivoiced, and hence representative, decisional process in both the theory and the practice of ethics and justice.

Three features of this book lie at the heart of its analysis and argument and deserve to be called to the reader's particular attention. The first is a description of a critical and specific public choice: the allocation of resources necessitated by the crisis in health care. As an example of how this choice is made, we will look at the Oregon Health Care Decision Making Project, a grassroots health care reform movement, an example of community allocation of public resources in contention with desperate appeals for autonomy and individual entitlement. This example was chosen not because it is a perfect health plan—it is not—but because it was a genuine moral gesture toward health care justice, a gesture rare in the American public sphere, both political and successful. I analyze and defend the philosophical base of the Oregon Health Care Decision Making Project *not* as a systematic critique of the economic, legal, and social factors in the allocation process, but as an illustration of how a theory of encounter works in a practical case study. I believe that while the focus of the case study presented here is medical allocation, the concepts and framing language are applicable to the allocation of other scarce social resources.

The second central feature is a description of the liberal theory that attempts to resolve the health care crisis and an analysis of selected challenges to the mainstays of liberal theory: individualism, autonomy, and personal rights.

The last feature is the search for a different language for ethical choice that emerges from a critique of liberal theory. Since I propose a solution from a different source tradition and theory, one that may be unfamiliar, I will carefully guide the reader through the Jewish texts and interpretation that frame such a language. This account of the Jewish tradition will of necessity be a limited and introductory one. I do not offer an appraisal of the entire Jewish tradition in ethics, and instead limit my analysis both in subject (resource allocation) and in quantity, using selected biblical and rabbinic texts to explore specific themes. We will revisit the philosophical and ethical debate surrounding selected texts of justice and do an exegesis of selected midrashic (narrative) and halakhic (legal) texts to seek ground for new ethical reflection on the development of alternative language to address the problem of the just allocation of scarce resources.

This book has two parts. The first is an analysis of the realities of the crisis in health care and the attendant crisis in language in the debate on reform. Chapter 1 describes the national crisis in health care and public policy as it unfolded in the 1990s in the United States. Chapter 2 introduces the Oregon health care access debates of that period and the problems of justice and allocation confronted therein, and Chapter 3 examines the reaction to the Oregon project in the ethical literature, as well as the broader problem of justice in classical source traditions. Chapter 4 describes the classical terms for debate concerning the theory of justice, offering a critical perspective on the traditional language of autonomy as individualism. Chapter 5 considers the notion of "the ethics of community" in the secular philosophical and sociological tradition, reviews selected feminist literature in which the language of community and relationality is developed, and analyzes religious traditions where the term "community" is a centerpiece of theology.

In Part II, I begin my argument for bringing Jewish ethics to the discourse. Chapter 6 discusses the Jewish ethical method and its suggestion of a different anthropology of the moral agent. The ethical theory of Emmanuel Levinas is introduced, and his proposals for our topic—an ethics of encounter—are considered. Chapter 7 is devoted to the responsa literature and the current debate in Jewish medical ethics among Jewish scholars. Halakhah is discussed relative to the contemporary crisis, using selected texts of responsibility toward the neighbor, of siege, of the *rodef* (the one who pursues), and of the flask in the desert. In Chapter 8, I turn toward a new, feminist interpretation of the Ruth story as the basis for common language. There I explore the language of encounter in the story of the stranger and her community.

It is through this encounter with the other that the Book of Ruth will offer us a new vocabulary for justice: personal, intimate, relational, and yet directly normative. And the application of this rediscovered vocabulary will allow for a different account of distributive justice. In the last chapter, we will return to the Oregon plan and ask exactly how it might look if we apply a theory of encounter and a shared language such as it suggests to the health care allocation discourse. That debate and that plan, although incomplete and flawed, still offers one of the best American attempts at justice in public health, and an emulative narrative for how the discourse of justice can proceed. At stake will be the problem of developing shared language, a language we can agree to hear, if not speak, in common, a language that allows us, in a cacophonous world, to attend to every voice with clarity, honoring the texts and the tools of each.

ACKNOWLEDGMENTS

•

I completed the research and writing of my dissertation, the first draft of what was to become this book, in the winter of 1992–93. As the days warmed slowly, I stooped to pick up the paper on the porch every morning and felt the end of the first rainy season in California in six years. For Californians, the end of the drought and the beginning of the new Clinton administration felt linked: perhaps the economy would turn again, ending the depression that had settled here like the dry brown grass had settled on the coastal hills.

Then the hills above my house turned green, and the paper was full of fascinating news. In Washington there was the first serious talk of health care reform in over a decade. Every day, my family pointed out a new article to me: "Isn't this about your dissertation?" they'd ask. Friends who knew my work for the last six years asked if I would finish the dissertation first or if the Clinton administration would solve the crisis first. Finally, one week before I turned in my final copy, the Oregon health care plan was approved for trial use.

At that time it was my fondest hope that the political system would work so smoothly that the crisis I had described in my dissertation would become an interesting piece of American history, like the shocking indignities of slavery. I thought that in time it would be unbelievable that we could have tolerated a system so transparently unjust and unwieldy. I could not have been less prescient.

A book takes a long time to gestate—longer than a child, and longer than the turns of history. In the three years since I finished the dissertation that became this book, I have given birth to a new daughter; the great teacher whose work animates this book, Emmanuel Levinas, has died; America has a new Republican Congress; and Clinton has been reelected. And the United States has a new way of debating the just allocation of health care resources. Because of changes in the system of distribution and payment, decent health care for the poorest, for any of the socially marginalized, and even for Americans with jobs, is in jeopardy. The language of the marketplace is now in the preeminent position, its claim the one that we hear most clearly in response to the crisis that surrounds us. The promise of health care for all hangs by a slender thread.

But the conversation that I have come to feel is central to an ultimate solution to the crisis will still have to be created. This is a book about what will be required to rethink the ideology that made such a crisis possible and about how a society constructs social conversation at all. It is a book about the process of the conversation, the call to hear every story, the call to reflect on the justice issues that are at the heart of any public policy decision: how do we provide for one another?

In this book, I have attempted to have all the intellectual discourses that I hold dear occur in the "same room," as it were. My theory was that if I could create such a conversation, then the language that would emerge would allow radical shifts in public policy. My life is a little like this work. There are several worlds that I try to reconcile: the world of clinical work in bioethics; the world of relationships, friends, family, and Jewish communal life; and the world of the theoretical academic study of philosophy. Such a life is, of course, only possible because of a moral community that supports my own work, and such work, about community, reflects the conversation of my generous, tolerant, and rigorous family, friends, and colleagues, who are mutual participants in my moral community.

I want to thank first my dissertation committee of extraordinary teachers, Karen Lebacqz, Clare Fisher, Carol Robb, Daniel Boyarin, and Elliott Dorff, for their support and insights throughout the process, and for their critical review of my work. Each of them, especially chair Karen Lebacqz, contributed generously of their time, enthusiasm, and considerable talents. They serve as models of careful scholarship and attentive mentoring. Larry Churchill and Baruch Brody also were supportive at critical stages in the process. Larry Churchill's persistent support of this manuscript throughout the editing process was remarkable. Daniel Matt and David Winston gave extremely important criticisms to Chapter 5. Lord Immanuel Jakobowitz and Rabbi Moshe Tendler were generous with their ideas for research.

Many others have helped. My closest colleague, Susan Rubin, collaborator in all my clinical work and constant friend, has not let me get away with a thing. Mary Pinkerson and Dena Seiden provided long distance assistance. The wonderful community of the Kaiser Permanente ethics committees, in particular chairs Martha Snider, the late Nancy Radosovich, George Peters, and Eric Cornwall; the thoughtful members of the Children's Hospital Oakland Ethics committee; and others too numerous to name individually have participated in the actual case work that makes my ideas tangible. The nurses and the physicians of the intensive care nursery at Kaiser Oakland have assessed the reality of my first ideas about bioethics by the bedside of many desperately ill newborns, many night shifts ago. Jeanne Friedman; Deborah Gerson; Vicki and Stuart Kelman; Leslie Valas; Alan Finkelstein; Toby, Ezra, and Kenneth Henden; Susan and Harvey Kayman; every single Resnikoff; and my other friends in the Berkeley Jewish community have always been generous with their intellectual and spiritual support, not to mention the years of Shabbat lunches. Becca Brown contributed her careful support as well.

At the UNC Press, Ron Maner, Sian Hunter, and Stephanie Wenzel all contributed their talent and energy to the work.

My family has been extraordinary. My wonderful parents, Helen and Art Zoloth; my aunt, Martha Cohen; Steven Zoloth, a public health scholar and brotherly supporter; Cathy Zoloth; Joan Zoloth; and Tom Dalzell have consistently encouraged me, delighting in every small victory. My eldest sons, Matthew and Noah, have listened to my theories, added their own ideas, told me never to despair, understood all lapses in mothering, and watched their baby brothers uncomplainingly. My baby sons, Benjamin and Joshua, whose arrivals blessed the years of research and writing, and Sarah, who made her entrance as this book was rewritten, reminded me constantly that relationship is prior to social contract, and that nothing is prior to the bonds of love. Finally, Dan Zoloth Dorfman—nothing about this life would have been fully possible without your presence.

•

PART ONE

A Crisis in Health Care and a Challenge in Ethics

•

CHAPTER ONE

LANGUAGE, NARRATIVE, AND DESIRE
What We Yearn For

The Reverend James Lincoln,[1] a big man at seventy-three years old, independent and proud, worked by day as a janitor and by night as the preacher in a small, tightly knit neighborhood Baptist church. On the weekends, he and his wife and family were on the road, singing their way home at night after long Sundays spent in bitter, dispirited, farmpicker towns in the Central Valley. Their work was to preach a faith in the power of miracle, in God's ability to heal even the most desperate, drug-addicted, or broken individuals. "We're good at it," he would have told you, "because we never give up."

When Lincoln was admitted to the hospital in early fall for prostate surgery, everybody who knew him expected a full and speedy recovery. But his recuperation was complicated by pneumonia and by a sudden, severe cardiac arrest. Lincoln rallied after these setbacks, teasing his daughters and holding on, hard, to his wife's hand. But he needed acute renal dialysis on a daily basis. A week later he unexpectedly choked, aspirated, and collapsed in the arms of his family. Despite a full resuscitation attempt, Lincoln did not regain consciousness. After a month of intensive care, he remained on full code status and total life support, including artificial ventilation, artificial nutrition and hydration, renal dialysis, dopamine to support his blood pressure, and a variety of antibiotics. His neurologist described him as "less than a vegetative patient" and in fact stated that he met "most—but not all—of the criteria for brain death."

The nephrologist who was giving the dialysis had heard enough. She came to the Ethics Committee asking for permission to discontinue treatment. "This patient no longer fits the criteria of acute dialysis, nor does he meet the community standards for chronic dialysis. Why is it ethical to continue this treatment? Isn't this futile based on outcomes, based on fairness? Don't you people have standards for quality of life?"

When pressed, the hospital administrator shifted uncomfortably in his seat.

"I'll be straightforward about the cost. This care is tremendously expensive. It costs $3,000 a day for all this care and the use of one-to-one nurses, and then there is the blood products. We are just pouring blood and chemicals down this guy. All of these are limited resources. Frankly, what is the point? Is it justifiable, given all the ways we need to spend money in health care?"

The family listened in quiet horror. Mrs. Lincoln spoke, and her daughters nodded in firm agreement. "Doctors shouldn't try to play God. When God wants Reverend Lincoln, He knows where to find him." They pointed to the minister's continuing survival as evidence of a miracle already in progress. "We know you are thinking about the money, too, even when you don't tell us. But how can you place a money value on a human life? Would you do it on a rich white man's life? Would you think about cost if it was your father?" His wife simply shook her head. "Here's my husband, worked all his life, built the shipyards and then cleaned them every night, paid his insurance dues. I know you don't think that is so much, cleaning toilets and emptying your trash. But you sure took our money in those premiums every month. Now all we want is what is due. You doctors, do what you have been trained for. And that is to save lives, not to turn our lives away."

Paulie Gallo is four years old. One afternoon, when he was two, the families in his neighborhood gathered for a picnic. His father was the kind of man who could fix anything, so everyone called on him when the barbecue needed starting. And everyone thought that somebody else was with Paulie. Suddenly, though, Paulie was gone; he wandered unnoticed into a neighbor's pool. Although he was found minutes later and was promptly resuscitated on the scene by his father, an Army medic who knew CPR well, he never recovered consciousness.

Now Paulie has been in a persistent vegetative state for two years. He lives at home, fed with a gastronomy tube and breathing through a tracheostomy, with a large green oxygen tank nearby. The machines whir quietly all night and all day at the Gallo house. His big family likes to bring him right to the center of things. He sits strapped up in his wheelchair at the breakfast table, staring at nothing, as his brothers and sisters fondly kiss the top of his head as they run out the door to go to school. He goes on church outings with his cousins, packed up in the van— machines, oxygen, and all. Whenever anybody gets a cold, however, Paulie seems to pick it up, and three times in the past year his colds progressed to pneumonia. He was taken back to the hospital, put on a respirator when he could not breathe well enough on his own, and given intravenous antibiotics. The nurses and doctors tended his silent body; watched his mother, who slept at the bedside; and just shook their heads.

His pediatrician comes to the Ethics Committee. He is a young man; it is his first year out of school. No one else on staff will care for Paulie. "Do we have to keep readmitting this child to the ICU [intensive care unit]? We don't have the space or the beds for kids like Paulie. Can't I simply tell these parents that intensive care is just not appropriate, that it is futile, and send them home with Paulie to let him die in peace? What a waste of money this is, when our clinic can't see the kids who need immunizations, when we have to cut back on prenatal care appointments."

But Paulie's parents insist that everything be done for their child. His father and mother want to be heard. "To you, he is just a vegetable, but to us, it's our little boy in there."

It happened quickly, the way that freak accidents do. One minute friends were hiking in a remote area of Tennessee on vacation; the next minute James McElveen slipped down a thirty-foot cliff. When his friends found him in a pool at the bottom, the water was bloody, and James was unconscious, pulseless. His best friend, Benny Millagan, carried him up the mountain, and the group drove frantically to the nearest town. But on the dash for help the friends were anxious. It was not only the apparent severity of the injuries that troubled them. Employed as a house painter, James still had no health care coverage. Articles the group had read in the local press made them uncertain that the emergency room they were headed to would admit him. They made a desperate decision. When they carried James to the emergency room, they gave Benny Millagan's health plan card to the clerk. Millagan had health coverage as a federal government employee. Tammie Millagan signed the papers verifying that she was the wife of the injured man. James was transferred twice, to ever more sophisticated care centers, and was operated on. His spine was fused to prevent permanent paralysis. He emerged intact twelve days later, having survived a life-threatening injury with a residue of only occasional headaches. James was a very lucky man. Those twelve days cost $41,107. It is much more than most Americans make in a year of work.

A year later, James McElveen and Benny and Tammie Millagan began to face the real costs of their desperate gesture of friendship. All three were convicted of fraud and conspiracy, and the two men were sentenced to serve time in federal prison, Millagan for nine months, and McElveen for seven months. Tammie Millagan, for her part, would serve a house arrest, presumably because she must care for the couple's three young daughters. Their sentences were similar to those served by child abusers and armed robbers in some states.

Did the Millagans and the others who crouched over their friend's body that day overreact? Were their fears that their friend would be "dumped" or receive inferior or no care absurd? Were their actions criminal? A federal law passed in 1986 stipulates that every hospital that receives Medicaid money must provide emergency care to any patient in a life-threatening situation. At their trial, an attorney from Legal Services of Mid-Tennessee serving that region's poor and uninsured thought the fears of the friends were justified: " 'I absolutely know cases, since the law, where people in life-threatening situations are refused treatment,' said Gordon Bonnyman, who testified as an expert witness at Mr. Millagan's trial last summer. 'I had one where a guy with acute ketoacidosis went to the hospital, but when the attending doctor found out he had an unpaid bill, he dragged him out to the parking lot and dumped him under a tree, where he died within 12 hours.' "[2]

The federal law covers life-saving care and immediate stabilization. It is not designed to cover the surgery and rehabilitation that made it possible for McElveen to work again. "This is really what our public policy decrees," said Bonnyman, "even though it's not the morality of most Americans."

That Mary O'Connelly knew her own mind, all were certain. When she developed an indolent form of cancer doctors described as "slow growing," her family— an adult daughter, her husband, and their son—were told O'Connelly would probably outlive them all. But the disease was complicated by her diabetes and her history of smoking and resultant emphysema. Her recovery from surgery was slow, and she was unable to maintain any oral intake. O'Connelly simply could not keep "anything down." Despite aggressive surgery and several highly technical interventions, she continued to decline. She remained conscious and alert, "but so mad that we can't get her to speak," reported the nursing staff. When asked directly, O'Connelly stated flatly that she did not want any more surgery. After several months, she was being maintained on hyperalimentation and had a tracheostomy, which needed frequent suctioning, some of which she could do herself. But intravenous access was a major problem.

When the case came to the attention of the Ethics Committee, a femoral line was the last port for the nutrition and hydration that were keeping her alive. While the surgeon and the family wanted to continue aggressive care, the main motivation for such a plan was embodied in her statement, "I will not under any circumstances go to a nursing home!" The Ethics Committee considered the case. After a silence, several people wanted to speak at once.

"Isn't it unjust to be giving such aggressive care when we really think the care is useless? Do we have to do what the patient wants even if we don't do it for others? After all, what if every patient told us they didn't want to be in a nursing home? We can't keep them all here indefinitely, doing the most technologically sophisticated interventions, simply because such technology exists. We cannot afford to."

The social worker spoke slowly, shifting in her chair. "I think there is something else here," she said.

Mary O'Connelly lives at home with her daughter, son-in-law, and grandson. Her son-in-law is disabled after a major accident at work, and he has been out of a job for five years. Her daughter is diabetic and only works part time. And now it seems she is four months pregnant. If Mary goes into a nursing home, she is only covered by long-term care benefits for three months. After that she'll have to "spend down" to qualify for benefits under Medicaid, which means that she'll have to sell the house the family all lives in. They can't afford to keep it. As long as she stays here, her care is fully covered by insurance, we take care of her until she dies, and her home is still hers. She is worried about her kids—they'll end up on the street.

"There is no moment like this one," said Carry Johnson, a single mother of three girls. "You wake up at night to hear your kid's cough. You lie rigid, thinking, 'God, please don't let that baby be sick. Let her just go back to sleep, let it be nothing.' Because if she is sick, if she wakes tonight with a bad sore throat, an ear infection, there is no money, no insurance, and no doctor to see."

And when the baby awoke sick in the night, Carry Johnson was in an emergency room in the morning. For Carry Johnson and a growing number of America's working poor, emergency room care is the only health care available. The wait is long; eight hours is not unusual. The county emergency room is full: gunshot wounds, drug overdoses, and industrial accidents from the refinery. Carry Johnson held her baby and sang to her as she waited her turn. "It wasn't serious," she was relieved to say after the doctor saw her. "But," she wondered aloud, "what if next time it is?" She knew she was lucky to have any job at all. Health care insurance had somehow become a luxury that would have to wait.

Ray Cates, a state assemblyman from a big California district, represents Carry Johnson and the county hospital where she waited for her child to be treated. In 1990 Cates held hearings on the problem of access. He listened to clinical staff, weary physicians, angry community activists, and hundreds of people like Carry Johnson. The hearings continued all day.

"The need was overwhelming, and this was when the economy was theoretically stable in this state," he recalled, "and the problems in funding, in access, in allocation, simply massive." He shook his head. "The problem is that we treat health care with policies that presume that we could do with 'less' of 'it,' that we could do with less home care support services, for example, or fewer well baby check-ups. The reality, that I heard testimony to prove, is that we need more services, not less. Because of the ongoing budget problems we have slowly whittled away at prevention, education, and long-term health programs. This will, of course, cost us more in the long run. It is almost as though we are trying to fool ourselves: that if we trim health care around the edges, maybe people will get less sick. But people are simply waiting until they are sicker to come in for care. Even if we were not in the economically desperate situation we are now, can we adequately address the totality of change that will be needed?"

These cases are ordinary scenarios showing how a crisis in public policy comes home, literally, to American families. They render us speechless, which is to say, we have no speech, no talk that allows us to answer the questions that they raise. In the aftermath of the 1994 midterm election, amid the wreckage of attempts at fundamental health care reform, it is critical to talk. It is critical to make meaning of the collective failure to address the crisis in the social arena that such a moment represents. What do all the cases that I have described have in common? All give a human face to the health care crisis in America, the leading and most personally felt of all the crises in the problematic arena of public justice. It is not that we have not noticed or talked about this before; such stories were the commonplace of news shows throughout the early 1990s. The failure to restructure the health care delivery system follows a period of extraordinary public discourse about the crisis in American health care. But this discourse itself has failed. It has failed to give us a compelling reason to pay social and political attention, which is to say, sustained attention, to how real justice ought to be achieved. Why? It is in part because this discourse has been primarily organized along the patterns of traditional language of bioethics and has thus been largely and carefully based in the principles of autonomy, beneficence, and the liberal tradition of justice understood as individual rights. Ethicists have taught the theory of Aristotelian and Kantian principle thoughtfully—they have been central, after all, in curtailing decades of unjustified paternalism and overtreatment—and such theories have framed the precedent-setting legal cases that established the tone and the agenda for American bioethics. But despite this debate, the health care system was not reformed by decisive legislative action, even though dozens of creative plans emerged. What went wrong in the debate around health care reform? What was flawed in the conceptualization and the language and theory of justice that inspired the debate, and perhaps most critically, how can such a debate in theoretical bioethics affect renewed efforts in justice and allocation?

•

The proposals for a just health care system insist on a shared vision of the common good, rather than a good deal for my interest group. This stance challenges altogether the notion of autonomy understood as individual rights, group identity understood as privileged, and what the role of the religious ethicist ought to be in giving leadership to that national policy debate. My point here—and it is a frankly argumentative one—is to challenge both the existing substance of the debate and the process by which the debate is organized. At stake will be the restructuring not only of the content of publicly available health care, but also the restructuring of the public reflective process that can engage citizens in the making of deeply meaningful, and deeply public, moral community. To speak of such a task means to take seriously the premise that the midterm elections cast into the forefront: that a popular and populist debate about the nature of fairness is not only possible, it is prerequisite to the shaping of federal policy.

To prepare for this debate, we need first to understand the current justice literature and address the ethical tasks of the classic justice discourse on health care. Why? Because in contrast to the focus on the mesmerizing economic and technological questions that have captured the forefront of the discussion around health care, we need to reflect on the moral meaning and justice choices that ought to underlie the first premises of the discussion, not the technical "how to" of health care reform. We need to (re)think about reform and understand why, unless we reflect carefully on this, we will continue to fail and fail and fail again in this basic task of justice.

At this juncture, a question arises for some readers. Ought there to be particularized religious responses to the health care reform debate? And what does a Jewish response offer a non-Jewish or secular reader? This book is a long answer to that question. In short form, that answer emerges from what I believe are the tasks and purposes of the religious community in America. In part, these are to organize and focus inchoate public outrage into collective moral action. This mobilization of public conscience and moral habits has been lacking in the public discourse, and we ought to expect that theorists of morality, ethics, and obligation should have a coherent response.

But this is not a book primarily about organization. It is an academic reflection on the importance of language and power. The cases tell us that the careful debate of liberal theory, the discourse of individual rights versus social justice, is no longer able to provide the philosophical means to a moral resolution, one that makes compassionate practical sense in the actual world. For this new discourse is needed—a discourse of conscience in concert with community, a discourse that resituates the embattled self within a community that then reflexively constructs a self that possesses a conscience alert to the necessities of the other.

In the argument, the contention, that we call social ethics, there are other voices that have urged us toward this path. Communitarians, feminists, theologians, and religious theorists have argued for the restoration of a tradition other than rights based theories, that of the common good, and the revisioning of the commonweal as a paradigm for public policy. To be sure, these voices are critically important. But they have not been enough, as any witness to the congressional budget battles has seen. To this argument, this table of debate, I bring another voice, one that has hardly been heard before, or it has been marginalized as "merely" religious. This is the voice of a reinterpreted Jewish tradition. Bringing new Jewish language to the table is more than bringing sweetly decent theological vocabulary or a plea for multicultural inclusion. This is the language of necessity, of prophetic urgency and exilic responsibility. It is a voice that bears the weight of the tradition and history of a cultural and religious worldview that is distinctive. It belongs here and calls attention to itself because neither the largely secular nor largely Christian conversation has gone far enough in insisting that public policy is a matter for each of us, and that a good society needs an inescapable encounter with the other. It takes as a premise that the flight from the common ground of medical necessity is not an option for a just social order. And it proposes that the language that we will need to use as we speak in the vernacular of the medical commons is a language that takes careful account of faith, and of meaning, in American life.

This book reflects one Jewish response to the call for the reconsideration of the common good and the moral community in health care reform. I consider some of the failed proposals for reform and present a response to the various aspects of the plans that were presented. Was it the politics of health care reform or the money poured over the debate, tenacious and tempting as honey, or was it that the theory behind the reforms could not capture any of the passion or the pain of the meaning of justice in the ordinary life of the citizenry? Ethical analysis of and reflection on such a social problem require a consideration of method, of vantage point, and of philosophic terrain.

Ultimately the relationship between public policy and the prophetic voice must be considered. How ought the community of academic religious scholars contribute to public policy and bioethics? Is there a role for the prophetic that can be addressed by this community? What in particular can religious scholars, as opposed to scholars of good will in other disciplines, add to the discourse? And we need to do more, if academic discourse is to mean anything in the world. We need to reflect on the nature of the correspondent obligation in order to participate in the public discourse on the shaping of religious citizenship. How are religious scholars shaping the moral sense of ethical choices in American life?

The last several years have been marked by a profound crisis and a sharpening debate in the United States about both the inflation of health care costs and steadily increasing medical expenditures and the scarcity of health care resources and lack of access for a growing number of the nation's poorest, and even the working poor, in the national health care system. To describe it is predictable, even liturgical. It is commonplace to recount the horrific details: the nearly 40 million people who have no access to health care, the 20 million more who are marginally covered by health care benefits, increasing numbers of children without immunizations, and the number of women who receive no prenatal care. Another list chronicles the chaos for the people within the system:[3] a growing litany of ills and epidemics; lack of adequate resources to address fundamental health problems, drug addiction, and illiteracy; and daily losses from the simplest causes, such as infant diarrhea, malnutrition, and asthma. Yet another description of the health care system portrays the enormity of the business of the health care marketplace and the steadily rising cost of care, technology, medications, research, and physicians' fees.

Though such a crisis is described as occurring in the arena of health care, it can be found in other social sectors as well. What is inescapable about modern American health care, however, is that in this arena we play out our most profound fears about life and death and about the meaning of human flourishing. Because the response to the blood of the neighbor has become not a social and theological response but a medical one, we tend to use the language of medicine to describe a crisis in health care that might have been characterized in other historical periods as a crisis of the social order, of the moral integrity of a people, of a people's relationship to God: Look, the widows and the orphans go untended! "The tongue of the sucking child cleaves to the roof of his mouth with thirst" (Lamentations 4:4).

Why begin a larger work about justice in the health care system with the particularity of case narratives? The chaos in health care access and distribution can be expressed in a volley of statistics. But to actual providers and patients, policymakers, and citizens each statistic is a particular story, and every gesture of health care, even the simplest, that is made or withheld is a rationing decision. Although it is a crisis of large numbers and a crisis involving millions of people, each decision cannot be objectified or abstracted.

Yet another reason is to locate the language of the analysis itself. Ethicists who consider the problem of justice and access are themselves situated, morally, socially, and, possibly most important for the discourse of bioethics, physically, in specific and limited bodies. Classically, the ethics of the dominant liberal tradition teaches dispassion, disengagement, disembodiment, and the critical importance of the rational will as central to the possibility of moral reflection itself.[4] Moral reasoning and policymaking are of the intellect; the search is for the language that will allow the expression of a shared, mediated objectivity and the development of a shared discourse.

The problem of health care reform, however, resists the pull toward the displaced observer; it awakens in us an awareness of the face of the teller of the story, the specific call of the child in pain. Ethics and the just application of ethics in health care reform must be embodied. They must start with the corporal and limited selves we are—all patients, all doctors, and all policymakers—all fragile and marvelous in our detail and complexity, all yearning, uneasy in loss, and limited by our own death.

This may seem overly dramatic. But the effort of this work is to keep in the foreground the exact nature of the problem. It is exactly at the meeting of the specific with the theoretical that critical work must begin. The language of health care reform must be rooted not only in the notion of the commonweal but in the actual encounter with the specific face of the other, with the story that could well be ours. If the language is not rooted there, health care reform is merely an arithmetic calculation or a stubborn economic problem. The answers, complex as they are, can be technically mastered without addressing the actual human pain that must be heard.

The crisis of health care not only has various effects; it not only defines and names us as a society by declaring just where the parameters of our energy and compassion lie. It has various sources as well. Hence, both analyzing and addressing the crisis has multiple dimensions.

Inflation of need is one aspect of this crisis. First is the growing number of the vulnerable poor, the immigrant poor with high health needs, and the newly poor of the recessionary era of the 1990s. Second is the inexorable aging of the American population. Third is the rise in recently recognized infectious diseases, auto-immune disorders, and cancer rates. In short, one aspect of the crisis is an increased demand, in real terms, for health care services. In the words of the California assemblyman, "We need more, not less, of 'it.'"

Increasing expenditures, inflation of costs, and an explosion in technology are another set of cascading factors in the crisis. This series of linked events represents a precipitous increase in per capita dollars spent on health care. Economics does not stop at the insurance company's door. The problem is not only how to pay; it involves deeper questions about the power of the free marketplace, what cost is just, and how to limit profits that are judged to be excessive.

A third factor, one that has been less reflected upon, is the shift in ideology that leads to the social creation of health care "wants." The social creation of desire, the need to have health as one would possess any other commodity, has been an expectation that has inflated as surely as costs have increased. Americans expect to live longer and to be fit, disease free, and perfectly able for longer and longer. How did this work in the national debate on health care reform? Two 1992 campaign bumper stickers come to mind when reflecting on the issues of expectations; their language makes them interesting in this context. The first was a Democratic slogan, OUR FAMILIES WANT HEALTH CARE THEY CAN AFFORD. Note the language of commodification and the ideas that (1) one can buy health care and (2) one must get it cheaply, like a sale item. Imagine if the slogan had been OUR FAMILIES WANT FIRE PROTECTION THEY CAN AFFORD. Note the assumed link between income and health care, the implication that the rich can simply buy more health care, and that is fine. The second slogan was from the populist health care reform movement. It said simply, GIVE 'EM GOOD HEALTH! This is even more striking. Note how some larger force is addressed as "you," as in "you ought to give 'em." Note also that "'em" may mean some others but is also curiously detached from any actual selves. The poignancy associated with this phrase is striking: One cannot be given good health; it is a complex matter of genes, germs, social status, and luck. Even people with normal lives have to expect periods of illness and weakness and, ultimately, mortality. The demand for accessible health care, while large, cannot be large enough to include an Edenistic account of health. Justice can be demanded, even organized for, while good health, despite eager preventative plans and despite jogging and oat bran, unfortunately cannot.

I offer one further bit of evidence of the trend toward constantly rising expectations for extended good health. My father, at seventy-two, looked at his reflection in a pane of glass, straightened, and laughed. "Can you imagine Grandpa caring how he looked in a bathing suit?" I cannot imagine my grandfather without shoes. I knew his desires. They were for being a Jew, studying Torah, doing his hard work (as a house painter), and having healthy children and curious American grand-children. He expected his body at seventy-two to be an old man's body, and every morning he was gratified at waking. My father's point was that a generation later the desire for external beauty as a marker of health was so deeply a part of our culture that no one, even men in their seventies, escaped the gaze.

Our understanding of good health and our expectations in its pursuit have changed enormously in the last century. In his book on medical triage, Gerald Winslow notes how Civil War soldiers waited for doctors; without systematic triage, they queued up, waited with patience, and took their turn.[5] Justice was in temporal sequencing. Now the consideration of triage is more complex. What is need-based medical triage? Who constructs need? Who decides the need?

Linked to the issue of the creation of desire is the difficulty in conceptualizing the ill self. If health care decisions must be formulated in advance of illness, the well self must make a probabilistic judgment about a self that does not exist at the moment of decision. Yet it is that latter self that will confront medical scarcity in the future. There is unease in America about the ill and the aging body. The enterprise of advertising and the world of image creation itself rest on the desirability of a body that is eternally young, fit, and almost oddly thin—in short, the body of a healthy fifteen-year-old. In a society where the ill or vulnerable self is so feared and mistrusted, it will be conceptually difficult, if not impossible, to formulate justice.

Yet another problem that shapes the crisis is the uncertainty of health care providers themselves. Is this a field that can be maintained? In the area of internal medicine, largely as a result of this crisis (the fear of AIDS is speculated to be the greatest cause for alarm)[6] there has been a significant decline in applications for residencies in urban hospital centers.[7] The 1980s marked the longest continuous period of a nursing scarcity since World War II. Growing fears about tuberculosis, and drug-resistant tuberculosis, and frustration at the inability of medicine to treat basic diseases add to the sense of despair.

At the federal level, a push for a national health care system and regulation of technology and fees have met with little success. Despite the political pressure, which reached a crescendo in 1992, for changing the way Americans receive health care, the political process failed to achieve even the slightest hope for success. Many of us had renewed expectations in 1992 that in the palpable, Clintonesque future, health care financing and restructuring would become a reality. Even had a sophisticated and wrenching, hard-fought battle for health care access been successfully waged, however, the problem of rationing would exist to unsettle the most careful political compromise. Rationing waits just behind the most optimistic plans. It exists today. Even for people with fully funded health care, every gesture of care is rationed, less strikingly for the wealthy and more starkly for the poor. We ration by exclusion but also by waiting lists, by quickening the pace of the medical encounter, by increasing co-payments, and by ever more tightly "managing" care through a growing list of gatekeepers. In health care, we use the market metaphor, which, by definition, is a language of limits, of allocation and exclusion.

We cannot provide medical care to all—not endless amounts of care and not on the demand of each. The basis for decision making must rest on some theory of justice or moral imperative. There are not enough organs for transplant, even if unlimited sums were available to pay for the operations. Any new technology— the first ventilator, the first MRI, the first trial of AZT—is, for a time, in limited supply. This is a fact about the human world that will stand, regardless of political will. Our amazement at its continuing veracity speaks of our distance from the boundaries of mortality and from the sensibility of the natural world itself.

Our surprise also reveals much about the acceptance of the concept of autonomy as the cornerstone of philosophical bioethics. This issue speaks to a deeper problem with the ideology of health care reform. In the arguments about resolving the crisis in health care, the ethical principle of autonomy and its association with individual rights and the philosophic claim of entitlement have become central. But this is precisely where, as a society, we run into the deepest trouble. It is the concept of autonomy understood as individualism and limitless entitlement *itself* in moral philosophy that must be challenged. Addressing the problem of justice requires different language, the language of communal obligation and community responsibility rather than of autonomy, individual rights, and entitlement. The nearly unlimited principle of autonomy has successfully trumped the voice of justice in bioethics and collapsed the principle of beneficence into the unlimited social and medical support of the demands of the patient as true and final expert on the inhabited and vulnerable body. I do not intend by this work to suggest that this expertise and the needs of the vulnerable and individual patient in the medical context should be ignored—far from it. It has been a victory for the discipline of bioethics that this voice is so strongly heard in the clinical encounter. But a new balance must be struck. The principle of autonomy must be balanced with principles of justice and community as society struggles to create new paradigms for health care reform.

In what follows, consider the problems that I have raised in light of a process for resolving them rather than for giving a pat or quick answer. First consider the philosophic premises used when justice is discussed. Then reflect on a compelling example of how one state addressed justice, and analyze its assumptions. In light of this, consider how our available language falls short of understanding the potency of the encounter between the stranger and the self that the health care reform effort necessitates.

In 1996, 1997, and 1998 the American public watched as all the proposals before Congress that sought to address the crisis, particularly the problem of access for uninsured Americans, were allowed to die. The proposals tended to focus on the issue of universal access to health care services and, later, on the new systems of managed care but, as a whole, did not address the ethical or social problems of the social construction of need, the issue of how much money it is just to provide for health care services, the question of what is making Americans ill, or the matter of who ought to care for the vulnerable. Thus, while the problem of access was addressed and while the debate flourished over the issue of who would pay for access, the reality of allocating the finite amount available for health care services that will be available *after* the access issue is resolved (as it has been, frankly, for most Americans) was never truthfully examined. This issue of rationing, and the justice of such rationing, is the focus of this work. Unless that issue is faced frontally, the skirmishes around payment will never be resolved.

While the federal government has been unable to construct the political compromise that could lead to federal health care reform, the states have begun to act on their own. Since state governments must share the cost of, determine eligibility for, and bear the brunt of outcomes of federal social welfare programs, several states have taken leadership in this debate. Since states are limited in how they can change the rules of federally funded programs such as Medicare and Medicaid, most state initiatives will ultimately need waivers of these rules to manipulate the structures for funding and allocation of public monies that form the basis of the care of the poor.

Despite the collapse of the federal reform effort—according to a popular joke, Elvis is more alive than health care reform[8]—all is not moribund. Oregon is among the states that have begun to develop solutions to the health care crisis. The Oregon legislature has created and passed controversial legislation that would guarantee universal access by establishing *both* medical and funding priorities in a basic health care package available to all the state's citizens, and it has been quietly operating this plan despite the controversies of its birth.

In August 1992, at the height of the presidential election campaign, this legislation was reviewed by the federal Health Care Financing Administration (HCFA), the agency that grants waivers of its regulations about how Medicaid funds can be allocated to the very poorest citizens. The waiver was denied, thus blocking at least for a time the implementation of Oregon's plan. Early in the spring of 1993 this action was reversed, and the Clinton administration approved the waivers, allowing the Oregon experiment to proceed. In 1994 the plan began, with thousands of Oregonians flocking to register for new benefits: access that is universal in that state. In 1995 Oregon's experiment continued tenaciously, while all around it health care reform at the federal level collapsed and the marketplace forces accelerated their Procrustean restructuring of health care delivery. Oregon seeks to resolve the terrible dilemmas that I presented above. Just how and just why that solution is important is the point of much of what follows.

This book is a complicated project, rather unlike a straightforward publication about policy or about religious studies. I present several conversations about justice and attempt to engage in their levels of discourse simultaneously, and simultaneously to see if disparate venues of conversation about the crisis in justice can, together, provide what one conversation has failed to deliver. I look at theory, practice, and new theology. At stake is our shared ability to hold all the narratives to be of equal worth in a search for a new ethics: an ethics of encounter.

I start with an actual encounter: the face-to-face, citizen-based Oregon prioritization process that led to a new attempt at reform in that state. This story is historical, and it will ground our search for the alphabet of ethics in the real losses that such an ethical encounter demands. For Oregon citizens, the hard talk of reform involved rationing, both the setting of values on which to base allocation decisions and the provider-based process that led to the prioritization process itself.

What is the point of starting an argument for new language in a detailed history of such a specific and limited reform? Basing a critique of the philosophy of encounter on an analysis of the Oregon project is methodologically parallel to beginning this chapter with actual stories of the most vulnerable. It allows us to situate the principles and policies in the awkward and difficult unfinished world, the embodied, political, passionate world of the public arena.

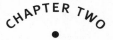

OREGON

A Conversation Once Entered

When the national crisis in health care deepened, first darkening the lives of the most marginalized poor and then shadowing the lives of more and more of the American middle class,[1] it began to substantiate a public feeling of unease, startling even professionals with a glimpse of the chaos generally veiled by the system, and invoking a passionate response in the electorate. In Pennsylvania and then nationally, the debate about reform began to spill out of the private world of kitchen table desperation to create an ongoing national discourse about how to reform the health care system. But before the debate was quite so public, before the campaign platforms were written and the *Journal of the American Medical Association* declared reform "inevitable,"[2] a quiet citizen-based discussion had been opened in the northwest corner of the United States. This discussion in Oregon began as a search for values that could guide physicians and families in making difficult decisions about withdrawing or withholding life support and developed into a discourse on the best and most just use of the dwindling health care dollar offered by the state-run Medicaid program. It became a discussion about the ends and goals of health care for all citizens, about scarcity and obligation, and about a vision of responsibility and the limits of the capacity to heal. Looking at this process closely enables us to see precisely how an altered language is critical to rethinking the moral enterprise of health care justice.

The adoption of the goals of this citizen-based process, and the official, codified embrace by legislative bodies of the values expressed by citizen activists, has had far-reaching, national implications. Despite failures at the federal level, the citizens of Oregon have reshaped the very terms of the discourse and brought to the table that long-avoided reality: the fact that health care, even in the most science-driven, medically advanced nation in the world, is rationed at some level, by some entity. Moreover, if we are to continue as a democracy, health care will have to be rationed under some system of justice. Oregonians took the commitment to democratic justice—that everyone is entitled to a basic package of care, not just last-ditch emergency care, and that that care must be openly and fairly distributed—as the centerpiece of their work. Thus, the commitment was both to universal access and to open, rational planning. Discourse was conducted in the language of the daily in light of the narratives of the actual.

•

Why Care about Oregon?

The Oregon example is remarkable. It allows us to understand how the call for new language for talking about justice can be understood as a call for reflection on the nature of human community itself. It is an example of how practical judgment and the theory of justice collide. What happened in Oregon is indicative of how democratic politics and discursive ethics create a complex terrain in which to locate both the theory and the praxis of justice.

The citizens of Oregon addressed not simply one question but two linked ones. First, they addressed the problem of ensuring universal access for all citizens. A key feature of all reform plans, universal access involves finding technical and economic solutions to the problem of resources once the basic moral commitment to provide such access has been justified. Second, they addressed the far more difficult and challenging problem avoided or glossed over by many reform plans, namely, the makeup of the basic benefits package itself—the question of "access to what?"—that ought to underlie much of the discussion of health care reform. This was unique to the Oregon plan, because other reform proposals have merely expressed a hope that the problem of allocation would disappear by virtue of reshuffling available resources. Thus, the question of the limits and the justification of an ethics of limitation created the furor that surrounded the discourse itself. The notion of naming the limits, calling them out, was controversial *in and of itself.*

The citizens of Oregon made a final, extraordinary gesture in addressing the issue of health care reform. By their very process of discourse they raised the central question of *who* should decide health care policy. For the first time, it was neither the politics of particular interest groups nor the postulates of theoreticians that were the engines of reform; rather, the circles of citizens' diverse, face-to-face encounters drove legislation to completion. The ethics of this encounter, the language of the naming of the limits, is the template for the larger discussion of justice. To understand this language and the persons who spoke the narratives that named the issues in this "ethics of encounter," it is important to recount the narrative of the process itself.

•

Oregon Faces the Economic Downturn

Oregon is a rural state with a relatively small population, 2.5 million people, mostly clustered around the major city of Portland and along the lush Willamette

River valley, a valley so surpassingly lovely and so fertile that it captured the imaginations of the thousands of migrants who struggled to reach it via the Oregon Trail in the 1840s and 1850s. These people came not for gold, but for the land itself—its deep topsoil and well-watered meadow grass. Near-mythic images drawn by Western artists were handed out in hometowns in Missouri and Ohio, portraying the "good life" in the sweet, unspoiled, and abundant land. Everywhere in Oregon there are still green-black forests thick with old growth, and on this timber land the state's economy was built. Themes of abundance, of the frontier, of the settler families who traveled to Oregon in community because they could not have traveled alone continue to dominate the political landscape, as the forests dominate the natural landscape.[3]

The timber-based economy of Oregon began to falter before the rest of the U.S. economy during the recession of the 1980s. In that decade, while much of the nation was still enjoying an economic boom, the economy of Oregon contracted. Oregon comes close to being a one-industry state, and a loss of jobs in milling and timbering affected an entire workforce dependent on lumber-generated revenue, a workforce whose unemployment is frequent and seasonal even in the best of times.[4] Employers struggled to cope with new economic realities by offering union contracts that retained jobs but drastically cut retirement benefits, then health care benefits for dependents, and finally health care benefits for workers themselves. Others reduced expenditures by direct layoffs or by the reduction of hours. Despite long and bitter strikes, Oregon unions could do little to reverse these trends, and they faced a situation similar to that experienced by labor unions all over America: workers' confidence that a union job meant full health care coverage began to be undermined.

•

Provision and Community: How Health Care Is Organized, or Working for Health Benefits

The basis of this confidence has a long history. Health care benefits in America, unlike in most other modern democratic states, are tied to employment rather than to citizenship or personhood. This factor was of central importance to the entire debate about health care access. The securing of employer-provided health benefits was a major victory of the organized trade union movement. More than wage parity or on-the-job safety—two goals for which workers struggled with less success—the promise of health care coverage once seemed assured. Union victory appeared final when, as part of a medical welfare reorganization, Lyndon Johnson instituted tax exemptions for health care benefits. Still, since benefits were tied to employment, the loss of a job meant loss of health care coverage, and any change in employment contract could mean the loss of health benefits coverage for a worker or that worker's dependents.

Significant numbers of workers in the Oregon timber industry losing their health care benefits contributed to an increasing number of "the new uninsured": Americans employed, even working full time, but not covered by medical insurance as workers had been previously.[5] A run of drought that plagued the salmon fishing industry further affected the workforce in Oregon. And an overall decline in the health of family farms nationally had a negative impact on the state's small farm economy as well.

Just as steadily increasing numbers of working people began to turn to the state, wondering if benefits it provided could cover them, the legislature, like state legislatures throughout the nation, faced economic woes of its own. A contracted economy meant a diminished tax base and, hence, reduced revenues available for state spending on all social welfare programs, among them the Medicaid program. Oregonians rely completely on property and income taxes for revenues and reject a state sales tax as a matter of pride. Their income tax is also relatively low compared to that in other states. They have a tradition of "lean state and county budgets." "With the waste not want not attitude of their pioneer forebears, Oregonians constantly strive to live comfortably within their means."[6] Moreover, their mood was not expansionary. In 1990 Oregonians were also dealing with the passage of a citizens' tax relief initiative amendment (Ballot Measure 5) modeled after Proposition 13 in California to cut property taxes, resulting in even less reserve for social welfare spending.

•

Providing for the Other America: The Medicaid Project

Pressure applied to the state to provide for the health of its poorest citizens is not new. In the 1960s, the publication of Michael Harrington's *The Other America* increased insistence that the poor and disenfranchised should be accounted for, and the movement for justice and a concurrent rise of liberal theory created an optimism about and momentum for a radical change in health care financing. The American Medical Association opposed the initial calls for sweeping reform, but in the period 1965–70, several federal programs were instituted to address the most egregious problems of health care provision. First among these federal measures were the tax reforms noted above that allowed benefits packages exemption from federal income tax, and second was the passage of Medicare, which provided health benefits for all elderly Americans, whatever their income.[7] Finally, Medicaid was established as a joint state and federally funded and managed program intended to provide full health care coverage to Americans unable to work (the disabled, the blind, and mothers caring for young children). The provision plan, schematically, envisioned four scenarios, as follows.

1. Working qualified one for health care. Most people worked and had coverage granted to them by employment contracts and a variety of private insurance plans. Families of workers were also typically expected to be covered. The private insurance plan made a "bet" with the members of the plan each year—that the insured worker and his or her family members would not get sick or need major hospital care. Conversely, the members covered by the private insurance plan "bet" they would. The employers "covered the bet," such health care coverage being a benefit that was tax exempt. Hospitals and doctors took care of the workers, who, paradoxically, "won the bet." The fees to providers were paid retrospectively by the insurer. Thus, the risk of illness or accident faced by individual workers and their families was statistically spread among the thousands of individuals that each private insurance company guaranteed. Since, on a statistical basis, more people, especially persons healthy enough to be employed, are not seriously ill in any given year than are, the risk of everyone actually drawing on the funds was minimal. Hence, in what is known as "risk pooling," millions of dollars were taken in by these private companies each year as premiums, with very little chance that an equivalent amount would be paid out. Variations included self-insurance, held by the companies directly, or affiliation with Kaiser Permanente, the California-based health maintenance organization that pioneered the HMO concept. Kaiser Permanente used capitated (i.e., per head) prepaid premiums as payment made to one group practice that then provided health care.

The assumption behind these systems was that working full time allowed one to remain above the federal poverty line and thus not be in need of government assistance in obtaining adequate health care coverage. It was also possible to buy individual private coverage, but such coverage was not expected to be necessary in this vision of health care reform. Coverage was intended to be directly provided as a workplace benefit. The content of the coverage was not an issue in the original considerations. Whatever the physician deemed necessary to effect a cure was covered by the plans.

2. Those outside of production by virtue of their age would be covered by Medicare. Whatever was deemed necessary for a cure would be covered by the plan.

3. Those outside of production by virtue of their inability to work, expected to be a tiny minority based on severe disability or temporary commitments to the very young, would be covered by Medicaid.

4. Traditional means of providing for the poor had relied on cost-shifting. Doctors and hospitals assumed the care of a percentage of the poor of each city as an essential part of the mission of health care itself, shifting costs by charging a little more to those who could afford it. This would no longer be needed. All such care to the poorest members of society would be compensated by the federal

government. It would no longer be addressed by each physician or hospital as a matter of charity, but addressed by the newly empowered welfare state as a matter of fairness.

In an expansionary economy these assumptions held. Backed both by liberal ideology and by the philosophy of entitlement developed at Harvard by John Rawls and others, this patchwork coverage was intended to guarantee a physician-directed, and hence unregulated, response to the health care needs of all Americans. But when significant economic and ideological shifts led to disillusionment with liberal entitlement in the 1980s, a new libertarianism created a restructuring of the tax base that diminished the flow of public funding into the budget at the same time that it enhanced the call for greater defense spending that increased competition for diminishing tax dollars.

Meanwhile, not only did the economy worsen for the sector of the population closest to the margin, but the cost of unregulated health care began to spiral upward. Rapid advances in technology, steadily increasing remuneration for physicians, the development of new drugs, and a seemingly unlimited coffer from unquestioning third party payers expanded the percentage of the GDP devoted to health care to 13 percent by the late 1980s.[8] Pressure to control costs was felt most strongly in the public arena, as states struggled with Medicaid entitlements that eclipsed other portions of their budgets.

While Medicare is fully financed and administered by the federal government, Medicaid is a federal-state program. States are expected to contribute matching funds to provide for the poor. The federal share contributed to each state is inversely related to state per capita income. The program is state administered, but the federal government oversees the program with a variety of congressional regulations intended to apply to all states, regardless of income levels. To change any congressionally mandated requirement in what is offered as a part of the plan necessitates a federally granted waiver of the regulation, called an HCFA waiver.

Entrance to the program was determined by income criteria or by admittance to disability or Aid to Families with Dependent Children (AFDC) status. Originally conceived as meeting the needs of all the poor (i.e., those below the federal poverty line), the standards were tightened and eventually included fewer and fewer of the poor. The indigent poor, once they met federal eligibility standards as "poor enough," were given vouchers, renewable upon monthly recertification of poverty, that were submitted to physicians in lieu of payment. The combined federal and state monies were then given directly to the provider, who was reimbursed for a portion of his or her charges after services had been delivered. Thus, the traditional American fee-for-service system was maintained with certain key differences. First, the employer was replaced by the government as the provider of the insurance; second, admission to the group was determined by an accounting of exactly how poor the participant was. As in all fee-for-service medical practice, the insurance provider may not reimburse the physician for the actual and total cost of the service. This standardization of reimbursement was a relatively new development that resulted in the concept of diagnostic related groups, advanced as a cost-saving measure during the 1980s. The proportion of provider reimbursement had fallen steadily as that cost, too, was scrutinized in the budget cutting of the late 1980s. There were no legislative means to coerce physicians to provide services in response to the offered vouchers. Any individual provider could refuse to treat Medicaid patients.[9]

Until reforms were included in 1990 budget regulations, individual physicians were similarly unregulated with regard to how much they could charge for medical interventions, how many tests they could order, or what treatments they could recommend. Physicians, alone, decided what was a "medical necessity," who was a "surgical candidate," and when care was "futile." Cost was not part of the factor. Since all patients were theoretically covered, it was considered irrelevant and perhaps unethical ever to turn anyone away from care by reason of cost alone. The imperative was to cure or to keep trying, to the point of nil benefits.[10] Paradoxically, the entrance of law and philosophy into the physician-patient dyad did little to affect or regulate this arrangement; rather, it tended only to legitimize the patient as participant and, thus, add to the tendency to search even more diligently for medical solutions to presenting problems. As each technological wonder was deemed no longer experimental, it was added to the benefits covered by federal regulation. Recent evidence suggests, in fact, that even when patients wanted treatment levels to be de-escalated, physicians resisted despite an aggressive series of regulations intended to have that effect.[11]

As the 1980s progressed, a growing deficit and a stalling economy led to cuts in Medicaid funding at the federal level. The 1981 restructuring of the federal budget substantially reduced federal grants to states and allowed for "block grants" instead of dedicated programs, and individual states faced with fewer state dollars from tax coffers and from block grants responded by cutting eligibility and increasing entrance criteria. Since regulation prohibited reducing benefits offered to recipients, decreasing the number of recipients was the sole way states could respond to fewer dollars. Fewer poor people were judged truly poor, and the state obligation disappeared, in this budgetary sense, to provide for poor people who no longer appeared as a line item in the budget. It was a linguistic solution to the crisis: to redefine the margins of the poor, the meaning of "poor" and, hence, the obligation of the state.

There are 37 million Americans who currently fall into this category and perhaps more who "float" in and out of it. Maximum income for Medicaid eligibility is less than 50 percent in thirty-two states. In 1988 in Alabama, the worst-case scenario meant that a family of four could not earn more than 15 percent of the federal poverty level, or more than $1,416, in a year to qualify for Medicaid.

For the families who qualified, all was covered. For the many who did not, nothing was guaranteed.

Because there are no federal standards for eligibility, the capriciousness accentuates the inequity of the system: families eligible in some states are not eligible a few miles away, across the state border.

•

The Crisis Unfolds in the States

Oregon residents fared slightly better than poor people in the rural South. The eligibility level in Oregon was set at 52 percent of the federal poverty level. In its reimbursement to providers, the state ranked forty-two of fifty.[12] In Oregon in 1989, of 400,000 uninsured persons, 300,000 of whom were living at or below the federal poverty line, only 162,000 qualified for Medicaid. Of the 400,000 uninsured, 105,000 were children.

Providers faced a decreased ability to shift costs and to treat these uninsured persons (simply doing charity care for the uninsured using real income earned from paying patients on either public or private insurance) both because of a decrease in the surplus from entitlement programs and a decrease in persons carrying private insurance. This was potentiated by increasing poverty and its attendant health care risks. Further, and perhaps most importantly, a generation of physicians had grown up in a post-entitlement social order. Not since 1965 had there been a frank call for the ideological commitment to active charity as an expected part of medical practice. At the same time, physicians' real income relative to the real income of the rest of the population had increased dramatically. Twenty-five years of Medicaid and Medicare had changed both the sensibility and the notion of obligation as central to the daily work of a medical doctor as the shift from private to public solutions had been theoretically realized by the health care provisions of the Great Society.

Paradoxically, Medicaid was expanded in other ways. Medicare does not cover the cost of long-term care for the elderly. Few private plans cover this cost either. As the nation aged, more and more of the marginalized elderly were forced to "spend down," using all their money to provide for care. When they reached a level abject enough to be considered poor, then these costs were covered by Medicaid. Long-term care is expensive. The cost can vary, but it is seldom less than $20,000 a year. This means that most Medicaid benefits are actually dedicated to the elderly, accounting for 75 percent of the entire budget. AIDS patients gradually swelled the ranks of the medically indigent. Since states have restraints on how to determine the Supplemental Security Income (SSI) to the disabled and little restraint on how to distribute AFDC, here again children on AFDC received the fewest services (dependent children under age twenty-one make up the largest group of Medicaid recipients).

Under considerable pressure every year, Congress has responded to a variety of lobbying efforts aimed at expanding services within the plan and, to some extent, attempted to expand eligibility as well. As a result, state expenditures for Medicaid increased by more than 60 percent between 1984 and 1989.[13] Despite the increasing desperation of state governors, forty-nine of whom in 1989 at their annual retreat signed a formal request to urge a two-year moratorium on Medicaid expansion, Congress continued to respond to pressures to expand coverage. In 1990 there was a recognized crisis in children's services. Immunizations fell to an all-time low. For the first time since the availability of vaccination, measles and polio were making a resurgence, and infant mortality became a recognized problem as international ranking of infant mortality became widely known. The United States ranked fourteenth among industrialized countries. In response, and as a result of a political call for attention to families, a mandate that covered all pregnant women and their children up to age six in families making up to 133 percent of the federal poverty level was enacted. This mandate meant that all children born after 1983 in poor families receiving Medicaid would receive care until they turned nineteen. There was no limit on the cost of services, only the proviso that services were to be "medically necessary."

In other states, as both private insurance and entitlement programs have shrunk and the number of uninsured has risen massively, the county hospital system has picked up the surplus as a "hospital of last resort." But Oregon has no such county system. Access in Oregon was dependent on exactly that expectation of largess, that *caritas* upon which it had become so difficult to rely. And in Oregon, as in all states, the political will for tax increases to cope with revenue shortfalls or escalation of human demands has been minimal. Short of raising taxes, there has been no other source for the needed funds. Legislatures in every state debated the same choices: shift monies from schools, infrastructure, security, environmental protection, or other welfare programs, or continue to do the only other allowable thing—namely, define even more narrowly the meaning and syntax of the language of poverty.

•

The Oregon Narrative

In early 1987, facing a $20 million shortfall in the state welfare budget, the Oregon legislature took a different direction. The thought of cutting more people off the Medicaid rolls seemed unacceptable. The Joint House and Senate Human Resources Subcommittee of the Joint Ways and Means Committee recommended and the legislatures of both houses approved a selective reduction in benefits rather than an across-the-board budget cut of its Medicaid programs. The legislature's action meant eliminating public funding for the most expensive, highly technological procedures: heart, liver, lung, and bone morrow transplants, which were mandated but technically optional under Medicaid regulations. Further, these disappropriated funds would be reallocated to expand prenatal care for the Medicaid population, another optional item. They would not cut eligibility any further. The stage was then set for a major debate.[14]

The action of the subcommittee in response to the crisis in Medicaid funding was only one beginning of the story of the Oregon health care restructuring. The forces that led to the decision were as yet unaffected by several significant elements in the state that would play critical parts in the formulation and articulation of the process. The most central of these organizations was the Oregon Health Decisions Movement (OHD).

•

The OHD: A Commitment to Civic Discourse

The issue of health care reform had long been the passion of a particular group of dedicated health care activists throughout the state. Since 1982 Oregon had taken the lead in a process of direct citizen discourse in a grassroots "values discussion" project known as Oregon Health Decisions. It was then that Ralph Crawshaw, a psychiatrist, and Michael Garland, a theologically trained ethicist, first met to discuss the frustrations of trying to plan health care in the ill-fated councils that were established by the Federal Health Planning and Resource Development Act of 1974 and the Health Services Agency Project (HSA) of the late 1970s.[15] In the first attempt to control the costs of the ever expanding health care budget, "consumers" and "providers" of health care met to debate how many hospital beds ought be allowed per city and how many new technologies were appropriate in a given community. The council meetings held by the 200 HSAs were spectacularly unsuccessful, and the project broke down in 1983 after spending over a billion dollars nationally. But the network in Oregon remained, largely because of the commitment of Crawshaw to the concept of citizen-based health care planning.

Crawshaw had a history of dedicated activism in health care reform in Oregon, and within the state he is recognized as the primary catalyst for talking about the legal and ethical dilemmas facing modern medicine. He and Garland spent hours discussing the essential problems associated with the practice not only of medicine, but of democracy in general.[16] Their vision of the creation of a network of discussion, a concept they called "a wisdom machine," inspired the notion that health care policy should be set for and by the citizens.[17] In 1982 Crawshaw invited former HSA members to a Governor's Conference on Health Care for the

Medically Poor. At this conference the concept of a citizen-based, democratic ranking and prioritization of all the public goods and services that affect health and human flourishing was first discussed.

> The conference heightened participants' concern about two major questions: 1. What are the relative values society places on the curative and preventative services? 2. Given that an implicit rationing of health care already exists, what is the possibility of making such rationing explicit and congruent with community values? It also resulted in a recommendation . . . to form a task force to develop public awareness and consensus on bioethical issues. This task force developed into Oregon Health Decisions.[18]

Crawshaw and Garland self-consciously and carefully modeled this organization into something quite different from a health policy interest group. What they had in mind was meetings of engaged and responsible citizens alive to the possibility of radical transformation of self through the act of collaboration.

> The meetings facilitate group participation in the public examination of values declared by the participants themselves to be of major importance for defining the moral meaning of health care. At the meetings the participants collaborate to "hold a mirror up" to themselves in which they can glimpse their authentic longings for higher values and face up to their own—and through themselves—society's moral inconsistencies, hypocrisies, accommodations with injustice.[19]

Crawshaw and Garland were determined to construct "moral communities" where the notion of a public citizen reflecting on a public good would push a collective consciousness and, hence, a conscience, a sense of obligation to the other that could finally transcend the self-interest-driven politics that had begun to dominate the political landscape. It was not only the creation of a different kind of forum, but something far bolder. It was an attempt at reconstitution of not only the basic political contract between persons, but how the persons making the contract reflect on their place in relation to one another, something heretofore defended in American life as the most private of ventures.

The conference launched an ambitious project. Ethicists Joanne Lynn and Alexander Capron gave a formative seminar to the seventy-five leaders. Meeting in 300 small groups throughout the state, the Health Decisions Project developed a network of 5,000 citizens who had been active in a community of discourse, meeting in their regularly scheduled civic associations, ecumenical groups, college classes, senior citizen centers, nursing homes, and parent-teacher associations (PTAs). The OHD staff made every effort to ensure diversity and public access. Widely publicized, the meetings were held all over the state.[20] Surveys gathered participants' views on issues of autonomy, prevention, access to health care, cost control, and resource allocation. The assumption was made clear in each group: given that implicit rationing already existed, what was the possibility that such rationing could be made both explicit and rational and remain in keeping with actual citizen values?[21] In a state with a relatively small population, the impact of these discussions multiplied as each participant spoke to family and friends. Further, several other factors potentiated the impact of such small groups.

The state had a tradition of small town meetings. In the little towns and cities, people knew one another:

> The rural character of Oregon tends to play down class distinctions.
> In a small town the owner of a mill and the loggers may attend the same
> church. Nearly everyone knows a mother on welfare and understands her
> circumstances—generally how her husband abandoned her. This may
> account for the greater social solidarity than in more urbanized parts of
> the country. Moreover, a "moralistic" political subculture is attributed
> to Oregon, in keeping with the notion of public virtue already noted.
> Political Scientist Daniel Elazar observes that in Oregon, both the general
> public and politicians "conceive of politics as a public activity centered on
> some notion of the public good and properly devoted to the advancement
> of the public interest."[22]

The population is also more homogenous than that in other states.[23] Its workforce is concentrated in a few modes of production. It is predominately white (93 percent), Anglo Saxon Protestant, and unchurched. In fact, Oregon is the most unchurched state in the country.

The first round of meetings was a success, and what was first conceived as a one-time discourse emerged as an ongoing process, a movement. The OHD followed up the first round of meetings with another project, forums that focused on efforts to create new legislation to inform Oregonians about alternatives in the care of the dying and about the possibility of advanced directives and living wills. As well as organizing citizens without special "expert" status to think about these issues, then popularized in the media, the project trained leaders to lead laypeople in discussions about their basic values and beliefs about death, about personhood, and about quality and meaning of life. A fundamental goal of the project, according to Joanne Lynn, was to empower people to consider directly affecting their own health care options.[24]

By 1985 and 1986 the movement in Oregon had begun to attract national attention. Crawshaw wrote of the experience in the *Journal of the American Medical Association*.[25] Brian Hines, an early and influential leader in the group, wrote a widely read article in the *Hastings Center Report* that detailed the goal of the project as raising public awareness and consciousness, determining public values, and influencing policies. "What distinguishes 'health decisions' efforts from traditional public interest lobbying groups is that no preset policy positions exist. Stands on bioethical issues are founded as purely as possible on 'the will of the people' as revealed through a broad-based process of grass roots citizen involvement."[26] Hines called for the expansion of this work to other states and offered to coordinate the formation of an American health decisions resource center. If the Oregon legislature had set the stage, the OHD had been rehearsing with the players for years. Oregonians had been thinking long and hard, and collectively, about the inevitability of a crisis in health care delivery.

•

Saying the First No: The Legislature Takes the First Turn at Prioritization

In 1987 the agenda for health care discourse shifted dramatically in response to the Oregon legislature's action. The lawmakers on the subcommittee had turned to the proposal of eliminating funding for transplants, in part due to the frustration of allocating a budget that tried to fund $47 million in requests from Medicaid, juvenile corrections, child welfare, and other services.[27] They had $15 million in available appropriations. Jean Thorne, director of Oregon's state Medicaid programs, recalled in a later interview, "Well, they ran out of money before they got to the transplants. . . . So out of the session came coverage for additional people who had not been covered up until that time, but we dropped transplant coverage except for kidneys and corneas for those who were already Medicaid eligible. . . . Anyway, it was done quickly and in the closing days of the session which is always crazy."[28] But in a burst of last-minute activity, the plan passed the full ways and means committee and then both houses. It was supported completely, though not initiated, by the president of the senate, John Kitzhaber. Kitzhaber's vision of health care as a social project with social imperatives—that some limits on health care treatment were not only necessary, but were required in the name of justice—led to the construction of the essential argument that developed later to justify the decision. The goals were to increase access, stabilize funding, and distribute the most necessary goods in the manner that would effect the greatest good for the greatest number. The initial argument went as follows: $2.2 million to be spent on thirty-four transplants expected to be necessary over the next two years would be of dubious gain. Some surgeries had a low success rate (nine of the last nineteen patients funded had survived), and all involved years of expensive medical follow-up. In any case, predictably and exponentially, since the Oregon Health Sciences Center was about to become a regional transplant center, each year slightly more people would need transplants. If the $2.2 million was used to provide prenatal care to 1,500 pregnant women each year, then their pregnancies would theoretically result in healthy, full-term infants who would avoid costly, extended hospital stays. Thus, the plan was designed to *generate* revenue and not just save that year's budget. Kitzhaber, a practicing emergency room physician, spoke not merely about the utilitarian principle of greatest good for the greatest number served, but about using hypothetical monies saved from this plan to fund transplant operations in the future. The oft-quoted figure was that "for each dollar spent on prenatal care, three dollars would be saved on neonatal intensive care."[29]

The algebraic ingenuity of Kitzhaber's argument began to crumble under the starkness of individual children's needs. In the early fall of 1987, under the new guidelines, Howard family members were among the first Medicaid recipients to seek permission for a bone marrow transplant for their son Coby, an appealing, personable six-year-old with leukemia in remission. Jean Thorne denied the application. Desperate, the Howards publicized their son's problem and sought donations to fund the transplant. They raised $85,000 from Oregonians who were troubled and puzzled by the boy's plight. When he relapsed and died right after Thanksgiving, many wondered whether his life might have been saved had the money for the transplant been immediately available.

The Howard case was not the only highly visible one. That fall the *Oregonian*, the state's major newspaper, ran stories on several Medicaid patients who faced exclusion. Among them was fifty-five-year-old Kay Irwin, a gift store clerk with a sudden and devastating liver disease who became eligible for Medicaid when her illness forced her onto disability, and sixteen-year-old Chris Patrick, whose small-town neighbors had raised $100,000 in the late summer of 1987. All were desperate.[30] The *New York Times* ran an article that aroused the same doubts about the fairness of the plan. One who did not wonder was Oregonian Sheila Holliday, who had seen the Howards on television and read about the bake sales and the tin cup Coby Howard had carried in public. When her child faced chronic myelogenous leukemia, a life-threatening illness, he also needed a transplant. She told the *New York Times* she was moving to Washington State. "This little guy is not going to sit around and wait for the law in Oregon to change. . . . He's dying. I was fleeing for his life. I wasn't about to go through that fund-raising dance, competing with all the other kids. David Holliday is not going to be another Coby Howard, he is going to live."[31]

In the press and in the popular imagination the children of the poor were asked to balance the state budget on their backs. Posters appealing for help appeared in churches and community centers. The political outcry was remarkable: suddenly the poor had faces, narratives. Little had been said about the 105,000 children without any health care coverage who were eligible for nothing—not a transplant, not prenatal care, and not a doctor's visit or a polio shot. Little was said about the private insurance coverage that in many cases excluded transplants as "experimental" and therefore uncovered. And little was said about other, less visible forms of aid that were denied. Transplant denial clearly touched an important nerve in the public perception of health care. The mythic symbol of the transplant was the ultimate symbol of rescue medicine, the rescue that could outwit death when death seemed inevitable. The metaphor of human replaceability, the linguistic connection to a machine evoked by parts replacement and the implicit hint of theoretical immortality made this technology irresistible. To deny transplants meant to deny the unbounded possibility of American medicine itself. In January 1988, faced with mounting public outcry, the Emergency Board of the legislature (a subcommittee that meets when Oregon's part-time, biannual legislature is not in session) called the Joint Interim Committee into special session to reconsider their legislative decisions in light of public reaction.[32] The Oregon legislature, which prides itself on being a group of "citizen politicians," most of whom hold other jobs, meets biannually for six months. They were unprepared for the ferocity of the reaction, a packed hearing that went on for two days.

Sheila Holliday spoke, as did a member of the Howard family and Craig Irwin, an articulate and energetic spokesman for his mother, who was being denied a liver transplant. The session was emotional and embattled. The Emergency Board did not change the budgeting but agreed to listen to ideas about interim measures to help with the immediate crisis. Among the many recommendations was one from John Golenski, an ethicist and Jesuit priest, who represented the Kaiser Permanente Medical Group and Health Plan. He was unaware of the work of the OHD "wisdom machine," and so suggested a project virtually identical to the one that Crawshaw, Hines, and Garland had been working on for several years.[33] Golenski testified that the Kaiser plan did cover such transplants for its non-Medicaid members and had no way of making the distinction without tagging these patients, something the plan's ethos would oppose. As provider of record, the plan had a stake in any changes in coverage limits for Medicaid contracts it serviced. Golenski recalled the hearing as chaotic: "Everyone with their kids in wheelchairs, lined up and screaming. The press, special interest groups—it was a zoo."[34]

Kitzhaber made the difficult point at the hearing that he continued to make in print and in public throughout that year: the statistical and unseen deaths he witnessed daily as an emergency room physician that were caused by lack of access to simple care routinely denied were as significant as the highly publicized appeals of people who sat before them in need of transplants. By insisting that all the effects of denial be seen, he made tangible the faces of the excluded and began raising the issue of a more generalized rationing plan. "While arguing against restoring funds for transplants then and there, Kitzhaber called for a subcommittee to 'stand back and look at this issue and say if there was more money available, where should these next dollars go?' "[35]

In his role as president of the senate, Kitzhaber began to play a central role from the moment the budget was passed. In July, just after the legislature closed its session, Alexander Capron invited Kitzhaber to speak at a conference he had convened in Princeton with ethicists and social scientists interested in the idea of prioritizing by consensus, an idea then emerging in several states.[36] Hines, Garland, and Crawshaw of OHD were present. Over August, September, and October they developed OHD's response: statewide forums designed to set priorities the state legislature could use in the next session when considering citizen values.[37]

•

The OHD Project: The Second Prioritization Discussion

As their third major project, OHD organizers scheduled a new round of discussions for the early spring in communities throughout the state. This time they would ask participants three major questions: First, what priority should health care hold in relationship to other social "goods"? Second, what general allocations should be set within the health care budget? And third, should the state representatives fund transplants for Medicaid recipients? There was a guarded willingness to allocate. Everyone understood that difficult trade-offs would have to be made, that some participants would refuse to become involved on moral grounds, and that all of this would contribute to the community process facilitated by the OHD leadership.[38]

At issue was the question of *need*. In small groups, and in telephone surveys that followed, citizens debated the issue of what was needed in a health care system and what "good health" meant. This discourse was at the heart of what made the Oregon project full of the stunning possibility that the health care system itself could be radically transformed. It was precisely this face-to-face encounter that made the discussion so compelling. Rather than listening to an abstract dialogue among political leaders and faceless aides about health care policy, group participants were invited to form a moral community, to describe to their neighbors their fears and desires about their embodied self, their flesh, and their vulnerable, fragile lives. Asking questions about what to value about this embodied life created a shared text, a terrain that needed its own language for negotiation and trade. For making trade-offs requires the language of the shared public space. This process brought into public the most private of all intimacies— sexuality, birth, and death.

The small-group process had a further component. Each forum elected representatives to serve as delegates to represent the group's consensus at a health care decisions parliament and to help craft a list of Oregon community values about health care. This statement of principles was then circulated and promoted as a guide to the establishment of moral authority/moral vision in the state. Hence, the group was not only a moral community; it was a democratic community of civic discourse. It is this combination of intimacy, acknowledgment of desire, and democracy that created validity for the process and the parliament. Thus, the values were based not only on reason, the traditional terrain of decision making, but also on passion and were widely perceived to reflect actual needs, a workable consensus, and an authentic political will.

That spring Kitzhaber, Thorne, and the committee continued to meet, and the national press attended nearly every conference. There was an abortive effort at raising volunteer money to be matched by the state. Kay Irwin had obtained a free transplant from a brand-new transplant center that had opened in San Francisco and was looking for a first patient. Coby Howard had died, and his aunt donated the money collected for his bone marrow transplant. Craig Irwin agreed to work for the fund. Since Oregonians were generous when their neighbors needed help, it was thought practical to request general donations to meet this need. But generalized donations did not materialize, again proving the maxim postulated by ethicist Albert Jonsen in his "rule of rescue"[39] that the most highly visible, desperate case will usually be addressed over statistical cases even if more people are affected by the statistical danger. This effort was called the Oregon Transplant Fund. The goal was to establish clinical criteria for eligibility and allocate money on a case-by-case basis. The project was shut down in September 1988, when it became apparent that the donations would not cover the flood of requests. That same month, the OHD project, which had met throughout the spring and summer, chose its delegates from each community. In late September they developed a consensus that was to become the Principles of the Health Care Parliament—principles that would direct all further attempts at allocation and the legislative process itself.

·

The Fred Meyer Trust Project: The Third Prioritization

In the meantime, others were at work to influence the process from different directions. John Golenski had been interested in the rationing process since his testimony. Jean Thorne had asked him to consult on the failed Oregon Transplant Project. In June 1988 he addressed the Oregon City Club, proposing again his ideas about allocations. He met Garland and Hines, who told him about the work the OHD had been doing. It was an essentially analogous project, they explained, and had been in place for the last five years with broad citizen participation.[40]

John Kitzhaber also had rethought the crisis and developed a proposal for legislation based on his analysis of the problem. In late summer the Bioethics Consultation Group[41] invited Kitzhaber to explain his concept and the proposed legislation. Kitzhaber was eager to share his ideas with a wider audience. At his trademark slide show for an annual conference for members of ethics committees (among them Kaiser Permanente's) trained and served by the consulting group, Kitzhaber focused on explicit rationing (called "Using the 'R' Word" at the conference). Kitzhaber's detailed proposal was received with fascination.[42]

In January,[43] working under a grant from the Fred Meyer Trust, a private philanthropic organization, Kitzhaber asked fifty senior physicians and some associated senior nurses and social workers[44] to determine whether a comprehensive evaluation of existing health care services could be accomplished and, if so, how the services might be ranked, as suggested by Kitzhaber's proposed legislation.[45] Brian Hines and, later, Michael Garland joined the group, presenting it with the extensive surveys and evaluations they had gathered and the consensus statement they had formulated in the community meetings about this topic throughout the preceding year.[46] Once the ordering was completed, the list was prioritized.[47]

At issue, the project proposed, was the capitation of the care at varying levels of provided services and at varying proportions of covered populations. Thus, there would be a vertical axis (all services described) and a horizontal axis (all uninsured Oregonians covered). What remained was to determine the extent of the political will that would translate angst over lack of access and efficiency into dollar amounts and garnered tax revenues.[48] Priorities in the project were set by both "provider judgments," admittedly paternalistic and beneficence based, and grassroots social values generated by the OHD. It was the inclusion of the OHD principles, in particular the principle that insisted on universal health care access, that was key.[49] Eventually, however, neither this procedural model for the ranking process nor the substantive model for the content of the services ranked was used in the final Oregon plan. In fact, it was, in large part, the widespread political reaction to the perceived "elitism, provider subjectivity, and political exclusion"[50] of the model that led to the demand that citizens' values and voices be included at all stages in any subsequent legislation.

There would be no more "closed door decision-making."[51] The issue of citizen participation, citizen values, and citizen voice in the prioritization process became the centerpiece of all subsequent rationing plans.

•

The Citizens' Principles

The principles named by the OHD as central had been developed through a long and careful process. The structure of the citizen discourse itself created the possibility for face-to-face directness in the articulation of values that were then argued for and chosen as representative from each small group. In other words, the substantive concerns and ethical choices created in the process of the discourse further created the language of the discourse. The list of the principles follows.

Principles for Health-Care Resource Allocation Purpose of Health Services:

1. The responsibility of the government in providing health-care resources is to improve the overall quality of life of people by acting within the limits of available financial and other resources.

2. Overall quality of life is a result of many factors, health being only one of these. Others include the economic, political, cultural, environmental, aesthetic, and spiritual aspects of a person's existence.

3. Health-related quality of life includes physical, mental, social, cognitive, and self-care functions, as well as a perception of pain and sense of well-being.

4. Allocations for health care have a claim on government resources only to the extent that no alternative use of those resources would produce a greater increase in the overall quality of life of people.

5. Health-care activities should be undertaken to increase the length of life and/or the health-related quality of life during one's life span.

6. Quality of life should be one of the ethical standards when allocating health-care resources involving insurance or government funds.

Why priorities need to be set:

7. Every person is entitled to receive adequate health care.

8. It is necessary to set priorities in health care, so long as health-care demands and needs exceed society's capacity or willingness to pay for them. Thus an "adequate" level of care may be something less than "optimal" care.

How to set health priorities:

9. Setting priorities and allocating resources in health care should be done explicitly and openly, taking careful account of the values of a broad spectrum of the Oregon populace. Value judgments should be obtained in such a way that the needs and concerns of minority populations are not undervalued.

10. Both efficiency and equity should be considered in allocating health-care resources. Efficiency means that the greatest amount of appropriate and effective health benefits for the greatest number of persons are provided with a given amount of money. Equity means that all persons have an equal opportunity to receive available health services.

11. Allocation of health-care resources should be based in part on a scale of public attitudes that quantifies the trade off between length of life and quality of life.

12. In general, a high priority health-care activity is one where the personal and social health benefits/cost ratio is high.

Who sets what priorities:

13. The values of the general public should guide planning decisions which affect the allocation of health-care resources. As a rule, choices among available alternate treatments should be made by the patient in consultation with health-care providers.

14. Planning or policy decisions in health care should rest on value judgments made by the general public and those who represent the public and on factual judgments made by appropriate experts.

15. Private decision makers, including third party payers and health-care providers, have a responsibility to assure their use is consistent with the values of the general public.[52]

•

Assessing the Values of the Discourse

Of the fifteen principles that were adopted in 1988,[53] the project seemed to craft a strategy based on six: responsibility and limits, quality of life, longevity and meaning, greatest good for the greatest number, equity, and public good. While these six are among several concepts articulated, it is my understanding that these are the key factors that underlie the process that makes these principles possible. The first principle that was strongly articulated throughout the statement was the notion of *responsibility and limits*.

> This first principle addresses a basic question: why does government exist? And, more specifically, why is government involved in providing and paying for health care services? The short answer to both questions is that people live not only as individuals, but as members of a community. Thus governments should serve us by using public resources in ways that improve our quality of life beyond what we could accomplish by acting on our own. . . . Obviously there are limits to those resources available to government. Tax revenues rise and fall with the economy and changing political philosophies . . . so the notion of limits is central to the issue of health care resource allocation.[54]

Note how the language of this goal statement acknowledges that the extent to which individuals can go to achieve a reasonable telos is limited and can (and ought to) be potentiated by a social structure that is itself limited. Not only is this social order limited by the availability of public funds and resources (including political will and collective energy), but the notion embedded in the language of "quality of life" is inherently limited as well, for "overall quality of life is a result of many factors, health being only one of these. Others include the economic, political, cultural, environmental, aesthetic and spiritual aspects of a person's existence" (principle 2).[55]

Thus, the social relationship honored by the government as the American expression of the social order is for human flourishing,[56] not health care service per se: "Allocations for health care have a claim on government resources only to the extent that no alternative use of these would produce a greater increase in the overall quality of life of people" (principle 4).[57]

Limited by default and by design, then, the health decision parliament advocated a primary focus on what it defined as quality of life. This category, while exceptionally problematic for theorists (what does this mean, in any case?) is nonetheless consistently evident in community-based discussions.[58]

Principles 3, 6, and 12 develop the value of *quality of life* as a cost-attributable benefit that is measurable ultimately only by the individual (i.e., "no single definition of 'health-related quality of life' is possible"),[59] but it can be "brought down to practical terms [and] described in detail . . . to be objectively measured." While the notion of having some objective standard is inherently problematic, the democratic process must cope with the actual language that emerged from the groups. As noted before, quality of life occurs as a theme. Hence, the parliament tried to come to terms with this by providing a specific description: "how well persons could care for themselves: dressing, eating, bathing, shopping and so on."[60] The basic articulated value was that priority of a health care intervention was in direct relationship to the "personal and social health benefits/cost ratio."

Connected with this basic value was a general value on *longevity*. The parliament described the quality of life by weighting the value system with the "fact that almost everyone would be willing to trade off some portion of their *length* of life for an increased *quality* of life."[61] Yet extending life certainly was of value to the group. The use of the quality-adjusted life year (QALY) reflected this tension between length and quality of life. This scale adjusts the chronological length of life for the quality of life. Deeply value driven, it is based on particular values derived from accumulated surveys of the national public.

Recognition that there was some possible conjoint notion within the shared hermeneutics of the debate on public health led to an acknowledgment, both implicit and explicit, of a type of rule utilitarianism—the formulation of *the greatest good for the greatest number* as public policy:

Since enhancing the quality of life is a prime goal of health services, this should be one of the most important criteria used to allocate health care dollars. For it is imperative to use limited societal resources so that they do the most good for the most people. Health care that does not demonstrably improve quality of life is ineffective and inefficient, and should be reduced to a minimum. The only way to accomplish this is to focus on the values of the benefits which health services bring to people. This principle calls on those entrusted with community health dollars—insurance companies and government—to assure that services produce "the most health for the buck."[62]

The value expressed (the greatest good for the greatest number) was translated into a protocol for ranking actions based on the greatest good. "Good" was defined as length and health-related quality of life, and majority (the "greatest") as people whose funds had been pooled for use in common.[63]

Equity, meaning that "all persons have an equal opportunity to receive available health services,"[64] was the fifth value that can be lifted out of the principles statement. The commitment to equity was revealing and important on two counts. First, adherence to this value was pivotal in creating the OHD model of complete access to health care services. The commitment to equity is what distinguishes this plan from current systems and other attempts to change health care services. If all persons are to be served, then scarcity is a constant should tax revenue be fixed or only moderately increased. Without radical root and branch change of the medical *and* social systems, rationing becomes a variable. Second, it is remarkable that the participants in the community of discourse could envision a theoretical system of equity that would involve them in concrete ways.[65]

The last value that emerges from the document is optimism for the concept of *public good* as more than the aggregate of personal individual choices and life options. Throughout the document, the assumption is put forward that a general public will exists, and therefore a common polity can express its values.

> Linked to this principle is the conjoint one of *strong democracy*. The value placed on this principle is clear: . . . throughout society there is often a wide gulf between people and the institutions which attempt to serve them, but the life and death nature of health services makes it especially important to bring about direct citizen involvement in the area. What is indicated is a shift toward "strong democracy." Citizens should be expected to do more than simply select representatives who make decisions for them. This is weak democracy. *Strong* democracy involves citizens directly in practical policy choices.[66]

The value of strong democracy is linked to another value, a *process* or *methodological* value. This is the emphasis on the small-group, face-to-face structure of the discourse. It is the social interaction that creates the level of discourse, the rhetoric of intimate exchange itself that is rare among strangers. It is precisely this level of intimacy that is the first step toward building a *moral community*. Only in moral community can the language of the collective vis-à-vis the language of individual ownership and marketplace make sense.

•

The Oregon Legislature's Response: The Fourth Discussion of Priorities

It was in this climate that the next step in the process began. The biannual legislature met and considered Kitzhaber's proposed legislation and, among other appeals and proposals, Golenski's project, which had been released to a firestorm of swift, and nearly universally negative, press coverage.[67] Meanwhile, other citizens' groups had become increasingly involved, confronting lawmakers with questions about continuing and legislated citizen involvement. Among them was the Oregon Health Action Campaign (OHAC), a grassroots coalition of ninety-six different agencies representing labor, senior citizens, minorities, women, children, and the disabled. Religious groups, among them an active Catholic coalition, were involved as well. Ellen Pinney, executive director of OHAC, had seen the list generated by the Golenski group and was wary. She worried about her constituency—the elderly, the poor, and the disabled—and felt excluded by a process that had been provider driven and that had generated lists largely in private. As an advocate for groups served by the Medicaid budget, and thus particularly affected by cuts in the Medicaid package, she wanted a stronger voice in shaping the legislation for the groups she represented.[68] Pinney was invited to join the working group, advising Kitzhaber in drafting legislation. Senate Bill (SB) 27, Kitzhaber's proposal, retained the concept of a ranking and allocation of benefits and a basic benefits package that was then sent to actuarial services for capitation. The working group also drafted SB935, a "play-or-pay" employer mandate for small business to increase workplace benefits. The group that drafted the legislation represented a somewhat reluctant coalition. Not everyone was completely satisfied with the results of the compromise package, but nearly everyone agreed and later defended the legislation as the first step in a long process of health care reform. All participants were eager to "try the experiment."[69] What was critical, they agreed, was to establish consensus on the objectives and principles of the plan. Kitzhaber had drafted a series of four questions to be addressed by the legislation: (1) Who is covered? (2) What is covered (who decides who is covered, and how is it decided)? (3) How is it financed? and (4) How is it delivered?[70] The working group addressed these issues by agreeing on a set of principles and objectives, as follows.

1. Allocations for health care must be part of a broader allocation policy which recognizes that health can be maintained only if investments in a number of related areas are balanced.

2. The resource allocation policy must include a mechanism to establish clear accountability for the allocation decisions themselves and for their consequences.

3. There must be universal access for the state's citizens to a basic level of health care.

4. It is the obligation of society to provide sufficient resources to finance a basic level of care for those who cannot pay for it themselves.

5. There must be a process to determine what constitutes a "basic" level of care.

6. The criteria used in this process must be publicly debated, must reflect social values, and must consider the common good of society.

7. The health-care distribution system must offer incentives to use those services and procedures that are effective and appropriate rather than those that are of marginal or unproven benefit.

8. The distribution system must avoid creating incentive for over-treatment.

9. Funding must be explicit, and the system must be economically sustainable.[71]

The committee had learned the lessons of the hastily constructed transplant decision the session before. Therefore, the resulting proposal was thoroughly and publicly debated. Ten hearings were held in the state senate, four in the house, and five in the Joint Committee on Ways and Means.[72] The working group proposed a package of three bills, two of which drafted new language for a basic benefits and funding package, and the third proposed amendments to a bill passed in 1987 that addressed the issue of a statewide high-risk pool. The first, SB27, addressed the issue of rationing (i.e., limiting services that are deemed necessary).[73] This bill established the permanent standing Oregon Health Services Commission (HSC), a governor-appointed committee with representatives from a variety of backgrounds. It was to base its findings on the widest possible hearings from the communities most directly affected. The bill read, "The commission shall solicit testimony and information from advocates for seniors; handicapped persons; mental health services consumers; low income Oregonians; and providers of health care, including but not limited to physicians licensed to practice medicine, dentists, oral surgeons, chiropractors, naturopaths, hospitals, clinics, pharmacists, nurses, and allied health professionals."[74] Four of the eleven panelists were to be laypeople; the remaining seven, members of the health care professions. Its job was annually to review a ranking system that would assess the relative value and standing of health care services provided to recipients of state funding in light of social science and outcomes data. The bill directed the HSC to make its first report on prioritization to the governor and the joint legislative committee no later than 1 March 1990. It was to provide a list of health services ranked by priority from the most important to the least important, representing the comparative benefits of each service to the entire population to be served.

Further, the bill increased Medicaid eligibility to at least 100 percent of the federal poverty level. Hence the bill, while it did not assure coverage for all uninsured persons, attempted to add 77,000 of the poorest uncovered Oregonians to the pool of covered persons. The horizontal axis was not complete under SB27, but the bill provided coverage for many more persons than ever before. The jump from 58 percent to 100 percent was a singular promise of the bill. No other state currently funds to this level. However, the vertical axis was restricted. Not all services already funded by Medicaid continued to be covered. A basic minimum standard would be set according to the funding granted by the legislature each year. Whether additional services would be covered beyond those the HSC deemed essential and how far down the list of services the legislated funds would reach became dependent on political will. SB27 also directed the state to seek waivers from the HCFA to restructure (reduce) the federal benefit package for the state. Several waivers would be required, among them permission to include people with incomes above the financial parameters for Medicaid eligibility but below the federal poverty level, and permission to restructure benefits.[75] The bill further mandated that the state seek prepaid, managed-health-care services contracts for the provision of all necessary services, except in rural areas with insufficient providers per capita to provide for such a plan. The bill also required an independent actuary to determine the funding necessary to cover the capitated costs of services that were part of the package. It promised a cost-based reimbursement to physicians for services rendered and immunity to physicians who refused care to a patient who needed it if the patient later sued the physician for nonprovision. Finally, the bill prohibited the state from reducing the percentage of persons eligible in the event of funding cuts. If cuts were made, legislators would be proscribed by law from decreasing the number of persons covered by public funding, but could allow for a benefits package of services starting from the most essential and the most necessary and descending down the prioritization scale. Benefits, not beneficiaries, would be cut in funding shortfalls. Restricting reimbursement or capitation rates was also prohibited. The bill was designed to make tangible to the legislature and to the public actual limits relevant to services lost, thus creating a specific mandate to raise taxes or increase revenues to re-include services deemed essential. A second bill, SB535, addressed the dilemmas created by the insurance crisis. It appropriated state funds to seed a state insurance pool for medically uninsured residents and authorized the HSC to levy an assessment on insurance companies for additional funds for this pool. Hence, applicants previously excluded due to preexisting medical conditions would have a refuge.[76]

A third bill addressed the problem of employers who did not offer health insur-

ance benefits by using a combination of incentives and taxes, called play-or-pay
plans. Hence, tax credits would be offered for five years to employers who began
offering health benefits. Beginning in January 1994, a monthly contribution, based
on percentage of taxable payroll, would be required of all employers who did not
provide health benefits. The capitation-managed health-care-coverage plan that
was available to the state would also be available to employers and individuals.
SB935 also established the Insurance Pool Governing Board to provide a benefits
package substantially similar to the one prioritized for state beneficiaries.[77]

This plan, then, sought to address the need for health care services for the
entire uninsured population. Of course, the mere existence of a state-mandated
minimum plan would affect the health care services offered to those already insured as well. In some cases pressure would be created to drive up covered services that were already part of negotiated contracts, and in some cases there would
be pressure to drive them down. The legislature was ready to move ahead, based
on what Michael Garland called "three central ethical commitments which its
methods seek to serve."[78] "First, that it is more equitable to assure everyone basic
health care than to offer a larger but unevaluated collection of benefits to some of
the poor while excluding others from anything but emergency care; second, that
explicit, publicly accountable choice is better than the hidden rationing that now
occurs; third, that health care priorities should combine authentic values of the
community with expert technical judgment about health care services."[79]

The legislation passed overwhelmingly in both houses. Reaction was immediate. The Oregon proposal included a plan to draft a prioritized list of health care
services (1,600 in the May 1990 plan, 808 in the February 1991 plan, and 709 in the
final plan submitted to the Bush administration, to be covered by existing funding
levels). That list generated the first and most immediately negative response.

Kitzhaber's working group was prepared for controversy. The release of the
Golenski project pilot list had been greeted with a firestorm of criticism. Oppo-
nents at the national level attacked it as "rationing the poor." A group formed to
reflect on the next steps and to advise the governor about composition of the HSC.
The commission, called "Friends of 27," represented a major cross-section of state
organizations that, along with OHAC and OHD, nominated members of the HSC.
Each commission member had an impressive record of citizen involvement and
commitment to the poor. This commission, then, became the "moral community
of record" for the final drafting of the Oregon plan prioritization list.

•

The HSC: The Fifth Discussion

Commission members were nominated by the governor, who considered suggestions from citizens.[80] Terms were staggered in four-year blocks. The commission's

tasks were to rank and rerank the basic listing of service every two years. There was a small staff.

The first HSC included a labor representative, a member of the Black Women's Health Project, a senior citizens' advocate, an owner of a wood products business, a public health officer for migrant farmworkers, a social worker, a public health nurse who managed a refugee clinic, a pediatrician who was medical director of the Oregon Board of Medical Examiners, an HMO provider, an obstetrician and advocate of prenatal care, a family practice physician in private practice, and an osteopath living in a rural area. The latter was one of the few commission members who served Medicaid populations. It was a diverse group, and several members had been active in the OHD process the previous year. "When the Commission was formed the members had only the vaguest notion of what their task was, and were largely unaware that prioritizing all medical interventions had never been done before. The Golenski project had convinced the legislature that prioritization was possible, but the Commission soon abandoned Golenski's approach as not detailed enough to allow prioritization of distinct services."[81]

The commission organized itself into three subcommittees. The first focused on the special problem of the exclusion of mental health and chemical dependency services in the prioritization process. It included one commissioner and thirteen members, drawn equally from providers and clients of both constituencies.

The second subcommittee was the social values committee, formed because legislation required the HSC to "actively solicit public involvement . . . to build a consensus on the values to be used to guide health resource allocation decisions."[82] The intent was to institutionalize the OHD process as a part of the law. This process was, in turn, supported by volunteers from various citizen action groups. The democracy and fairness of the project rested primarily on the active participation of all citizens. The organizers were intent on countering the criticisms already being hurled at the process that alleged that the middle class was rationing health care services to the poor. Oregon Fair Share, an activist group with OHAC, canvassed door-to-door. Radio and television stations urged attendance at public meetings. All Medicaid recipients received notice of the nearest meeting. The commission (recognizing that not all people would find any one forum comfortable) decided to hold three types of meetings to hear the citizens' opinions. Fifteen hundred people attended twelve community forums held as formal open hearings for the commission members. A telephone survey of 1,000 people was conducted among a statistically balanced control group. Further, in the winter of 1990, the OHD held forty-seven more meetings for the HSC that were attended by 1,048 people around the state.

The goal of the community meetings was to generate for the HSC publicly examined statements about what makes health care "important to us" as a common good. Participants were asked to think and express themselves in the first person plural, namely as members of a statewide community for whom health care has a shared value. They were not asked to think hypothetically about what might make health care important to some other group, but to think concretely and discuss among themselves what makes health care an important aspect of the common good of the community in which they live and to which they feel themselves morally bound.[83]

The OHD had been asking since its inception that citizens struggle with the question of the values held in common and of the notion of "the commons" itself.[84] Thus, once again participants were asked to reflect on scenarios and judge the relative ranking of interventions in each case as essential, very important, or important. The point was not to obtain an aggregate listing of participants' arithmetic; it was not a voting process. What was sought was a common, ongoing discourse that could lead to a reflexive sense of values that were justified, shared, and actively examined. Once again, common values did emerge.

Two themes emerged at every meeting. These were the expressions of complex values surrounding the issues of prevention and quality of life. Prevention was taken to include "a potential for achievement and cost effectiveness, for enhancing the quality of individual lives and improving community life, for benefiting many and having the promise for saving resources in the long run." Component meanings for quality of life include "enhancement of productivity, social functioning, emotional well-being, restoration of vigor, reduction of pain and suffering, and capacity for independent living." Quality of life and length of life tended to be intertwined rather than opposed.[85]

Themes that emerged with frequency were a concern with cost effectiveness and a concern with equity. These were the very issues that had marked the 1988 OHD parliament.

Commission members were clear. They did not view the work as creating a solution to the health care puzzle; they considered it only a first step in a long experiment that had begun with a list of available services, ranked by some combination of the values the hearings had generated and some way of assessing actual outcomes of medical interventions. On this last point the work became more difficult. Harvey Klevitt, HSC member and physician, remembered, "At the first HSC meeting, the chairman, who was a businessman, Bill Gregory, said to us 'You mean you doctors don't actually know if your medical care *works*? What are your measures to see if it works? How can you prove it to me?' He would not accept that way we had been ranking up until now, with a sort of intuitive 'sense' of outcome. We needed to find some measure that accounted for cost, real time, and quantifiable results: tangible outcomes of the care."[86]

This concern started the commission on a process of struggling to incorporate cost data into the values listing. By all accounts, the first attempt was not successful. The commission used Robert Kaplan and John Anderson's Quality of Well Being (QWB) scale to try to measure how quality of life was experienced by an individual in terms of how he or she functioned independently and felt normally as opposed to during an illness. Because using a cost-benefit approach requires figuring some measure of benefit, the question then focused on the linguistic meaning of benefit. The idea was to create a "quality-adjusted life year," a formulation economist David Eddy created, to express the relative value of suffering over time on the merit of an experienced period of time. If the individual experienced the time as miserable, it was "worth less," even if it lasted longer. Cost was then factored against that unit of benefit. The commission developed a new concept at this point: the idea of coupling all medical interventions into treatment pairs so that problems and solutions were linked. As in the Golenski project, provider groups were asked to categorize their interventions and then to estimate the probable outcomes using whatever outcome data they could find to measure their results. These outcomes were then tested against public reaction in the telephone poll. These quality-of-life-linked-to-cost formulas were the most troubling to advocates for the disabled. The inclusion of these categories led to the most significant setback in the entire process.

The initial list was long, extremely detailed, and complex. There were 1,600 treatment pairs by the time the list was leaked to the *New York Times* and published. And that list seemed incomplete. The reaction was no better than the response to Golenski's list. Critics found much to attack; some rankings seemed so counterintuitive as to be nonsensical. The commission itself was unsatisfied. "In the judgment of the Commission itself, the formula produced a ranking that gave inadequate weight to life-saving treatment and to social values (such as preventative care and number of people served by a treatment), suggesting deficiencies in the measure of effectiveness and benefit."[87]

The search for cost effectiveness and quantifiability had overridden the commitment to a values-based list. The commission tried again to prioritize, and this time the list would not be computer generated.[88]

> The commissioners created a system of sixteen categories to organize the
> items logically and after putting the categories into priority order,
> distributed the condition-treatment pairs logically among the categories
> and finally ordered the items within each category. The categories are
> fashioned around values. . . . In transmitting the list to the Legislature the
> commissioners recommended that categories 1–9 be considered essential

components of basic health care; categories 10–13 be considered very important elements of health care; and categories 14–17 be considered valuable to individuals, but significantly less likely to be cost effective or to produce substantial benefits.[89]

Several elements of the process enhanced the way that the reflections of the "moral community" (the citizen-based discourse itself) affected the final list generated in the HSC. First, the commission was encouraged to consider the list of services and rank them from "intuitive habits of thought and literature on health care." Second, community values were stressed and categorized according to relative value to society, relative value to an individual, and how essential they were in relationship to basic equity—what ought to be basic to health care service. Third, each commissioner reflected on his or her own "sense of the list" and then held an open discussion (this was called a modified Delphi technique).[90] The collective process of justification allowed for an opportunity to alter scores, which were then averaged for the mean.

The commission retained the provider-outcome data from the original fifty-four-member panel of health care providers who had addressed the first list. Providers were asked to respond to a list of twenty-four symptoms and six measures of activity taken from the QWB scale. They were then asked to give estimates of probability for success, duration of treatment, probability of actual use by patients, typical age at onset of symptoms, and cost to the payer both with and without treatment.[91]

Unlike the first listing, a net-benefit formula based on cost-benefit ratios was used only in the relatively few cases in which items had an identical listing or there was confusion about "reasonableness" in placement. The final listing was then rediscussed. In that open discussion the final changes were made, in a process the commissioners called "hand adjusting."

The final list was given to the legislature in June 1991. There were 709 conditions/treatment pairs. The actuary estimated the amount necessary to be paid per person per month to prepaid plans at funding levels that included 100 percent of Oregonians below the poverty line at various levels of benefit. The cost ranged from $700,000 (to cover the essential services for the first year) to $40 million (to cover the entire list for the entire population). The legislature, as directed by SB27, conducted more hearings on the level of funding and decided to draw the line at item 567. In actuality, this benefit package was surprisingly rich, covering not only virtually all current Medicaid mandates, including all preventative and screening services, but many services that had not previously been covered. Unlimited hospitalization, hospice care, dental care, physical and occupational services, prescription drugs, and new diagnostic and screening services were not covered. Most transplants were covered. Highly experimental treatments or treatments with a very low success rate, such as heart-lung transplants and liver transplants for active alcoholics, were not. Despite this, and despite the painstaking care that the HSC underwent to achieve consensus, the same national outcry greeted the final list. It was clear that the concept of prioritization by any methodology was antithetical to some conceptions of distributive justice.

Much more activity followed in the year between June 1991, when the final list was drafted and the funding levels established, and the late summer of 1992, when the Bush administration rather unexpectedly denied the HCFA waivers to the Medicaid regulation that would have allowed SB27 to go into effect. This was a period of intense debate and political maneuvering at the highest levels.[92] But the work of the citizens of Oregon had been well begun. The bill called for a biannual renewal of the assessment process, which would mean thoroughgoing discourse on health, values, and the medical commons every second year. While in Washington, D.C., and in the national ethics journals experts heatedly debated the list, in Oregon in PTAs and lodges, in labor unions and churches, something fundamental about the discourse with the neighbor had occurred.

At its heart the discourse about the Oregon plan is a discourse about justice and the language which with we speak as Americans about justice in a time of real scarcity. The Oregon plan, with its complex and riveting history, is a good example, but finally only one example of the various ways that this issue can be addressed. What makes the work of the citizens of Oregon critical is the philosophic enterprise they embarked upon, with the voice of their neighbor to illuminate the journey. The discourse of justice and the place of the citizen had long been debated, however. It is to the philosophy and the language of the discourse that we now turn. We must ask a deceptively easy question, the central question of ethics: If what is being attempted in Oregon is good and if it is right, why is this so?

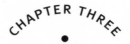

THE EMBODIED
DISCOURSE OF HEALTH CARE
Oregon Reconsidered

Does the close analysis of the history of the Oregon project help us in a search for the language that will enable us more truthfully to address the larger crisis of meaning that the health care crisis exposes? In Oregon the process the citizens engaged in reflects a practical application of the theory of the discursive community. This application then sets in motion the practical consequences that can result if close attention is paid to language and if new sources for language are sought. As I wrote the final draft of the dissertation that was to become this book, the radio was announcing the granting of the waiver for the Oregon state experiment, after years of delay. As this book moved to completion, the plan was enacted. Scores of Oregon citizens flocked to the offices that would enroll them, eager to try this new kind of coverage. In 1995, as federal efforts to achieve full access to health care collapsed, Oregon stood far in advance of what had looked like a tidal wave of reform. In 1999 the rest of the country still struggles with growing numbers of uninsured, and Oregon's effects still remain visionary, even with inevitable limits, failures, and false starts. The story of the plan is continually being written. But the evaluation of the citizen process continues to be the most significant and most neglected aspect of the remaking of the ethical discourse.

In their conceptualization of the plan, the citizens of Oregon first had to address the question of definition: What is justice, and what is health care? This was a remarkable event in the world of public policy, even more so considering that political interest or pragmatism so often defines the initial if not the sole framing question. Next, Oregonians addressed the question of norms: What should follow from this construct of justice? What was controversial was the attempt of the moral community created in this process to address the question of actual public policy reform. The ranking and rationing of health care in the open public arena is an original application of this experiment in participatory democracy. In the use of the reclaimed language of community in the discourse of justice in the arena of health care, both the constraints and the possibilities of this language were revealed.

•

Addressing the Normative Problem in Justice:
Health Care as a Case in Point

Questions about the use of particular language constitute the first problem in applying a theory of justice to the actual world of scarcity. But after definitional problems are addressed, then normative ones emerge. How does a theory of justice actually work itself out in the clinical world?[1]

Is there a need for a separate theory of justice in health care? Can a general theory of justice be applicable in all situations of scarcity? If what is at issue is scarcity of *health care*, is there a greater obligation to provide it than to provide for other social goods? How is the distribution of health care different from the distribution of clothing (which uses stark free-market principles) or the distribution of education (which is rooted in egalitarianism) or the allocation of infrastructure (which is rooted in utilitarianism)?

The initial question is rooted in an analysis of the nature of health care itself. Health care services belong to a category of goods that are of necessity social. A heart transplant, like other industrialized processes, is the kind of task that cannot be performed without the cooperation and time of a great many people. Even without raising the technological stakes to the level of a transplant, the simplest act of caring for the vulnerable ill person is a social encounter, and this act has been considerably potentiated by the routine concentration of such gestures in hospital settings.

Further, it can be argued that the provision or absence of health care affects more than just an individual because of the nature of the fear of, and actual risk of, contagion.[2] This is the difference between dying of hunger and dying of multi-drug-resistant tuberculosis. It is sad, and perhaps spiritually diminishing, if the man on the bus is hungry. But if he is carrying active untreated tuberculosis, his condition has an impact on a different social and physical level. It affects my body as well as his. The provision of health care is a *necessarily* social good; it cannot be otherwise.

Related to this point is the embodied quality of the discourse. At every breathing moment, the text of the corporal self intrudes on the text of the discourse of justice; it cannot be otherwise. The challenge that all health care workers face is the gripping certainty, which is routinely denied in the clinical setting,[3] that the body seen as object could, at any moment, be one's own. We are our breakable little selves; we do not simply live inside them as we speak the words of justice. Our bodies are the subject of the discourse of the just distribution of the "share."[4]

Further, health care is in that category of necessities whose withholding can be a matter of life and death, as opposed to a category of social goods whose withholding would have grave, but not fatal, consequences. Hence, it is also a *necessary* social good. It is not the only social good that is necessary to prevent death or that involves the passions and desires of the embodied self; the provision and distribution of food, water, and physical protection are also included in that set of goods.

Health care services also have a particular relationship to production and distribution of goods in the economic context. Health care services have a monopoly character. If one needs a mitral valve replaced in one's heart, for example, the surgery cannot be competitively bargained for; unlike growing tomatoes, it cannot be performed by just anyone. The surgical profession, with the support of society, controls, limits, and directs entrance into the field. The tools, the drugs, and the authority of medicine all are controlled by persons with particular roles, with role-specific duties, and in American society, with special power and special monetary reward. In exchange for the granting of this monopoly license, then, society is supposed to enjoy the beneficent care of the profession to which it grants these special privileges. As such, the goods that are offered could then be seen as having a special status, by virtue of their monopolized character. These points argue for a special status for health care.

But while all of these points make the discourse passionate, they hardly make it the only social good of central importance. Other, strongly contrary arguments can be made that demonstrate the similarity between health care and other needed provisions. Fire protection is also both necessarily social and necessary, and fires, like health catastrophes, are communicable, injurious to persons, and potentially fatal. Police protection, water provision, sewage treatment, and emergency disaster services (during hurricanes or earthquakes) are "like" health care services—they are necessarily social and socially necessary. For this discussion it is interesting to note that different languages of justice, and hence different allocation fact patterns, are used when a society, specifically the American society, discusses these other services. And in a way, the question of comparing health care justice to other theories governing other goods is suspect. Posing the question competitively articulates a forced decision that suggests that a lexical ordering of social goods, irrespective of context, is possible on theoretical grounds alone.

There are other perspectives. One might argue that there are socially distinctive spheres of justice, and in each a discourse emerges that must be respected on its particular terms. In urging us to look at the health care debate both as interpretive of the union in a given community and as substantive as well, Michael Walzer begins with a review of the history of health care services, suggesting that the history of the need for health care must be examined.

In addressing the specific provision of health care in the modern welfare state, Walzer notes how the linguistic meaning of health as a necessity had been changed, in part, by historical reality. Prior to the modern era the provision of health care was simply not entirely effective, and thus health care was seen as "mostly a matter of free enterprise," private, and relatively marginal based on the limits of its efficacy. Doctors were not considered a necessity. They were employed by the houses of the royal court, serving the poor only as an occasional charitable exercise or in emergency situations. In ordinary times, Walzer points out, the lack of communal concern on the part of the guild that controlled medicine was hardly noticed, partially because there was little that could be done to cure the afflicted human body beyond careful nursing. The care of the afflicted soul was another matter. The public acts of restoration were what counted, and such public acts were religious. The private acts of healing and care were a family matter. Today, comments Walzer, the situation is reversed. The energy and the attention, the yearning for salvation, are shifted toward expectations of longevity rather than redemption. This shift in what is construed as "necessary" and "needed" has a critical influence in what is first yearned for, then demanded, and then expected by communities.[5]

Further, the concentration, institutionalization, and secularization of care itself changed the focus in medicine to an ever more scientific method. As the belief in Enlightenment science became central to healing, the spiritual aspect of healing came to be seen as unreliable, based in superstition, and even dangerous. With this shift came an expectation that since causes could be found for illnesses, cures ought to be found and then administered. Illness was not to be endured or seen as a spiritual journey or as an inevitability of the human condition of mortality, because illness could be fixed. The post-Enlightenment sensibility could cope with a loss of faith, a sense of the random and capricious nature of the universe, and an existential and unredeemed loneliness. Infectious diseases, however, and pain, illness, and even death itself were not to be coped with; they were to be eradicated.[6] The eradication of disease became progressively more difficult, once antibiotics eliminated many common acute illnesses, and hence prohibitively expensive for one individual to undertake. The provision of sophisticated research and more complex cures, such as organ transplants, became a matter of expensive communal pursuit. The "want"[7] for health care services was then expressed not only as a community project but as morally necessary to the individual's ability to live a life of full human flourishing. To be cut off from such culturally shaped desires, claims Walzer, was to experience a denial of the right of any person. It was not only physically threatening in terms of the new expectations of health and longevity, but emotionally and socially degrading, as though one had been denied entrance to the elect.

Once this shift was made, however analytic one could be about the process, the result was the construction of an actual social and medical need that was then deemed necessary, scientifically verifiable. Now that a needed good existed, the idea of whether it was properly a commodity ceased to become an issue.[8] This description of the natural history of desire in medicine has become a common-place, and some analysts have called for a reconsideration of the goal of longevity itself. This is important because it recalls for us how the specific *language* of the communal shaping of the experiences of health and illness is at stake, rather than a fixity about what is properly required for a medically stable life. There is no marker of this apart from geography, history, and sociability.[9]

One participates in the discourse of health at an intense personal level. But justice concerns are not relevant as a result of a special status for health care. The language of justice is useful to understand more clearly how to integrate the persistent appeals for health care into a larger context of a theory of justice. The general linguistic concerns in the justice debate addressed in this chapter ought to be recognizable in the discourse that surrounds the allocation of any scarce social good. The vocabulary, however, remains distinct. The particular narrative of the vulnerability of the ill and the complex relationship between caregiver and patient must be reflected in nuanced and specific language. When theorists address the specifics of health care justice, the details of this narrative must be constantly before them.

•

Framing the Scope of the Problem of Justice in Health Care

Oregon citizens have suggested a specific thesis to achieve justice in their state in light of this particular narrative of rationing health care services. They tell us that the solution to the problem must begin with frank discourse about the ethics of rationing—how to say "no" to some and not to others. To speak of rationing health care is to make the linguistic assumption that not only will shares have to be apportioned justly, but also that in the "usual justice conditions of moderate scarcity," either some person will not get shares or the content of the shares will be less than desired.

Meanwhile, in the clinical world, despite the theoretical niceties, rationing happens at every level of the American health care system. Every clinical gesture is a rationing decision; every need addressed represents some other competing need that has gone unanswered.[10] And the rationing is mirrored at the highest decision-making levels—during the budget battles of 1996, rationing first spoke its name aloud in public. The Oregon process merely first uncovered this process and insisted on accomplishing it in full public view.

Behind any decision to address the clinical cases described in Chapter 1 lies a complex set of rationing decisions that must be considered. Thus, the public dis-course of justice must address several levels of concern. For example, how many resources should be allocated to this particular social good—for example, health care generally as opposed to defense, education, parks, libraries, the arts, transportation, and preparedness for natural disasters? How many resources should be allocated for any specific aspect of the social good, such as specific health care services (transplants or prenatal care, acute crisis care or preventative care, research or chronic care)? Which individuals meeting what criteria ought to be served first if not all can be served?[11]

But it becomes immediately apparent that it is only possible to address the final distributive choice after other choices have been addressed. At every level, a theory of justice is needed to validate why a particular choice is ethical. How should resources be distributed among individuals who will receive the social good; on what basis should health care services be provided (universal access, a basic decent minimal, a free market competition)? *At each level of decision, the language that expresses and is created by the choice must have shared and common meaning.*

Further, central to the debate confronting liberal theories of justice as they address the issue of health care rationing are fundamental questions of rights language. The question about rationing and its justification is ultimately grounded in an assessment of this language and its relationship to the question of justice. First, is there a right to health care, grounded in justice, or is the allocation of health care services properly based on the market first, then on charity and compassion? If health care is a right, is it an inalienable and unlimited right? From what source does this right derive? From social citizenship? From inherent personhood? From simple humanness? From the minimum rules of the entrance into a discourse?[12]

For liberal theorists, the answer to these questions will determine the response to specific proposals. Every right must have a correlative obligation. For example, if individuals have an unconditional right to health care, does society have a correlative obligation to provide a basic minimum?[13] To provide every service that can be described as medically needed by a neutral health care provider?[14] To provide any service that is perceived as necessary by the patient or family?[15]

Is the obligation limited to the necessity of allowing equal access, or is society committed to equality of results?[16] If there is not an unconditional right to health care, or if the right is conditional on the general aggregate utility being served, then other problems emerge. What does a society do with the unlucky minority who do poorly in both the initial lottery and in society's assessment of their place in the aggregate outcome (the problem of utilitarianism)? What does a society based on the uncoerced charitable response do if the charity cannot properly care for everyone (the problem of libertarianism)?

Finally, is it just to ration/limit health care services in any theory of justice? The language of liberal theory is based in consent theory. As such, it is limited in its ability to look beyond the formal contract of informed consent to address the vocabulary of relationship. Similarly, the narrowly defined classic rights language offers limited solutions when facing competing rights from persons with claims that are essentially of equal weight.[17]

•

Justice and the Problem of Scarcity

The astounding crisis in social goods and services within the health care arena is mirrored by this second crisis in moral language. Social ethicist Larry Churchill, in detailing with great specificity the dramatic collapse in health care, describes the increasing pressure to ration. But how can we ration if the language that surrounds each choice is so deeply committed to the sanctity of the individual self alone in a world full of competing strangers? The problem of scarcity forces this discourse.[18] As Daniel Callahan and Churchill point out, the progressive success of the medical field itself creates an escalation of desire for health care.[19] As Walzer notes, how can we ration if the provision of health care is associated with both spiritual redemption and membership in community itself?

The Current Debate: Two Schools

There are two general responses to the problem of rationing social goods and services. The first arises out of the liberal tradition and reflects its strengths and its essential weaknesses. According to this response, rationing of health care is un-ethical in any circumstances. Choices about health care are value choices, reason proponents of this position, and, as such, properly belong in the realm of patients' choice and patients' rights. The literature of autonomy, of beneficence, and of rights is reflected in the criticism of plans such as Oregon's rationing scheme as inherently suspect for individuals and their rights.[20]

The other response, that rationing is ethical in some circumstances, challenges reliance on these philosophic principles and language. This response justifies rationing as part of a larger discussion about the allocation of goods in the health care system. This position is based on the notion of a "medical commons" and uses the language of citizenship and discourse.

Autonomy and Beneficence: Rationing Is Not Moral

Traditional approaches to the allocation of scarce resources in medicine focus on the relationship of the individual physician to the individual patient. Because this is the critical encounter in medical ethics, all that follows from it is relative to the role-specific duties of the encounter. In the classic bioethics literature[21] the key task for the provider is defined as fidelity to the patient, and the key task of the patient is defined as the articulation of his or her need. In this context, the needs of a third party (any third party) are seen as secondary. The medical encounter is thus driven by either autonomy (seen from the perspective of the patient) or beneficence (seen from the perspective of the provider). This sounds simple-minded. But much of the argumentation that surrounds opposition to a priori rationing plans rests on a commitment to these two principles.

Patients' ability to direct their care, to accept or to refuse suggested interventions, and to be directed to the help they ask for, is at the heart of the medical commitment to human flourishing, which is the core of the enterprise itself. The argument for the promotion of autonomy of the patient is a direct parallel to the model of autonomy of a rational moral agent freely consenting to the obligation of a social contract in a liberal state. It is mirrored in the legal theory of consent that arises from that core liberal supposition. It is as follows:

1. A patient who is competent has the unconditional right to refuse or consent to any medical intervention.

2. This right is grounded in the notion of bodily integrity dating back to common law and codified in *Shlondorff v. The Society of New York City Hospital* (211 NY 125, 19–130, 105 ne 92, 93 [915]).

3. Autonomous consent is the basis for all treatment decisions.

4. The patient is the final expert on his or her own treatment, and it is consent itself that is the warrant for the doctor-patient relationship. Without the need for the provision of this consented care the doctor would not be a doctor.[22]

5. Thus, the patient has the right to refuse, and the doctor has the obligation to desist from, medical interventions.

6. The converse is true: the patient has the right to insist on medical intervention, and the doctor has an obligation to respond to the patient's affirmative desire.

Autonomy understood in this form has nearly unchallenged sway in the teaching of bioethics. Since the discipline of bioethics grew coincident to the U.S. National Commission for the Protection of Human Subjects of Biomedical and Behavioral Research, it was the first intent of the discipline to focus on the rights of the individual relative to the demands of essential medical research. The question arose primarily about how to protect the rights of the individual, how to maintain the protected space around every individual, and how to keep persons at the center of this medical interest both safe from manipulation and free from all conditions that violated their ability to exercise their complete human liberty and dignity.[23] The construct of the strongest possible protection against abuse of the person in this context was then applied to persons in all positions of vulnerability in the medical encounter.

An older tradition grew out of the principles of beneficence and nonmalefi-cence that are a centerpiece of the Hippocratic oath. Here, too, the warrant for a focus on the individual encounter of the provider with each patient led to a distrust of both prior societal and bedside rationing.[24] The philosophic tradition here is clear.

1. Human life is of infinite value.

2. The physician is entrusted with the special and exclusive knowledge of poisons and narcotics and with the use of patients' bodies as the training texts of his or her internship, of his or her very craft itself.

3. Hence, the physician has a role-specific duty never to do any harm to the patient and, further, to seek to do good for the patient.

4. Withholding medical intervention for any reason other than to promote the direct welfare of the patient is not, by definition, in the patient's best interest and might, in fact, lead to harm being done to the patient.

5. Hence, the duty of the physician ought to be identical to the best interests of the patient: to ensure all services and interventions that the patient might benefit from and to defend each patient's interest.

Paul Ramsey, Robert Veatch, Ed Pellegrino, David Thomasma, Tom Beauchamp, James Childress, and LeRoy Walters—as well as the members of the national commission, Karen Lebacqz and Albert Jonsen, the ethicists who shaped the initial thinking of the emerging field on this point—urged clarity on this critical issue of beneficence. The patient's interest, not interests external to the patient, ought to be considered primary to the informed consent encounter within the physician-patient relationship. The needs of research, the financial health of an institution, the demands of families, the convenience of staff, the desires of physicians—all these are secondary to patient-driven need. The primary virtue of the compassionate physician was loyalty. To listen sincerely, to be sensitive to what the patient needed, and then to defend those needs, was the call of nearly all early work in bioethics.

The Commonweal: Rationing Is Morally Necessary

The reality of a changed economy forced the rationing debate to center stage in the medical profession in the late 1980s.[25] Prior to this time, the world of insurance and government-sponsored safety nets was bountiful enough to keep most Americans shielded from the harshest aspects of rationing.[26] The material conditions of the recent period have forced ideological rethinking, but the ideological framework that structured a discourse on the relationship between justice and the common good[27] had roots in an older tradition. The idea of a community, of the citizen, and of the "commons" can be summarized as follows:

1. The ends and goals of medicine, like the ends and goals of all human endeavors, are to promote the flourishing of the individual as he or she exists in an actual society.

2. Hence, the fate of the social order itself will have a real and quantifiable effect on the health and well being of the individual.

3. Further, the just use of resources held in common means that attention ought to be paid to all possible human needs that present themselves in a particular context.

4. Hence, the moral moment of medicine is not limited to the informed consent relationship within the physician-patient encounter but includes the social surround of the commonweal: history, location, obligation, and community.

5. Hence, the physician must take the issue of justice into account to promote the actual human flourishing of his or her patient.[28]

6. Further, the role-specific duty of the physician demands that he or she consider the needs of the patient that is subsequent, and the patient that is previous, in the allocation of every gesture of medical care. All medical enterprise is bounded by relationship to a larger community.

This position grew out of the communitarian appeals that I have described as having essential criticisms of many aspects of the classic justice language, and especially the liberty language, of the dominant liberal tradition. In addition to Larry Churchill, bioethicists Daniel Callahan, John Hardwig, and Norman Daniels, among others, have been prominent in suggesting greater attention be paid to the commonweal. They have proposed changes in the language of ethics and justice that might direct approaches to the problem of rationing scarce health care resources. What follows is a brief selection of their current work on the general problem of rationing and justice in health care and their efforts to use the language of the common good as part of the discourse in health care reform.

Callahan's books on setting limits in medicine have been the most widely discussed, primarily because his first attempt focused on possible justifications for limiting care to the elderly. The politics of this reaction was telling and immediate.[29] Callahan suggests that all-out efforts to extend life at the margins are contrary to the purpose of medicine and *prohibit attention to the true needs of the elderly*. He argues that the true needs for companionship, long-term care, and decent housing are not being addressed because attention is paid only to end-stage, high-technological "saves" of limited temporal effect.[30] His argument is based on the assumption of a commonweal—that the resources available to all are not unlimited, that an appropriate decision can be made about broad classes or groups of persons, and that the individual desires of the one do not trump the overall health needs of the community.

Later books focused on how to make the true goal of medicine responsible to a communal vision and based in a collective understanding. Broadening the problem from the rationing of care to the elderly, Callahan's latest work focuses on the larger educational vision of rethinking the ends and goals of the enterprise of medicine itself. Hence, it is the notion of limits as inherent to the enterprise of the human act of healing that Callahan would have his readers remember. In this work Callahan's use of language is central: the imperative is not to *ration* per se, but to question the hubric construct of unbounded progress and omnipotence that stood at the heart of the post-Enlightenment medical quest.[31]

Larry Churchill defends rationing health care after he identifies a key problem in medicine itself. Medical rescue, he argues, is based on the language and the shared account of the story of the "Good Samaritan." But this account, in addition to its obvious anti-Semitism, is limited by its attention to the rescue of the one and the invisibility of the moral appeals of the many. What if, Churchill asks, the road is littered with wounded travelers? What is a Good Samaritan to do? Churchill develops two metaphors for the responsive "language of the commonweal" that he suggests. The first emerges in his book *Rationing Health Care in America*. Churchill, like others who criticized liberal theory, notes the tendency of liberal language to suggest an "absence of the social."

> Life in the modern liberal and libertarian state, based on enlightened self-interest, rational calculations, or the norms of an ideal observer, provides only enough social cohesion to support a very modest form of social justice. We might eventually develop a sense of belonging if we were lucky enough to have the same goals and life plans as other individuals, but this would inevitably be a thin sense of affinity based on nothing more than expedience and similarity of interests. . . . Without an undergirding and "given" set of experiences which we hold in common, the ideal of respect for the autonomy of others will be empty of content, and civil relationships—including justice—will depend entirely on a grudging respect for a *form* of relationship.[32]

In contrast to this language, he argues, the central theory at the heart of Aristotelian thought is the assumption that humans are social before they are individual. Churchill urges a "recovery of the social" by several routes. In Churchill's view, the human necessity for interactive speech is the first proof of constitutive sociability.[33] Second is recognition of embodiment: "The first sign of sociability is our bodies, for they link us inextricably to a natural succession."[34] In Churchill's view, it is not only the generative link that is critical, but the embodied realities of aging and the constancy of gestation, which are human reminders that human freedom, self-reliance, and individuation are inevitably circled by the necessity of dependence.

> It is not just the body in general but several characteristics of our bodies that suit us for social life. The upright posture, for example, brings us face-to-face with others, freeing our hands for shaking (or, no less social, our fists for fighting) and places us at a visual and metaphysical distance from

the earth. Speech, to cite another instance, makes sense only within a plurality of speakers and hearers. In addition there are what Kass terms "special social passions," such as sympathy, shame, pity, friendliness, gregariousness, esteem, and affability, which "permit and are cultivated in community."[35]

Beyond the fact of our creatureliness, proof of our constitutive sociability is demonstrated by the way that moral argument itself is framed and justified. To give reasons, states Churchill, is "tacitly [to] affirm the essentially public and social nature of morality." Further, the actual experiences of the "lived world," paying attention to social ethos, are another way that humans are persistently social and must seek justice choices that affirm rather than deny this.

Churchill roots his first attempt to find a language of social justice not simply in the vocabulary of embodiment, but in the concept of *sympathy*, as representative of the social passions that link us to others.[36] Sympathy, argues Churchill, is the capacity that makes justice possible.

> Sympathy works in our moral judgments of ourselves through our ability to judge our own behavior as if it were someone else's, through the eyes of the "impartial spectator." . . . The spectator is a way of appropriating a social relatedness or admitting into account the common moral sentiments of a community. . . . The impartial spectator acts as a way of evoking an alternative or counterbalance in actual choices, a mirror which carries the larger social sentiment and is roughly synonymous with social conscience.[37]

With this insight, Churchill seeks the recovery of an earlier formulation to inform the problem of the conflicted Samaritan. The importance of this language lay in the insight that "the range and depth of our sympathy [is] inalienably tied to social existence." Choosing to locate morality in "sympathy" roots the moral capacity not in an abstract realm of disembodied rational choice, of willed actions or assessment of telos, but in the midst of a complex and nuanced sphere that includes diverse aspects of human capacities. Moral action emerges from *both* the willed decision and the part of the person that is "uncalculated . . . a human endowment essential to our self understanding."[38]

Churchill ends his book with a further question: "Are we willing to care for the needs of strangers?"[39] Churchill responds that the framing of the answer must begin with a consideration of "ourselves as social" rather than as individuals, calculating the ends of our individual efforts. Hence, the commonweal is made possible by Samaritanism, "a sign of our social nature" enhanced by a principle of justice, naming the social context of our motives and "extending the range of our action to those beyond our immediate life."[40]

In an article published in 1991,[41] four years after his book was published and four years later into the ever deepening crisis of health care resource allocation, Churchill and Marian Danis wrote again of the problem of allocation, using the word "citizenship" to address a moral sensibility that would allow for reframing the justice problem. The authors argue that the crisis is potentiated by an ideology of critical care medicine. The evidence of this trend is found in reflecting on the wishes of survivors of critical care units. This evidence suggests that the experience of the potential restorative power of technology made a proportion of patients more likely to desire it again.[42] In this article, Churchill and Danis address the problem of autonomy directly and ask whether the concept itself needs to be questioned. "Ethicists have argued that the principle of autonomy justifies a patient's right to accept or refuse medical treatment. The impact of the individual treatment choice upon the distribution of heath care resources has been considered irrelevant. Because the right to self-determination was first used as a justification for refusal of treatment, there was no initial conflict between the individual's wishes and a fair distribution of resources. However, it is becoming increasingly evident that individual choices affect the resources available for others." Part of this problem is based in increasing demand for health care services. But the question of limited supply is also problematic. "We face a paradoxical situation in which the power to make individual treatment decisions exists in the absence of any guaranteed access to medical care for all citizens. The result is an almost unrestricted right for those within the system, but no guarantee of initial access."

Churchill and Danis's critique is that the consent implied in the physician-patient relationship is based on the wrong construct. It results in a forced-choice situation, in "divided loyalties." Since the traditional language of bioethics establishes the choice between allegiance to the autonomous desire of the patient that one serves and the best interests of the patient as understood by the physician, the resolution is usually made in favor of patient autonomy. Behind this attitude lies the theory of *ethical individualism*,[43] according to Churchill and Danis. Ethical individualism is limited by the possessive pronoun and by the habit of mind that sees patients one by one—the Samaritan on the road.

Churchill criticized Veatch's stance in A *Theory of Medical Ethics*, particularly Veatch's call for a return to the Hippocratic oath. "The idea that physicians have general, social obligation as well as special, patient ones is, to be sure, not absent from historical codes or contemporary theory. Past ethical codes describe general duties, such as public health measures, that can be exercised at a remove from patient care. . . . Yet the possibility of conflicting moral obligations with regard to the cost of care has generally been addressed by advising exclusive concern for the needs of the patient at hand."[44]

To come to a different resolution and to continue the discourse begun in Churchill's book, Churchill and Danis suggest a return to other duties also spoken of in such codes as the American Medical Association Code of 1947. These are the duties of public health and general welfare. Churchill and Danis develop the idea of *citizenship* to describe the relationship that is necessary to redefine the physician-patient encounter. This concept is novel because it calls for a reflective concern and a moral obligation on the part of *both* health care provider and patient. Both are citizens possessed not only of rights, duties, and protection, but citizens in the sense that they have civic responsibilities and relationships.

> Our reliance on the concept of citizenship is intended to invoke a sense of belonging to something larger than self, or particular individual relationships. Citizens are persons who perceive allegiances as extending beyond self-interest and beyond patient-specific professional duties to a sociopolitical order. . . . The sick individual is not only a patient with rights but a citizen with duties. The right to make health care decisions should not be seen as an absolute without a context, but is bounded by the limited resource of society and the competing rights of others.[45]

Churchill and Danis are realists. They understand and write eloquently about the random nature and horror of the "patchwork medical system" now in place. They are aware of the magnitude of the paradigmatic linguistic shift they are proposing. Nevertheless, they make this call to "give voice to a basic moral conflict and engage it realistically."

Churchill calls for such a moral bond in medicine because he suspects that appeals to theory and rationality do not suffice to address the current crisis in health care. Rather than basing the physician-patient encounter on the establishment and maintenance of the boundaries and rules which are themselves based on the need for protection in the treacherous encounter with the other, Churchill's language reflects the possibility of the largest discursive relationship.

I agree with his premise—in fact, I began this book in part as an answer to his call for new language. Why not, I thought, seek in the Jewish tradition, and seek for an ethics of encounter that insists on the wounded other and the choosing self to be in dialogue? In suggesting an attention to this kind of language, I argue for another kind of discourse. The language is anthropological; the anthropology of the person in the encounter must be described prior to the normative tasks he or she is given. For the first moment in ethics is the recognition of the other as a self in relationship to self.

This account of the theoretical response to health care rationing emerged largely as a hypothetical debate: What would happen if a society began to use rationing as a solution to the health care crisis? The Oregon health care reform plan dramatically changed the tone of the debate. In Chapter 2, I recounted the history that led to the legislative decision to ration public funds and restructure access to both public and private health care services. I offered that history as a dramatic account of the intensity of the crisis. But I also suggested that it was precisely that history that created the alternative vision. The discursive communities described in that history were the attempt self-consciously to create moral communities called for in the work of communitarian theorists. The Oregon plan demonstrated not only the crisis in health care, but the possibility of a solution, not because of the specific ends settled on, but because of the initiation of the discourse itself. What was the point of my elaborate recounting of the history of the Oregon plan? What was the point of retelling again and again the many attempts to meet, to meet again, to prioritize, and to reprioritize?

In the first place, while much has been written about the project, participants' motives and intents seem to have been missed, given a reading of the criticisms of the plan. Many readings of the plan miss the clearly intended, transitional nature of the work. Some analysts seem only to react to the rationing component of the comprehensive plan. Still others do not seem to grasp the plight of the uninsured, the lack of a county safety net in Oregon, the rural nature of the state, or the fact that benefits would be increased not only for those not currently covered, but also for those who had been covered. Some critics seem to blame the HSC for essential problems—for example, that no real outcome data exist for much of what we do medically. Most especially, most commentators miss the bold and far-reaching attempt to create significant *communities of discourse and encounter* that are at the heart of the OHD's ten-year project. It is precisely this community encounter that creates the possibility for new language with which to address a crisis that affects all citizens in every state. This encounter is the focus of my interest in the Oregon process. I argue that despite its many substantive flaws, the community created is the process model for all health care reform. That is why it is critically important to keep the argument about new language and new ethics and the real effects of language on public policy in tension. I will go back and forth between two tasks throughout this book—the tasks of "doubling," of seeing the other, of seeing the self, of seeing the private reflection, and of seeing the public choice.

•

Assessment of the Oregon Plan

Since the first decision to eliminate funding for some transplants, made in the first legislative subcommittee, not only has political response to whatever is attempted in Oregon been swift,[46] but the reaction in the ethical community has been intense, thoroughgoing, and largely critical. This is rather puzzling in light of the urgency to reform an existing system that few would defend as just.[47] But is the Oregon plan an ethical one? In light of the careful reflection on the nature of justice, and in light of the specific concerns raised in the discourse of bioethics about the question of rationing health care, ought the plan to be supported as right and as good? Two positions have emerged in response to that question.

What Is Wrong with the Plan

1. First was the response that any form of rationing was a priori a bad idea. Why ration health care, the argument went, when there was so much excess in the defense budget? As the end of the Cold War justified curtailing the defense budget in any case, the force of that particular issue began to erode, but it still had a certain familiar resonance.[48] The critiques could be made stronger by noting the cost in federal tax dollars of the rescue of the savings and loan industry, the subsidies for tobacco farmers, or the maintenance of a private horse-riding facility for the former vice-president. While this argument was made primarily by the left, the same argument was made by the right, but they targeted other entitlement programs.

2. A significant but related variant was that there was simply too much waste in the health care budget. This surplus could be "shaken out" by reducing the number of forms to fill out, simplifying billing, or reducing duplication in testing or technology. Arnold Relman and Norman Levinsky argued that rationing would be unnecessary if the "$700 billion expended on health care" were spent "sensibly."[49]

> Of the $817 billion that we will spend this year on health care, we will throw away at least $200 billion on overpriced, useless, even harmful treatments and on a bloated bureaucracy. . . . If the wasted money could be redirected, the U.S. could include those now shut out of the system— without increasing total outlay for health care and without restricting the availability of $100,000 bone-marrow transplants or $40,000 heart operations to those relatively few who need them.[50]

This last point is an interesting historical oddity, since many of the founders of the Oregon process themselves were veterans of the last attempt to reduce cost in the way described by Relman, the spectacularly failed Health Services Agency.

3. Many objections emerged that have targeted the basic philosophical theory of a plan that rations the health care of the poor based on a consensus of the middle class. In other words, critics charged, rationing for the poor was being done by those least able to understand or care about the effects.[51] Catholic ethicist Charles Dougherty wondered in print about the preferential option for the poor and clearly sought to make Catholic liberation theology's position a centerpiece of public policy. That position asked, Ought not the poor to get our social support and, in fact, preferential judgment that provides for their needs rather than being considered a source for revenue, a group whose services can be cut to save

money? "Social solidarity will have been undermined in an institutional and systematic way. An 'us versus them' mentality will have been legally established. The right to a basic level of health care will have been subjected to a political line drawing process in the Oregon legislature, a line drawn *by* us *for* them."[52]

Critics of the plan pointed out that it was the very nature of the citizen process that was worrisome. Due to the fact that citizens in Oregon were so homogenous, so white, they were a poor prototype in a country deeply and significantly divided by racial suspicion and hatred. Further, since the issue of race loomed so large in health care, and since the effects of race already played a significant part in precipitating and worsening illness, these critics argued, it was also unfair to institute a system of majority decision making for a minority that was marginalized and feared.

> The poor in many states suffer from deeper, more grinding poverty than do the poor in Oregon, and they are often separated from the majority of citizens in their state by deeper racial and ethnic gulfs. . . . Imagine the consequences for example if middle-class citizens of Queens and Brooklyn in New York—the majority of whom have health coverage through union contracts, public employers, or the private sector—were asked to help develop a package of services for Medicaid recipients whom they know to be largely African-American and Hispanic. Would sympathy overrule hostility? We know too much about the U.S. social environment to be confident that divisions in many states would not bring out the worst in people in a process designed to deny healthcare services to the poor.[53]

Critics have pointed out that since race was the single biggest risk factor for many chronic and acute diseases, further discrimination and marginalization based on race were practiced when health care was to be the topic of the "town meeting agenda" unless that town meeting included the persons most affected, the most vulnerable, and with the most to lose. Arthur Caplan and others have argued, further, that it was fundamentally unjust even to discuss such a plan while "some can afford facelifts and cosmetic surgery."[54] He suggested that it was ethically unacceptable to ration health care at all unless the health benefits of the wealthy were (somehow) rationed identically.

4. A different objection was raised by analysts who cautioned against the clause promising immunity to physicians who did not treat beyond the line drawn by the legislature. Might this be a cover for poor diagnostic techniques, an implicit signal to physicians that certain (poor) patients were not worth the trouble, that no one would care about such patients, and that even the last protection of the poor—the courts—would be removed? Further, was this denial part of the informed consent process?[55] Would patients be told they were participants in a "health care experiment" by virtue of their status as poor Oregonians? Could they

refuse such participation? If they were not told, how did that affect other aspects of the informed consent process?[56] What other information was it fair to withhold to protect the providers or to spare the patient? And how did this interfere with the Hippocratic notion of the doctor-patient relationship, built on advocacy and mutual trust in a mutual project to heal the patient?[57] In the view of these critics, it would be a fundamental distortion of this relationship to expect the doctor to make a utilitarian agreement regarding patients, as suggested by the plan.[58]

5. The Children's Legal Defense Fund consistently argued that the harshest burdens of the plan would fall on women and children, on AFDC mothers who were the least powerful and most needy.[59] Emily Friedman noted that women who at least had access to full medical benefits would experience a loss in these benefits. "So it can never come down to reallocating the embarrassment of riches in healthcare. We prattle about not being able to treat leg injuries in children while sitting in the middle of a $750 billion pig-out! Instead, it always comes down to cutting Medicaid, general assistance health funds, public health nursing, immunization. It comes down to who and what cannot fight back."[60] The blind, the elderly, and the disabled were not prioritized in the initial stages of the process and had coverage from other programs, whereas poor women and children, disproportionate users of precisely the services Friedman mentioned, had no other place to turn.

6. Even cautious supporters of the plan were uncomfortable with certain aspects of the quality-of-life determinations, especially those made in the telephone survey that assessed public reaction to the QWB scale.[61] For Bleich,[62] Dougherty, and others, any attempt at rationing was made even more odious because it relied on the concept of quality of life[63] and attempted to use external judgments to determine the quality of life in disease states that the subject of the questions was not currently experiencing.[64]

7. Other analysts have criticized the two-tiered nature of the plan as an unacceptable disruption of fundamental social solidarity. Health care and other social welfare benefit structures worked only because they were based on a relationship whereby the advantaged helped the disadvantaged in order that the fundamental social contract was fulfilled.[65] This contract allowed persons to move in and out of the disadvantaged position throughout a human life—through periods of relative dependence and independence. Over a lifetime the shares may equalize, but only if each person contributed maximally at the point of greatest productivity. Theoretically, the health care system ought to work in this manner, with individuals in upper income brackets providing for those in lower. It was a failure of the current system to achieve anything near such goals, but formal acceptance and institutionalization of reform based on this two-tiered approach, these critics said, would rectify it. True reform, they contended, must alter the two-tier concept entirely. True reform must begin with the best possible vision.[66]

8. More complete criticisms extended this line of argument. To "rationalize" current rationing served only to sanction morally an immoral system.[67] Even accepting the concept of a separate budget for the poor, suggesting that denial of care was just because the *rules* were justly chosen, was to deny the harsh judgment behind the rules.[68]

9. Providers were not affected by this system, many critics have pointed out. Only the patients were subject to rationing, while providers and institutions could continue to charge inflated fees for their services.[69] Once the cost of a line item was set, and it was set in large part by determining the "community standard" for cost, it became a "fact," a piece of unalterable data. Then the discourse focused only on whether this fact could be "afforded" by the state. No one challenged the reality of the price. Further, no one questioned exactly how much a physician or a CEO of a hospital should make, or the profit margin for the thriving drug industry whose profits had risen handily in the midst of a depressionary economy and whose research fees were increasingly paid by federal funds. In all the far-reaching discussions, no one seriously asked why physicians made five times as much as nurses, on average, and why many medical specialists earned several times more than the U.S. president. In fact, providers were arguably advantaged by this plan. Because they would have a capitated plan, physicians in the managed health care group stood to increase their margin of profit significantly from such fixed fees if they simply did their job well. If people were healthy and if preventative care was effective, then higher-cost procedures might never be needed in many cases.

10. Similarly, taxpayers were not affected. The nature of the exercise was such that lawmakers did not raise taxes or ask citizens to make further significant sacrifices. Rather, they could simply cut benefits back to a leaner level if a budget shortfall appeared. Taxpayers in Oregon were not taxed beyond those in other states. In fact, their rate of per capita tax was relatively low. There was no state sales tax, and the taxpayers passed a bill in 1990 that further reduced property tax rate increases for the majority of property owners. In fact, the state had one of the lowest Medicaid budgets in the nation.[70] Ought not the holders of property pay more so that the propertyless could be better served?

11. The question of rights was also raised.[71] Was there an essential right to life? If a life-saving therapy did exist, even if it was high risk or experimental, why should it be available only to the wealthy? Ought not a society to rescue each citizen equally?[72] It was one thing to ration nonessential things—preventative care, for example—but denying life-saving procedures such as transplants was like allowing someone to drown in full sight of the dock, especially in a plan linked to income levels. The critics argued that, surely, the basic right to life of each person could not be abrogated.[73]

12. Other critics argued that even if the ends were just, the means were suspect, and that the process ought to be rejected by individuals philosophically opposed to a utilitarian argument. In large part these critics focused on the language of the discourse itself. Did the process include minority voices?[74] How many mothers on AFDC were included in the OHD meetings? What of those too poor to own telephones, too marginalized to conceive of attending a public meeting, or too disenfranchised or demoralized to speak honestly at such an event? Critics argued that such meetings were held in middle-class forums and were run by middle-class leadership, and that the entire phenomenon of belonging to an organization held a class bias that could not be overcome with advance publicity. The discourse was inherently and persistently the privileged discourse available only to the middle class, who were comfortable with principles, positions, and the verbal use of power and moral suasion.

Children were not included in the councils that determined their fate; nor were the infirm, the frail elderly, the severely handicapped, or the chronically ill. The very conditions of vulnerability that necessitated their presence as "problem" also shaped their exclusion.

13. A more disturbing criticism could be raised about the fundamental utilitarian premise. Strong democracy was a basic commitment of the project, yet the results may not be fair—they may be discriminatory, fascist, or racist. The democratic process, even populist democracy, was no guarantee of decency. History, said these critics, was an example of this problematic untrustworthiness of democracy. These critics of the plan objected to the undermining of representative democracy and thought that public policy should be set by experts who could judge what a basic plan ought to contain, or by persons who might insist on equal treatment of a despised minority[75] or who might demand a cap on profits or taxes from different sectors of the population or who would do the unpopular acts that public policy requires rather than simply assessing consensus.[76]

14. Other experts in public policy suggested that the basic flaws of Medicaid itself—that it was an uneven, jury-rigged patchwork—were not addressed by this reform. Further, they contended that it prolonged the negative nature of the system at precisely the time when comprehensive, single-payer solutions were being sought.[77] They suggested that the Oregon plan had a desperate quality to it. All the existing parameters—public assistance for health, private employer-based insurance, and a high-risk pool segregated by disease—were retained. Only the quantitative facts were rearranged.[78]

15. Raanan Gillon had noted another problem with utilitarianism and commented that "utilitarian prioritization was itself an inappropriate and unwholesome method of looking at health care issues, suggesting as it does the loss of the individual to the common good."[79] Gillon argued that even if the process was just,

and even if ends in this case could be said to be just, the concept of the sacrifice of the individual to the common good was problematic. (Gillon mentioned the American slave system to illustrate his point.) He raised his objection on the basis that medicine is different from other social enterprises. He urged the consideration of essential duties that accrued to the gesture of medicine as a philosophic and moral, not political, system.

16. The question of experimental therapy was raised by many, especially activists in the disease communities.[80] When the president of the national right-to-life organization offered his protest to then-president George Bush, it was on this ground. He would have died months after his birth, he argued, were it not for aggressive experimental care and a courageous doctor ready to try what had not been tried before. Much of medicine has advanced in exactly this fashion, critics argued. The 500-gram premature baby born too soon at twenty-two weeks gestation, whose care was deemed experimental and thus below the Oregon funding line, may not survive treatment, but the experimental therapy could provide skills and a knowledge base that may eventually allow the consistent rescue of such children. This was how neonatology developed, as well as transplant surgery and hemodialysis. This, argued the critics, was the scientific method. It was the only way that medicine, faced with new diseases such as AIDS, could hope to progress.

17. Richard Steinbrook and Bernard Lo, among others, pointed out that the structure of the legislative response to the plan actually allowed for no guaranteed bottom line of health care support and no package of benefits deemed essential. Instead, the package could "float"—now generous, now lean, now insufficient—based on the public will to be taxed, lawmakers' fears of not being reelected, or the current ecological crisis the state had responsibility for repairing. Serious fires or other natural disasters could deplete state funds, and other social needs such as education could demand a larger share. Each, in turn, would affect health care benefits.

> Oregon's plan consigns to a lower standard of care Medicaid patients who need treatments that are standard practice but rank below the cutoff line. Because the line is financial, not medical, the level of coverage can rise and fall with budgetary pressures. This makes little clinical sense. It is one thing to cover new treatments as their effectiveness is proved or to exclude treatments that are shown to be ineffective or inferior to alternatives. It is quite another thing to call a treatment basic one year and not essential the next, depending on budget allocations.[81]

Lo called for a stable point at which the list of services provided would be fixed. Only in this way, critics argued, could the "clinical criteria" of medical science drive prioritization.

What Is Right with the Plan

1. Nearly all observers who supported the plan did so because of the radical experiment with strong democracy and public discourse.[82] The first gesture is the finest, in this view, and the nearly ten-year project of the OHD to elicit this discourse was the centerpiece of this approbation.[83] The ability of the citizens of Oregon to engage in far-reaching, face-to-face discourse was at the heart of all suggested social change in the health care system. Especially in the process of the allocation of social goods related to health, where questions revolved around the embodied self, it was the encounter with the actual face of the other in direct dialogue that was crucial and unique about this work. Trusting democracy is all that we have, said these supporters, and the process may be slow and difficult, but that is precisely the point. The process enabled us truly to face the other in ethical encounter.

Other proponents, such as Daniel Callahan, viewed the strong democracy as critical because it allowed for full citizen accountability.

> No longer can the consequences of limited funds be hidden or obscured by administrative obfuscation; the winners and losers will be known. The citizens of Oregon are being asked to accept a priority-setting system as well as to accept the pressure it will (and should) put on them to be more generous in what they provide as taxpayers. Will both the public and the legislators be able to stand this kind of bright, cold light of accountability? That remains to be seen, but it is in any event a unique way of making everyone aware of just what it is they are doing. There will be no place to hide.[84]

The citizen discourse was the single most important good of the plan. It was a step toward the civil community so critical to the process of justice and reform of the health care system that it ultimately can be said to outweigh even the significant criticisms discussed above. Strong democracy was the centerpiece of the plan. It was this encounter of the other in the context of a listening community that allowed the reclamation of the language of obligation that would enable serious discussion of social changes. The process of argument and encounter could not be avoided; it was the method that generated language beyond autonomy and individual rights.

2. This plan was committed to universal health care coverage. As such, it differed not only from other reform plans, but so dramatically from the status quo that it was commendable on this ground. The legislature could not cut off anyone from the basic decent minimum that was given to all. No one would ever again have to fear being without health care. As noted by Oregon governor Barbara

Roberts, "Our plan is an honest answer to the nation's health care problem. It recognizes that no state can afford to provide every possible medical service and that choices must be made. Where other states are able to make medical coverage available to only a fraction of those in poverty, the Oregon plan would make the most effective care available to *everyone*."[85] To critics who noted that no bottom line existed in the package of benefits set as a basic decent minimum, supporters answered that now there was no bottom line on how many persons could be excluded entirely, to meet political expediency.

To critics who questioned the impact on women and children, this universal expansion of benefits offered a clear answer:

> [Expanded maternal and child services] will be available not only to the women and children now receiving Medicaid, but also to the thousands of other poor women and children who currently receive no coverage because they don't qualify for Medicaid under any of the narrowly defined federal categories. Equally important, these women and children already served will no longer have to worry about losing coverage should they "fall outside" federal categories. The plan mandates that by 1994 all private employers must offer coverage for at least the Standard Benefit Package. This assures health care coverage to the growing number of working poor who do not qualify for Medicaid. These provisions guarantee all women and children in Oregon access to effective health care.[86]

If universal access was assured, all poor people would be better off.[87] Further, social solidarity, rather than being undermined, would be enhanced as more citizens shared similar benefit packages, and as no one was left out of the net of social provision.[88]

3. This was an interim solution.[89] While the process had been derived from the best vision of the leadership of health care reform in Oregon, the present plan was seen by all who shaped it as a work in progress, a partial solution to the most egregious problems. It was not a final answer because it was all that the political will supported at this time. "Unlike many reform proposals, the Oregon plan does not offer a final solution, but rather a dynamic process. . . . Neither the list nor its process is engraved in stone. The list, the demonstration project, and the overall legislative approach are intended to remain flexible in order to respond to particular needs and special circumstances."[90] To win consensus support from this many people for this much change was a major victory and was much more than had ever been done before, supporters noted.

> As with any public proposal that attempts to solve a complex social problem, everyone has something they would like to change about Oregon's plan. . . . But, however stimulating those debates might be, they

should not confuse the real issue raised by Oregon's proposal. That proposal is the result of years of work and political compromise, conducted under severe restrictions imposed by current laws and competing constituencies. The decision today is not how to fine-tune Oregon's plan, but whether the plan, as it is currently configured, deserves a demonstration. The main criteria should not be whether the plan is ideal. As Oregon's leaders are the first to admit, it is not. Indeed, it is highly unlikely that any plan that emerges from a political process ever will be ideal. The criterion should be whether Oregon's plan improves on what is currently happening.[91]

4. The plan represented the first time a serious look had been taken at clinical effectiveness.[92] As such, it represented one of the first tests with the newly developing outcomes research movement, in which clinical efficacy is comparatively measured and reflected on. All previous plans used other standards, usually what the physician believed was "medically necessary" or what compromises could be hammered out between various interest groups and regulators.[93]

5. The plan was responsive to the variety of factors that created "health." It was a strength of the plan, said supporters, that there was no fixed standard on health care. The health care budget, just like the budgets for other vital services, floated in response to the complex variety of forces that shaped a citizen's life and health. The provisions of protection, education, a clean environment, and arts all affected health. Each biennium citizens, and the lawmakers they elect, would be able to rethink priorities that they would place on various services, reevaluate effectiveness, and again face their neighbors and ask, "What are the ends and goal of the services we seek?" It was entirely appropriate that the benefit package should shift in response.[94] In fact, this was one of the strongest features of the plan.

6. The workings of the plan based good health in part on the relationship between the self and the other, the citizen and the state. The working of justice was related to sentiment, to sympathy,[95] and not simply to the number of services nominally offered. Making health care the topic of civil discourse changed everything: expectations, what was known in common, and what was desired. The process of attention that the work required was intended to be empowering; it questioned the very idea at the heart of health care—that there were experts who, because they knew more than the ordinary citizen about the Krebs cycle and coagulation time, also ought to decide the value of the medical gesture offered to any one person.

7. The small-group meeting limited the privatization that was linked with autonomy in health care delivery. It challenged the pretense that each one who was enmeshed in the health care system faced the encounter alone, that one's actions were singular and had no effect on others. It put forward a vision of

citizenship that involved some sacrifice and a voluntary acceptance of the other at your side who must share the commons with you.

Again we find ourselves led not only to epistemic questions (How do we define the nature of the justice relationship? How do we describe this relationship?) but to ontological questions as well (Who is it that we encounter? What are the parameters of personhood? Of citizenship itself?).

The Oregon experience is a practical model of this discursive community. But we need to reflect on how we justify the model, and how we can defend, and then use again, such a controversial, even radical approach to the problem of justice. We must begin where the citizens of Oregon started, by asking the question, "What is just?"

•

CHAPTER FOUR

NAMING THE TERRAIN

The Language of Liberal Justice
and Its Claims

The Oregon experiment is a complex set of ideas—a bold attempt to respond to the crisis that I described in the first chapter. But how can the power and the flaws of the Oregon process be evaluated? I am a partisan of the plan, and I use it here as an example of how thinking and speaking in the right language can make a difference in public policy. But a careful scholarly defense of the project must begin with an analysis of the theoretical claims I am making for it.[1] How does a society decide what is just? In a world of scarcity, how ought a society justly to distribute goods and services? In light of the particular and poignant crisis of health care described in the first chapter, what would be the language of such choices, the vocabulary a society would use to describe the choices, and the signifiers of justice? Centrally, precisely how is it that a state can be accountable for justice and a human society can reflect on justice? How is it that a society speaks of justice when a crisis in resources arises?

In his seminal book on distributive justice in health care and the problem of health care rationing, written long before the problem had become the subject of widespread public discourse, Churchill anticipated both the crisis in public health and a second crisis in language. There were limits, he argues, in the language of social policy and analytic philosophy to frame an adequate solution.[2] Churchill, a theologian, roots his founding premise in theology and, as mentioned earlier, poses the Good Samaritan story as the organizing metaphor of medicine.[3] In recounting the story, Churchill notes how the story was built on the ethical response of the principled individual's acting out of compassion but limited to ethical individualism. Such a gesture is the best that can be expected of one person, who holds both power and means toward another who is vulnerable or ill on the journey.

However, if the Samaritan were faced with the more challenging problem of distributive justice, asks Churchill, if he were faced with several pilgrims beaten on the road, and not just one, how would he respond? How would simple compassion lead him to a just solution? This is the problem of the current health care crisis, which has only deteriorated with a worsening economy since Churchill first published. Churchill calls for a search for the language to respond, a discourse on the nature of ethical individualism itself, as the crucial first step in the social policy mechanics of health care reform.

But the language that Churchill is criticizing must be described. What is it about the present justice discourse in classical ethical theory that is inadequate? Why does the language of rights and autonomy, which serves respectably to protect patients in the clinical encounter, fail when the particular public policy of health care reform is at stake? Before turning to the new language, one must examine the theoretical basis of the old. It is to these theories that Churchill addresses his critique, and it is in the scaffolding of this philosophic and linguistic construction that the new language takes shape.[4]

•

The Formal Principle of Justice

The concept of justice presupposes the problem that arises in any society where there are inevitable conflicts of interest as individuals press claims and justify them by rules or standards, general principles that regulate and validate both the claims and the distinctions among the claims that allow a society to meet or override them.[5]

The formal philosophic principle of justice first expressed by Aristotle states that equal cases ought to be treated equally and unequal cases should be treated according to their relevant inequalities.[6] When all else is equal, and no claims could be justified for treating people differently, they clearly ought to be treated alike, and when treated unequally, they ought to be treated in proportion to their inequality.[7] The general mandate is to be impartial and consistent. All classic liberal philosophic theories of justice share this language of rationality, impartiality, equity, and just deserts. In terms of the telling visual symbol in the United States, justice is expressed by the image of a blindfolded woman holding a balanced scale. This is striking. Justice is not portrayed as a warrior or an avenging deity. Blindness and evenhandedness, predictability and consistency are characteristic of the formal response to the question of how to allocate justly. In theory at least, the weight of claim from one person is not made greater by virtue of criteria such as wealth or status unless such properties are proven as morally relevant differences.

Impartiality under this formal theory includes the language of moral reciprocity—doing to others as one would have them do to oneself and giving an equal return for benefits received. The agent in a theory of justice theoretically places his or her own interests on the same footing as the interests of others affected by the judgment.[8]

However, the language of this formal principle of justice is minimalist. It does not address the disagreement that arises over the criteria for relevance. It addresses the widest possible spectrum of cases; lacking material content, it does not state any particular aspects in which defined "equals" ought to be treated equally, what equal treatment means, or how that treatment is distributed if not all can be equally addressed. Moreover, the principle does not offer answers to the questions about how to determine equality or who ought determine it, how to determine what an equal share is, or what share or proportion of the share constitutes equality. Lastly, it does not identify what the morally relevant respects are with which a person is to be treated equally when persons are not identical, as they certainly were not in Aristotelian society, and as they are clearly not in our own.

·

Beyond the Formal Theory

Material principles of justice are thus necessary to put material content into the language of the formal theory. By virtue of these principles societies can identify the relevant properties on the basis of which benefits and burdens should be distributed. Among the standard candidates for material principles are *numerical equality, need, individual effort, social contribution*, and *merit* or *desert*. Different theories of justice place different emphasis on these material principles, and some theories are crafted to accept combinations of material principles. Understanding of a particular theory of justice begins with a critical examination of the theoretical justification of the selection of material principles.[9]

Theories of justice have both historicity and social veracity. Each theory reflects, at least in part, a polemic against its predecessors; it reflects a changing understanding of fairness, of righteousness, and of the social spirit.[10] Further, each theory manifests a changing social view of the human as well. What is at stake in discussing justice is, at least in part, the idea of personhood itself—who is and who is not a person, who is entitled to live as a member of the social world that is bound by the rules that the theory of justice requires, and who lives outside the human community.[11]

The *language of the discourse*[12] is key. If we are to answer Churchill's question about distributive justice in health care, the theory, the material principle of distribution, and the anthropology behind each approach must be examined and the language critically analyzed.[13] In literary terms, not only the signifiers and their relations to the signified raise ethical issues; so do the semiotics of the text itself. What follows are three classic philosophic theories of justice. It is to the constructs and language of these suppositions that theorists in the fields of bioethics and public policy historically look first in addressing justice concerns.[14] Such theories can be divided roughly along the lines of an essential dispute in ethics, between consequentialism, with its emphasis on beneficence and non-maleficence, and its associated material principles that stress desert and social efficacy, and deontology and its association with the principle of essential moral equality of each claim for justice.[15]

•

The Libertarian Theory of Justice

The hallmark concerns of the libertarian theory of justice are liberty, private property, and entitlement. Thus, at issue in this theory is the problem of ownership and the rights of each individual to own his or her own resources. According to the classic Lockean theory, the labor power of individuals, their actual work, is "mixed" with the natural resources, land, and water to create wealth that the individual then owns. The ownership of the harvested crops is brought into being by virtue of the individual's creation of this commodity where none existed before. Locke described this process and its link to a particular social contract in the *Second Treatise of Government*:

> 27. Though the earth and all inferior creatures be common to all men, yet every man has a property in his own person; this nobody has any right to but himself. The labor of his body and the work of his hands, we may say are properly his. Whatsoever then he removes out of the state that nature has provided and left it in, he has mixed his labor with, and joined to it something that is his own, and thereby makes it his property. It being by him removed from the common state that nature has placed it in, it has by this labor something annexed to it that excludes the common rights of other men. For this labor being the unquestionable property of the laborer, no man but he can have a right to what that is once joined to, at least where there is enough and as good left in common for others.[16]

Locke, writing in the late 1600s, understood land for agricultural use as unlimited and uncontested: "33. . . . Nobody could think himself injured by the drinking of another man, though he took a good drought, who had a whole river of the same water left to him to quench his thirst; and in the case of land and water, where there is enough for both, it is perfectly the same."

At the heart of this theory is the anthropology of the free individual, the rational, discerning, choosing self who is at liberty to select all association and all work equally. The self at liberty is autonomous, making the appropriate rules that will best guide the work and achieve the goals that the individual desires. This autonomy is both the organizing principle and the goal of this theory.

Lockean theory has a strong claim on the modern American sensibility. It is based on a particular historical notion that, at the time of its development, was revolutionary in intellectual history—that the autonomous individual is a theoretical possibility. In other words, the notion that an individual could choose a plot of land, select his relationship to resources, and defend his choice was a relatively recent historical notion.[17] Further, it was confined to a particular class with access to the possibility of land ownership, and of course to men nearly exclusively.[18] But this claim of ownership is at the basis of the libertarian entitlement, as the ground for the idea of individual *rights* to social goods. Necessary for full human flourishing, according to this theory, is property ownership. A protected sphere of personal rights is a direct result of property rights. Rights to property translate into control of all uses of the wealth that is generated within this sphere. Locke's theory is at the heart of the contract that creates social relationship. Free association is secondary both to the individual and to rights of self and property.[19]

This anthropology grants that individuals exist, disconnected and free, and are able to choose association, ownership, and entitlement. Of course, once the premise of liberty is granted and free land of the wilderness is made into property that can be owned, the structural problem inherent in this moral description emerges. Can an individual possess everything that is gazed upon? Is everything for sale? And what happens when one entitled individual encounters another in pursuit of his or her particular human flourishing?

Locke postulated a condition of nature where individuals roam in competition for resources.[20] The state emerges as the minimal contract against aggression. In the view of the libertarian, however, the state is only minimally entitled to exert an independent will. The state was, in fact, constituted to exert a minimalist hand precisely so that the individual could define his own logical end and his rightful capacity.

Still, Locke can seem fairly removed from debates about health care. Libertarianism, however, exerts a powerful force, especially in the ideology of the Republican Congress. Robert Nozick, the modern theorist who best clarifies the strengths of this theory of justice, helps us understand the backdrop upon which justice struggles are played out. Note how this theory undergirds the current theory behind block grants and welfare reform:

> Individuals have rights, and there are things that no person or group may do to them (without violating their rights). So strong and far-reaching are these rights that they raise the question of what, if anything, the state and its officials may do. How much room do individual rights leave for the state? Our main conclusions about the state are that a minimal state, limited to the narrow functions of protection against force, theft, fraud, enforcements of contracts, and so on, is justified; that any more extensive

state will violate persons' rights not to be forced to do certain things, and is unjustified; and that a minimal state is inspiring as well as right. Two noteworthy implications are that the state may not use its coercive apparatus for the purpose of getting some citizens to aid others, or in order to prohibit activities to people for their own good or protection.[21]

Nozick's minimalist state emerges from the same justification as Locke's—the need for an existence that is as free as possible so that each person can pursue his own property concerns and yet be protected from the violence of others. There will be times, even in this minimal state, that an individual will have to give up some of his immediate rights[22] and thus need to be compensated if either an unconsented crossing of another's boundaries is permitted or if a crossing is prohibited to protect the state from potential harm.

Since the state is warranted only to protect basic rights of free choice in the marketplace and to protect individuals from aggression by others, it can compensate only for infringement of these rights. The state is not warranted or authorized to compensate for unfairness or inadequacy in distribution of goods. The rules for distributive justice arise from a justification different from those which evolve for a state; they are the rules of the free exchange of the marketplace and have nothing to do with a state's proper power, except as it would enforce a contract once agreed upon.

Nozick's premises are basic. Justice is marked by two tenets. The first is that disproportionate needs are unfortunate and not unfair.[23] The second is that allocation of resources is a matter of charity and not justice. Persons have no intrinsic rights to goods separate from their ability to acquire them through their acquisition of property. In fact, good health is based on the outcomes of two lotteries—the genetic and physical one, and the social one—by which material conditions are distributed. Bad luck, bad genes, bad parents, or a bad neighborhood are misfortunes, but not a violation of any entitlement. Health care dollars could be spent on the vulnerable ill by compassionate and charitable persons, but it always remains a free choice of any particular individual whether or not to offer this charity.

Taxes, or any other forced assistance of the disadvantaged, are improper and unjust in Nozick's libertarian state; to impose them is the legal equivalent of forcing someone to "gather acorns for someone else against his will." In both principle and result, it violates the most basic theory of *entitlement* for Nozick, and for Locke before him, that the rights and the property that results from the rights are intrinsic to the self and stand independent from society. While the plight of the poor may stir the libertarian, it does not compel him, and no state ought to force him to react.

It is important to Nozick that justice exists in the way that holdings are originally acquired and in the way that holdings are exchanged; he finds fault with the term "distributive justice" itself.[24] His point is that distributive justice is the complex net result of a set of gifts, exchanges, and trades within a diverse and quirky society that consists of different and free individuals making a series of choices based on values that are unique and not coerced. Justice has been done if three things obtain: first, if the original acquisition is in accordance with a principle of justice; second, if the subsequent acquisition of the holding from someone else entitled to that holding is done in accordance with a principle of justice; and third, if no one is entitled to any acquisition outside repeated application of the first two principles.

Thus, the *entitlement theory* is grounded in two concerns: historicity and justice of legitimate process. Acquired goods ("holdings") can accumulate to the clever but honest trader in any amount, and the foolish and unfortunate trader can slip to any level of despair. There are no limits on the amount on either side, as long as no one is harmed by the actions of the other—as long as no one steals, defrauds, enslaves, or excludes unfairly from competition. All other theories, contends Nozick, simply look at a current time or at an end result principle that cannot truly explain or describe how the world of what is currently real came to be. Knowing the origins of the real is as critical as accurately describing it at the present time. To ignore this point, said Nozick, is to ignore the principal place deserts have in a theory of justice.

•

Free Holdings and the Problem of Inclusion

Libertarians believe that the first gesture of self is free acquisition.[25] Persons do not have "shares" in a common system; they create for themselves "holdings" that are truly theirs. They wrest their share from the free earth; they mix their sweat with the land; they create possession. Secondary to that acquisitive gesture, the self, with its correspondent freedom, is intact. Humans could live, ideally, without a contract, were there not threats to their safety and projects of joint enterprise that require collective action. Given this, social contracts are a necessary and limited constraint on liberty. Society is a way to manage individual desire and passion, which, according to libertarian theory, overpower freedom itself by their cruelty and excess.

The persons held within this social contract are persons who manage to wrest out a holding, and some are simply not in the contract.[26] Hence, the moral appeal of these others is that of an order different from that of stakeholders within the minimum state themselves. This leads to a final problem with the notion of freely acquired holdings that was not tangential to the project of distributive justice. That problem is not the language Nozick proposes, which places so much stress on process, but the fact that in U.S. society much of the acquisition of the holdings is unjust, wrested from native peoples, bought under false pretenses, taken in unjust wars, or built with the labor power of slaves, whose chances for holding were never made actual. Much of what libertarians take as the givenness of the world rests on such unjust first division and relies on the value assumption that what is uncaptured in "nature" can be fairly taken by the most determined hand.

The language of this theory holds enormous appeal. For Americans, libertarian justice is foundational, merit based, and popular. One sees its use in the insistence on the protection of the free-market metaphor in health care, on the use of the managed competition mode, and in the linkage between health care benefits and their relationship to the means of production. Moreover, the insistence on attention to the historical actuality and genesis of claims rather than justice based on what obtains at present is a significant contribution to our understanding of the given.[27] Furthermore, nowhere does one find as pervasive a sense of desert, albeit covert, as in the notion of preventative health care. Beneath this concept (eat right, exercise regularly) lies a libertarian theme: work hard, play fairly, and what you "acquire" in terms of health is yours.[28]

What is critical about the language of libertarianism is its appeal to individual liberty and rationality and an insistence on the noncoerced consent of the governed. Additionally, it implies a basic optimism about the human spirit. First, it allows the acquisition of property as the basis of entitlement. Hence, the mythic possibility that the free marketplace is available to all who work hard remains intact. If things work out for single individuals (Nozick cites athletes), that is fair enough, and if things do not, that too is fair: all have the chance to pick up the acorns. Second, it is optimistic about charity. Theoretically "the bounds of reason" keep irrational greed in check, so one can be optimistic that the urge to help others would emerge.[29]

•

The Utilitarian Theory of Justice

Concern for the liberty of the individual is most commonly held in tension with the concept of the common good. The leading philosophic response to the problem of the shared and common fate of all is the theory of utilitarianism. Utilitarians ask, Does it really "not matter" how the system of fair exchanges manifests? Are there truly no limits on what "becomes actual" as exchanges, in and of themselves "just," generate power, wealth, and profit in a way that is quite obviously unjust, or at least unfair? There is a broad answer to this. It is consequentialist justice theory, which looks less at the rightness of the claims of competing individuals and more at the outcomes as they affect the generalized whole. One type of consequentialist justice theory takes as a basic premise that utility, named as happiness, ought to be the primary consideration of justice. Utility is judged by the evaluation of the outcome of a series of exchanges. This is the theory that most explicators of the Oregon process name as an inspiration, and it figures largely in the current managed-care debates.

Utilitarian theories of distributive justice are historically linked to an abiding concern with teleological or consequentialist considerations.[30] John Stuart Mill is one of the principal theorists associated with this approach. Mill believed in a language of rational discourse that led to a clear and objective consideration of consequences. "All action is for the sake of some end, and rules of action, it seems natural to suppose, must take their whole character and color from the end to which they are subservient. . . . When we are engaged in a pursuit, a clear and precise conception of what we are pursuing would seem to be the first thing we need, instead of the last we are to look forward to."[31] What is at stake is a notion of the aggregate general welfare of a population, in which all have both a stake and an obligation. Prior to any action, utilitarian theory insists on a consideration of the usefulness (utility) of the outcome of the proposed action. This language focuses on the end goal of utility and finds justice in the maximization of utility for the greatest number.

In this theory the hallmark concepts are general aggregate welfare and utility, generally understood by Mill, in particular, to mean "happiness." In maximizing the good consequences for the greatest number, and in minimizing the bad consequences, there is a recognition that justice of this sort may involve a loss of all goods for some minority if in this way the general utility is benefited.

Mill was not unaware that one of the strongest objections to his theory of utilitarianism was that utility took no account of justice.[32]

> In all ages of speculation one of the strongest obstacles to the reception
> of the doctrine that utility or happiness is the criterion of right and wrong
> has been drawn from the idea of justice. The powerful sentiment and
> apparently clear perception which that word recalls with a rapidity and
> certainty resembling instinct have seemed to the majority of thinkers to
> point to an inherent quality in things; to show that the just must have
> an existence in nature as something absolute, generically distinct
> from every variety of the expedient.[33]

But Mill questioned this intrinsic conception of justice. His language makes clear that the existence of a moral sentiment does not equate with the appropriateness of its use in society. "That a feeling is bestowed on us by nature does not necessarily legitimate all its promptings."[34] Higher reason required a clear examination of the consequences of social actions. Mill is clear in his choice of ends: "Pleasure and the freedom from pain, are the only things desirable as ends; and that all desirable things (which are as numerous in the utilitarian as in any other schemes) are desirable either for the pleasure inherent in themselves, or as a means to the promotion of pleasure and the prevention of pain."[35] Insistence on this principle, the greatest happiness principle, is fundamental. Mill makes explicit that the language of justice is to mean the best outcome for the society as a whole.[36] Each person may pursue in the private sector of his or her own life the conduct that will make him or her happy. In the public sector, however, two rules obtain.

> First, that the conduct pursued will not injure the interests of another, or rather certain interests, which either by express legal provision or by tacit understanding ought to be considered as rights, and secondly, in each person's bearing his share (to be fixed on some equitable principle) of the labors and sacrifices incurred for defending the society or its members from injury and molestation . . . as soon as any part of a person's conduct affects prejudiciously the interests of others, society has jurisdiction over it. And the question of whether or not the general welfare will or will not be promoted by interfering with it, becomes open to discussion.[37]

Societies can constrain behavior by legal means or by moral gesture. Mill mentioned "opinion" as an option in this regard and envisioned a society that shaped moral praxis by education and persuasion, a process whereby the help that persons "owe each other in distinguishing the better from the worse" would be facilitated.

Distributive justice, according to Mill's theory, must take into account the necessity of the greater good. In practice this means that the liberty of the one can be curtailed and the right of absolute unlimited choice can be limited by a claim of the many, on the basis of other, competing liberties or on the basis of the economic or general welfare of the aggregate whole. Whether the one is the least advantaged, the weakest, or the most able, the aggregate good trumps the claim of the one. The sentiment of justice as a "moralized social feeling" is a response to perceived threats to the whole "act[ing] in the directions conformable to the general good: just persons resenting a hurt to society, though not otherwise a hurt to themselves, not resenting a hurt to themselves, however painful, unless it be of the kind which society has a common interest with them in the repression of."[38]

It is critical in understanding Mill's language of justice to clarify that rights and liberty, the centerpiece of Locke's theory, have a specific and limited use in Mill's account of utilitarianism. "To have a right, then, is, I conceive, to have something which society ought to defend me in my possession of. If the objector goes on to ask why it ought, I can give him no other reason than general utility . . . the interest involved in that of security, to everyone's feelings the most vital of all interests."[39] Rights for equal treatment, and for reward and punishment to be meted out according to deserts, are contingent. They exist except when "some recognized social expediency requires the reverse." There are no "rights" that attach to any specific individual desire. Since all material benefits are understood and desired idiosyncratically, only collective security can be understood as essential, and only the demands of this collective security can be understood as primary. For Mill, this is the ground of justice. "The machinery for providing it [must be] kept unintermittedly in active play."[40] Even liberty is not a right unless it is justified by its utility to a society that is secure. Claims of merit, claims of prior social contract, conflicting appeals, and material principles of justice are ultimately subjective and hence do not give a consistent account of justice.[41] The language of this theory holds that arguments concerning the equality or relative inequality of particular individuals are capricious and "pretentious," based as they are on "imaginary standards not grounded in utility."[42]

This suggests a minimalist language of obligation as well as rights. "A person may possibly not need the benefits of others, but he always needs that they should not do him hurt."[43] This lends itself to a curious distancing from the subject in the language. It does not matter who the particular individuals are, or their context or passion. What will trump appeals are the external needs of a state that is girded at all times with the potential for violence and catastrophe.

American society, while libertarian in mythos, also uses the language of utilitarianism in its most basic civil relationships. It is the language of democracy itself, of voting and living by the result, of accepting payment if one's house stands in a freeway's path, and of understanding that while one may desire help for one's sprained ankle in the emergency room, the busload of badly wounded campers will get treated first. It is the language of first morals, of parents to children.[44]

This theory of justice requires stepping back to an objective "neutral vantage" to see if the manipulation of other forces results in a net improvement for all. It requires that less attention be paid to the legitimacy of each agent's competing claim and more attention to outcomes, specifically to both net and aggregate happiness and to the avoidance of harm. The language assumes objectivity, that one's own interest, narrative, or context will not influence this rational view. Reliance on this premise and on using the language of the rational participant as the standard for the measure of the terminology itself commits Mill to conclude that common sense[45] will rule out the most pernicious behavior just when (in fact) it is egregious.[46] There is a compelling methodological logic to this theory. In addressing the allocation of scarcities, the theory uses the vocabulary of outcomes, happiness, universalism, and some aspects of the common good. It is familiar, requiring no idealized thought construct. It is rooted both in the normative experience of democratic justice and in a certain sense of terror that is similarly compelling, suggesting that threat of social chaos ought to define the limits of our freedom.

The Problem of the Majority

All discussions of utilitarianism have major conceptual problems. The first is the issue of inclusion. Just who is included in the "greatest number"? Do we have an obligation to include every possible member in a given society? How broad does a consensus have to be? Is a clear majority, a simple majority, or a consensus needed? Whatever determination is made, the net result is that some group, larger than the other, is on the whole more satisfied (in what way is another problem) than the other. Majority trumps minority.

Did the majority in such an application set limits based on the aggregate utility of the security of the whole, or can a small group make such decisions because of a certain relationship to the apparatus of power? Does our assessment change if the view of the vulnerable minority is actually represented, but the deciding group still sets values and, hence, policy for the vulnerable minority?

The Implication of the Public-Private Split

Linked to this concept of majority versus minority is the implied notion of the "public" versus the "private" sphere. The language of utilitarian theory most strongly implies this critical tenet of liberalism. Dealings within the sphere regarded as private are relatively free from restraint unless they affect another. Then they are public acts and thus can be addressed by the needs of the state. The framing construct reifies the notion that there could be acts that were entirely private, thus socially invisible. Action can be either self-regarding or other-regarding. Because the groundwork is laid conceptually by means of this linguistic and ideological assumption, utilitarian theory is able to suggest that use of isolated and discreet persons as a means to a just end is permissible.

The Problem of the Good

The recognition that the aggregate utility is best rendered by a democratic process is an interesting, but not necessary, correlate of this theory. At stake is the very issue of "good." How are we to assess human flourishing? Is it the aggregate number of preferences that are satisfied? Baruch Brody suggests that there is a problem even with this formulation.[47] Perhaps there is a difference, Brody notes, between "true" and "expressed" preferences. Both may differ from "objective assessment of the good" or, in a social construct, "necessity" or "basic minimum standard." The utilitarian principle, while intuitively accessible, does not tell us what the normative answer might be in writing public policy. For example, it may lead to a decision either to assist or to cut drastically public assistance (for example, changes in Wisconsin and California health care budgets for the Medicaid population).

The Problem of Evil

What if the bad consequences cannot be minimized? The aggregate good, even the total consensus of the whole save for one, may be met, but the consequences for the one may be so terrible, so odious, or so unthinkably cruel that the good consequences are trivialized. This was the significant problem of the eighteenth century, when the aggregate good could clearly be enhanced for the majority by the use of slaves. It is also the central critique of all rationing: How can society deny any "good" if the consequence is death? At stake is, of course, whether it was ever right to use another person merely as a means to an end.

This was Kant's central concern. The Kantian critique of utilitarianism is foundational to egalitarian philosophic theories that base their source of essential rights on something other than the entitlement of property. The focus on the language of sublimation of the individual to society privileges some aspects of social obligation. The language of utilitarianism, that "each received his proper share and bore his proper share," works as long as the greatest good is served. The distributive justice suggested by this theory obtained only if all are, in fact, receiving and bearing within a shared moral system, with a shared moral vocabulary, so that the terms themselves, and the costs and benefits (the "ends") they describe, are understood and experienced as intuitively worth the loss of autonomy that is suggested.

The language of utilitarianism can be useful in addressing the concerns about the common good that arise in a consideration of libertarianism. But like that language, utilitarian theory has similarly proved inadequate in addressing significant justice concerns in the health care debate.

The critique of utilitarianism is based on a persistent disquiet about the fate of the individual in such a distributive system. Following the line of utilitarian reasoning logically, one encounters deeply emotional and principled reactions in the public sphere. These responses are becoming apparent now as health care planners cheerily attempt to use outcome measures or cost benefit analysis in reform efforts. A concern for the essential human equality of all persons, a concern for the individual life project of each and the voice of each, and a deontological concern for a sense of fairness are central to the major philosophic challenge to utilitarianism.

•

Deontology: Duties and the Matrix of Promises

Deontology (duty-based justice) pursues the question of obligations to others with a steady and compelling force. It assumes that the public world of ethics has at its heart the autonomy of the individual and rational choosing self, but that it is a self in a world of others to whom promises are made and to whom duties are owed. What matters most are the underlying norms and presumptions, the *means* of being, and the contexts of relationships and their attendant obligations that guide our acts. For some deontologists there are certain acts (truth telling, promise keeping) that contain moral worth distinct from their impact on consequences— independent of the net happiness, pleasure, or difficulties the fulfillment of the obligation would bring.[48]

For a careful look at this theory, scholars classically return to Immanuel Kant.[49] Kant acted on the premise that there is a categorical imperative that can never be violated.[50] This imperative, which demands that each act is universalizable, generalizable, and consistent, is the basis for the framing language of the deontological Kantian system. Not only must acts be universalizable and consistent with the categorical imperative, but they must be inherently consistent with each other. *Justice* implies that like situations will be treated equally, and that this will be both reciprocal and replicable.

Centrally, Kant assumed that this method assures that each rational being is an end in himself or herself. Persons cannot be used as "mere" means to an end. The language of *personhood* is central: Every "other" is also a "self" and is capable of the juridical power of choice and maxim creation—a source of moral norms, accountable and subject to the causation of others. Accountable, autonomous agents can be the subject of contracts, both social and private, and can be *bound* by the duties of the contract itself.[51] Without the assumption of obligation, of course, no contract is valid.[52]

In the creation of the current welfare state, deontological concerns played a central part. Contract egalitarian John Rawls creates much of the shaping language in the current debate around social contracts and distributive justice— distributive justice is the central theory of affirmative action, of entitlements, and of a strongly protective state. Embattled and still central to the liberal vision, the language of Rawls's approach must be explored.

•

John Rawls: The Promise of Fairness

Rawls argues that justice is the "first virtue of social institutions, as truth is to systems of thought."[53] Rawls is interested in the basic structure of social institutions and not simply in schemes of distributive justice, and he uses the language of the "inviolability of personhood" to describe the citizen in the just state. Rawls firmly rejects the utilitarian and libertarian premises:

> Each person possesses an inviolability founded on justice that even the
> welfare of society as a whole cannot override. For this reason justice denies

that the loss of freedom for some is made right by a greater good shared by others. It does not allow that the sacrifices imposed on a few are outweighed by the larger sum of advantages enjoyed by many. Therefore in a just society the liberties of equal citizenship are taken as settled; the rights secured by justice are not subject to political bargaining or to the calculus of social interests.[54]

Persons are not equal because they are entitled to equal shares in a system of distribution, argues Rawls, but because of this prior inviolability. Society consists of a "more or less self-sufficient association" of independent persons who recognize in their relationships the existence of certain binding rules and who act in accordance with these rules. It is social cooperation motivated by an identity of interests around a general goal of mutual gain and marked by a conflict of interest around the allocation of the benefits of that cooperation.

Rawls's goal is not to achieve equality of the resultant shares. It is to achieve "pure procedural justice," to establish the rules of the basic social contract such that the circumstances of choice are fair. The principles required for choosing the "division of advantages" and for underwriting the agreement are the principles of social justice. Further, they provide a construct for assigning rights and duties that correlate to the benefits of social cooperation. The outcome may lead to relative inequality of such shares and duties; but if the access to process is based on equality of persons and is freely chosen, if all know that the rules are mutually acceptable, and if the social institutions thus created satisfy the principles, then the outcome is fair and hence just.[55]

This language of procedural justice is predicated on the premise of deontology: the ability of *autonomous* persons to make rational choices. What is held in common is a shared conception of justice and "civic friendship" based on a "fundamental charter of a well-ordered human association."[56]

Each actor in such a system has his or her own distinct concept of the good, of happiness, and of a proper end, rendering a unanimous goal elusive. Equality of ends or the achievement of a overriding end that is agreed upon may not be possible in a complex, pluralistic society, claims Rawls; hence the language of justice must be based in the sense of fairness of the initial contract. "Those who hold different conceptions of justice can, then, still agree that institutions are just when no arbitrary distinctions are made between persons in the assigning of basic rights and duties and when the rules determine a proper balance between competing claims to the advantages to the social life."[57] The theory requires focus on how standards are chosen, who chooses them, and what follows after such choices.

The language is rooted in an extended thought exercise that takes place in a fixed, formal universe and envisions moral agents engaged in a joint act of social construction during which the rules of procedural justice are created. How ought one to construct the language of fair choice? All persons begin in an "original position of equality."[58] Rawls assumes essential features of this situation. First, autonomous moral agents are ignorant of their own situation, of their class, social status, natural assets, and strength or abilities (Rawls describes this as wearing the "veil of ignorance"). Second, all agents agree that "usual circumstances of justice prevail."[59] There is scarcity, conflict over distribution of shares, and conflicts of goals, and while choices are disputed, all agree that cooperation would improve the lot of all. Third, agents are "in history"—they know about sociology and psychology (having read Freud and Durkheim) and will not set up rules that are unworkable in this culture/society.[60] Fourth, they are mutually disinterested and rational. Fifth, as disinterested agents they "are conceived as not taking an interest in one another's interest." They further their own goals to meet their own needs, and once these needs are met, they are not envious of another's larger share.

With this linguistic construct as a metaphor, Rawls suggests that two principles[61] are chosen that characterize social actions. First, each person gets an equal chance for the largest set of liberties, right, and duties possible.[62] Rawls assumes that each person will rationally choose to acquire an equal share of that which is divisible—all social primary goods, such as liberty and opportunity, income and wealth—the material and social basis of self-respect.[63]

Rawls recognizes that in an actual social world there are differences among individuals. When the veils of ignorance are lifted to reveal our true places in the hierarchical ordering of a real society, some are old, some are young, some are wealthy, and some are poor. Given this, rational actors choosing the procedures of justice would permit social and economic inequalities only if they result in compensating benefits for everyone and in particular for the least advantaged members of society.[64]

This second principle of "difference" works to protect those who are least advantaged.[65] Moreover, since one does not know if one would be old or young, one will want to allow for the prudent use of resources and for systems of distribution that do not place lives and goods at risk for later generations in order to provide for those presently served. Rawls calls this the "just savings" principle. Since power and position are linked, it is also to the advantage of each person to make the process one that allows for changes in the hierarchy itself, so that all positions of privilege would be open to all.[66]

Rawls describes the actual world of distribution as having elements of both relative conflict and cooperation among various interests who are differently endowed. While the human status of each interest is equal in terms of the liberty to which each is entitled, the actual circumstances in which people are located are distributed rather randomly, largely on the basis of a natural and social lottery that must be addressed in actual systems of contracts and ordering.

Rawls draws our attention to the caprice of the lottery and to the desirability for social mediation of its effects by rules that are socially constraining.[67] A basic tenet of the language of this theory, unlike libertarian thought, is that the results of natural and social lotteries are undeserved and unjust.[68] Further rules that we presently operate under unfairly weight the lottery and disadvantage some still further. The inequity that results is real and measurable in terms of health effects.[69] This inequity must be socially redressed and not just lamented, in Rawls's ideal system, because it is not "rational" or "fair." It does not lead to a well-ordered society even if the inequality serves to enhance the utility for the greater good.[70]

Allocation of goods is a matter of the procedural rules of justice and not charity.[71] The most just system is likely to be fairly chosen under the rules of citizenship in the social contract. Like other deontology systems, the ethical primacy of justice is in the *rules* of the game, not the outcome.

Rawls, while concerned with *initial* procedure and locating his language of justice in these procedures, builds in an evaluative final rule of adjustment. Both the description of the initial contractual situation and the principles that match our considered judgments in response are assessed and reflected on in light of "particular cases which may lead us to revise our judgments."[72] The final rule of Rawls's theory, "reflective equilibrium," argues for the necessity for reflection and renegotiation of the critically important language of the social contract.

Rawls argues for the language of the contract as the fullest expression of our human liberty: this liberty expresses what it is about us that is fundamental. But his is not the only egalitarian theory. Egalitarian theories claim that as humans each of us has inescapable and essential rights and obligations toward one another that cannot be ignored, and that these rights, obligations, duties, and needs arise from something we share as persons, something that is common to all and, hence, respected by all. This commitment to equality and the ability to make rational choices that honor this equality are at the heart of this theory of justice. First among these duties is the notion that justice is rooted in equality, an equality due on the basis of shared human embodiment and participation in a mutually consensual human society.

The distinguishing language of this theory includes equality of access to shares in the good, to fairly determined rules of procedure, and to a basic decent minimum. This basic decent minimum is an assessment of a quantifiable human necessity that constitutes the share to which all persons are entitled by virtue of their personhood alone, not because of merit or desert.

•

Egalitarian Theories of Justice

Robert Veatch, a theorist whose work is formulative in the field of bioethics and in justice in health care allocations, explicates the language of egalitarianism, the pure application of which differs in important respects from contractarianism.[73] Veatch asserts that the basis for a belief in equality comes from faith sources, what he calls "the Judeo-Christian myth system."[74] All justifications for theories based on equality were "faith moves." All philosophic critiques of justice theory had covertly "bootlegged" (Veatch's term) these faith assumptions into place. Without them, the theory of equality did not stand, and the social contract was certainly not possible.

Veatch notes the three premises for this tradition of equality:

1. The first and most fundamental commitment of the Judeo-Christian [sic] tradition that leads to a commitment to equality is that God is absolute, the ultimate concern, the infinite center of value in comparison to which all humans are equal in their finitude. . . . In comparison to the Absolute, humans in their finitude are nothing, and the differences among us count as nothing.

2. Hobbes and Locke (or at least the secular versions of them), regardless of their differences, both share an individualism in which resources in the state of nature are originally unowned and, within certain limits, up for grabs. The Judeo-Christian creation myth is a way of challenging that view of nature and nature's resources. . . . The land (and by extension all goods) is a gift, a public good, a community resource, or if not, then a privately held trusteeship to be used responsibly according to the needs of others.

3. According to the Judeo-Christian myth system, it is not—as the modern libertarians would have us believe—that individuals originally stood isolated and alone in the state of nature only gradually building artificial and fragile links whenever it was necessary to avoid a life that was nasty, brutish and short. A duty of stewardship in such a context would be contrived at best. But with an understanding of human relations built on the model of brotherhood [sic] and common parentage, the linkages are bound in blood, making the community the corporate protector of the welfare of those in need.[75]

This is strong protection of the least advantaged, and it arises not out of charity, but on behalf of the needs of all for a strong contract based on equality. By offering this defense of individuals who are at greatest risk, egalitarians appeal to sympathetic and reflexive perspectives that are strained by faithful adherence to other theories that provide impersonal, acontextual, or structural accounts of individuals on whose behalf the contracts are created. Particular duties in roles and relationships are part of the justice assessment of this language. The role of the state as a strong center of welfare, as adjudicating conflict and reorganizing injustice, also emerges in egalitarian theory. Unlike Rawls, Veatch argues strongly for a shared set of ends—one of the characteristics of human uniqueness for Rawls is our idiosyncratic choices of goals and ends.[76] But language that focuses on equal rights, on a civil and contractual base for a society, and on only those inequalities that benefit the least advantaged have what Lebacqz has called "a strong intuitive appeal to many in our contemporary world."[77]

Deontology is easily challenged in the real world. Utility and proportionality heavily influence nearly every contemporary understanding of justice, and this requires close attention to outcome, narrative, and context. Deontologists note intention and duty, but when they consider the problem of narrative and context, they frame a response in the language of duties inherent in freely consensual relationships or in the freely chosen obligations of the contract itself. This language is not successfully applied to many clinical cases and ultimately is flawed when addressing the particular and competing appeals and rights of those who could claim our attention in a crisis of distribution.

Can any language of deontology adequately allow for critical reflection on the demands of the other, or is there a danger of the procedure itself failing to describe adequately the complexities of the actual situation?[78] While stressing motive, process, and obligation, can this language take into account competing cultural norms and visions of what constituted the "rational" being? In part, these questions can be raised as a critique not only of the language of deontology, but also of the entire enterprise of all liberal theory.

However the representative theories of liberalism differ, the language that each uses to address the issue of justice is similar. All three can be summarized as belonging to a unified hermeneutic: the discourse of liberal theory itself in which the concept of liberty has priority over all other values.[79] These theories share powerful central concerns and linguistic assumptions.

•

Summary of Justice Approaches Based in Liberal Theory

In summary, while the hegemonic theories have obvious critical distinctions, all three stress the language of equity and impartiality that marks the formal principle of justice and is distinctive to that approach. Justice-based approaches to the question of how to allocate scarce resources fairly differ in two ways: in their selection of material principles and in the weight given to rights and entitlement. All are theories not only of distributive justice, but of the operation of the liberal state.

All liberal theories share the presuppositions of the liberal tradition; they rest on the assurance of the primacy of the individual and share the idea that the individual "self," with liberty, rights, duties, and the ability to engage in voluntary consent, exists prior to the social contract. In fact, the social contract that is entered into by rational free agents operating from an original position, which is either historical or hypothetical, created the idea of the liberal state.[80]

•

Foundational Constraints on All Theories: Scarcity Is Prior to Theory

Common to all theories of justice is that they are based in the fact of scarcity. As David Hume pointed out, the consideration of what is just, and the passions and sympathies that frame this consideration, change as the impact of the scarcity affects the social order.[81] If there is no scarcity, there is no call for a philosophic theory of justice; each person would live in perfect abundance.

> It seems evident that, in such a happy state, every other social virtue would flourish and receive tenfold increase; but the cautious, jealous virtue of justice would never once be dreamed of. For what purpose make a partition of goods, where everyone has already more than enough? Why give rise to property, where there cannot possibly be any injury? Why call this object *mine*, when upon the seizing of it by another, I need but stretch out my hand to possess myself what is equally valuable? . . . We see, even in the present necessitous condition of mankind, that, wherever any benefit is bestowed by nature in an unlimited abundance, we leave it always in common among the whole human race, and make no subdivisions of right or property.[82]

The condition of limited resources forces rational individuals into public association.[83]

Beyond the general theory and the material principles, any application of a particular theory is rooted in specifics of power relationships that are both historical and located in a narrative of an actual social world. Any theory, to be ultimately credible, must address certain social imperatives: cultural politics, economic limits, and the power of the state.

•

Different Terms of the Discourse

The power of the central concepts embedded in the language of liberal justice theories—the priority of liberty, autonomy, universalism, and rational discernment—is such that these concepts have become the significant currency of all philosophical ethics since the Enlightenment. In a relatively new application—the field of bioethics—this language, in part because of its foundational philosophic quality, constitutes the "first principles" and, in some venues, the only principles of biomedical ethics.[84] It is striking that in the literature of clinical bedside ethics and social policy these core ideas are the presumed stance, prior to all debate on specific mechanics of reform. But they are not unchallenged ideas.

Significant critiques of autonomy, universalism, and even rationality itself have emerged strongly in recent years.

The language of liberal theory describes a world that is compelling but ultimately of little use in addressing the allocation discourse. The classic liberal theories offer a vocabulary of order and containment in the face of the health care crisis. Rather than allowing situational chaos or the mere survival of the fittest to dominate the clinical encounter and the arena of public policy, the classic theories of liberalism set some limits on what is permissible. However, defining the nature of rights that arise out of this contractual liberty ultimately does not address the problem of competing but legitimate rights to scarce resources.

The critics of this language challenge not only the efficacy of the terms, but also their very anthropology. The very image of the autonomous rational agent, choosing obligations out of an unchallenged liberty, needed to be challenged, argued these theorists.[85]

This chapter characterized the problem of justice and allocation in the philosophical debate between collective outcome and the language of rights—the classical grounds for this debate, the major theoretical methodologies, and the language they have in common. The next chapter examines what lies prior to and beyond this language of the source traditions. It is to the challenges to the language of autonomy, individualism, and rights that we now turn in our search for a way to speak justly to our neighbor.

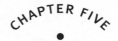

THE MORAL
LOCATION OF THE SELF
The Languages of the Alternative
Discourse

That the language of justice is constricted and lacking in key moral sensibilities is scarcely a new point. Nor is it news that such justice language has failed to address adequately critical social arenas such as health care, crime, or poverty. Many critiques of liberal theory and the construction of the self in the language of liberal theory have emerged in disciplines once removed from public policy and bioethics. The deconstruction of the language of liberalism and the critique of the project of justice as fairness has been extensive. Among these critiques are religious perspectives on the meaning of self, autonomy, and the language of community; the contribution of feminism in the recovery of the relationship with the concrete other as an aspect of moral life; observations of sociology and political science on social discourse in human communities; and the movement in philosophy known as communicative ethics, which emphasizes the language of the actual encounter in the philosophic project. It is critical to look beyond the traditional sources of debate and justice theory—the traditional terrain of debate, bioethics, and public policy—to recapture what is imperative in the construction of the self. The necessity to speak and hear a differently imagined narrative of justice allows us to move forward. Reclaiming that language implies attention to an ethical decision-making model that is contextual and narrative, organized around the principle of respect for community. This position further implies the following three elements.

First, there is an inherent link between private desire and decision and public acts of moral choice. Conscience (the individual, interior discernment of the morally appropriate choice) and human community (the interdependent relationships between the self and the other) are linked.

Second, not only are public and private acts inherently linked, but focus on community allows a shift in paradigm from the agent of moral action (defined as an individual actor) to the nature of moral agency itself as collective, invoking a language of mutuality and interdependence.

Third, independence as an organizing principle is not an ultimately practical mode, especially for research that takes sizable amounts of human social organization to mobilize, such as transplants or the production and administration of vaccines, intensive care, and trauma units. A different principle, the principle of community, is corrective and theoretically critical at this juncture.

Focusing on embeddedness in relationships and maintaining a principle of community in moral reflection means asking the questions presented in this chapter. Further, such a focus helps answer the framing questions "Who owes what to whom?" and "For whom do you care?" with the premise of mutual obligation as a requirement of personhood.

A different approach to the problem of justice raised in the previous chapter rests on a series of assumptions about the person and society different from those made in the classic debates. It begins with the assumption that the social in the person is prior to the individual. These texts argue that, in fact, only through society and in community does the self begin to emerge. In this alternative theory the fundamental paradigmatic shift made is that all individuals, by definition, are included in society. Sociability is not a willed choice; it constitutes personhood.

•

The Central Problem: Autonomy and the Entirely Free Self

Central to the classic liberal approach to justice is the conceptualization of the entitled self, autonomous and rational, freely choosing, and discrete. In the discourse of ethics, legal theory, public policy, and most particularly, bioethics, autonomy has a near trumping potency. In bioethics the construct of autonomy has served importantly to define and defend the ability of the vulnerable patient to choose freely among a variety of health care alternatives. The primary evocation of autonomy has not been in the service of distributive justice, however, but in the service of patients' rights. It has been a key principle in countering the excesses of physician paternalism in the last fifteen years and in reconfiguring the law relative to consent relationships. As such, the use of the principle of autonomy has been central to each detail of the physician-patient encounter. The prior operational agreement, based in paternalism and its association with beneficence, between the patient and the provider has been examined anew in light of this recognition.

The idea that an individual, freely consenting self with rights can be said to exist at this point in the history of intellectual thought (post-Freud, post-Kant, and post-Locke) is so automatically assumed that it seems to be a natural fact. It seems to be a notion as inherent to the idea of humans as furriness is to the idea of bears. Yet, the construction of the self as an autonomous self-legislator, belonging to no master, to no God, and to no a priori community, with an internal and privatized biography, is a post-Enlightenment philosophical and theological revelation. What made the Enlightenment so revolutionary was, in fact, largely, although not entirely, this premise.

But the language of autonomy, like the language of the marketplace, turns out also to be extraordinarily limited in its ability to handle the problem of justice between several autonomous and contending selves. The high-stake problems involved in the allocation of social goods in general and medical goods in particular do not lend themselves to solutions by louder insistence on the depth of autonomy for each person. The construct of autonomy is itself based on a particular social and cultural availability. As Charles Taylor has pointed out, the awareness of the independent, boundaried self, autonomous, freely choosing, nonreferential, and nonconstrained by tradition or social surround, is only possible because this self exists in this particular social order. The social order values this type of freedom and, in fact, constructs liberation and its metaphors in the language of the isolated self. Hence, this free self, at the moment of radical proclamation of self, is paradoxically constrained, committed, and "placed" in the defining society, in the reigning tradition, and in the accident of birth and geography. It is as likely that an American teenager will want to be free to do his own thing as it was that a serf would do the work of his lord. Both are framed not only by the dynamics of the economic marketplace, but by the dictates of the state and the ideology and vocabulary of their society. The very words used to utter freedom are constrained by the givenness of history.[1]

If the critical assumption of the language of liberal theory is the existence of a social contract made by persons who are "inherently, naturally and equally free,"[2] and the critical quality characteristic of a human is liberty, then the making of a social contract is somewhat paradoxical. The liberal social contract is a construct that will limit some aspects of one's freedom, but it is legitimated by virtue of its being freely chosen. The voluntariness of this primary obligation is what is defining in liberal theory. Nancy Hirshmann explains the point: "The only legitimate limitations are those that are imposed by the self: for if I am above all else free, a limitation of freedom can only be legitimate if it is simultaneously an expression of my freedom. Thus social contract is an expression of human freedom, of our ability to make choices and control our destiny."[3] The priority of liberty and the contract model of the association of separate, freely choosing persons describes a state where the common good can be conceptualized as the aggregate good of many separate and individual interests.

Ronald Beiner describes the ethos of liberalism, in a pluralistic society, as language secondary only to the language of democracy, and as persuasive and unified.[4] Beiner urges us to remember that all such theories are the result of the "theorist as storyteller," and that all are correspondingly placed in the particular story as the "moral vocabulary" of a culture. The very idea of the autonomous self is a construct of the particular moral vocabulary that emphasizes rights rather than the achievement of collective and social goods.

Baruch Brody raises a further problem with the use of the term "autonomy."[5] Kant's use of the word implied that the language was useful in establishing the ground for human flourishing, in finding the enduring human basis for morality. Kant would claim that the agent is both subject and maker of laws. Hence, in contrast to acting in whatever direction one will, the focus is on action that promotes and furthers freedom and rationality itself (thus, no suicide) and in making maxims that will bind not only the self, but others. At the very heart of this autonomy lies the notion of limitedness, self-imposed but chosen and rational, and hence honored. This use of autonomy, respect for persons as self-legislators, is not the common-sense application or the application in current use in the bioethics debates. Far more commonly meant is Mill's notion of privacy and nonmaleficent freedom: I can do what I will inside my sphere as long as it affects only me. Action is permitted if it is either entirely self-regarding or poses no harm to others. At the heart of this latter notion of autonomy is the idea that the human is naturally unlimited, offering some of this unlimited power only because of the desperate necessity for survival. At the heart of each individual is the unrestrained self, in an original position, with no prior commitments, truly free, and freely choosing.

•

An Alternate Model of Community and Citizenship

In rejecting autonomy and the validity of the social contract, calls for a language of *community* challenge the very notion of an independent self understood as prior to and apart from social organizations. The call for new language to address the health care reform debate had been previously postulated as philosophically imperative by communitarianism, a position articulated by several theorists as a critique of liberal theory. Emerging in the modern period largely as a response to Rawls's work, communitarians called on older theories—the Aristotelian tradition of both virtue and the common good, and the sense of the polis—as critical to the language of justice. Communitarians argue that the decline of community as a way of life in the material world is linked to the formalistic, ahistorical, and individualistic legacies of the Enlightenment. The language of these theories so constricts our imagination and impoverishes our moral vocabulary that we cannot even conceptualize moral solutions to current crises in social organization. This impoverishment is tied to a general loss of moral organization, a weakening of moral bounds, and a thinning of moral tradition. Without a shared tradition of the good, little can be passed generationally, claim the communitarians. Communitarianism urges a return to the Aristotelian model of phronesis, a practical reason that is contextually embedded, and to casuistic methodology that is responsive to the particulars of history, place, and culture.[6]

This perspective is explored by a number of philosophers, among them Alasdair MacIntyre, Charles Taylor, Thomas Nagel, Michael Walzer, and Michael Sandel. Sandel's formative work in response to Rawls remains the clearest statement of the communitarian challenge to liberalism. The language that Sandel proposes is a radical break not only with the notion of justice as fairness, but with the idea of an autonomous self that is able to make meaning or vocabulary in the absence of the existence within community.[7] Sandel defined community as "both constitutive of the shared self-understandings of the participants and embodied in their institutional life."[8] "If utilitarians fail to take seriously our distinctness, justice as fairness fails to take seriously our commonality. In regarding the self as prior, fixed once and for all, it relegates our commonality to one aspect of the good, and relegates the good to a mere contingency, a product of indiscriminate wants and desires 'not relevant from a moral standpoint.' "[9] A world with no telos, ungoverned by a purposive order, is a world "disenchanted," to use Max Weber's term, according to Sandel. Only in such a world is it possible to conceive of a subject prior to and apart from the moral purpose of world and community. Only in such a world are the principles of justice open to individual, consumer-driven choice, creating a marketplace of possible ends and of possible meanings. In such a world, the social contract is seen as secondary to self and requires the emphasis on the rational and willed self found in the language of liberal theory. A kind of entrepreneurial voluntarism, a subject eager to construct, takes the place of the epistemology of a community with a shared and developed goal and good.

Sandel is careful to note that the deontological universe, while devoid of intrinsic meaning, is not a world that is ungoverned, but a world that is inhabited by industrious, if individual, selves who construct a world in the void. This willed choice creates the priority of the right over the good. Such a deontological universe implies a freedom from all prior claims and from antecedents, traditions, and standings that emerged from prior conceptions and states, unchosen and unbidden. It is seductive, noted Sandel, but finally is a flawed account of our actual moral experience, as "less liberated than disempowered."[10] In the face of this he called for the institution of "community" rather than the social contract as the appropriate pattern for the discussion of distributive justice. The language of community allows the fullest description of the moral choices that actually operate in the application of justice.

What Sandel describes as the loss of a "common vocabulary of discourse and a background of implicit practices and understandings," sociologist Robert Bellah and his colleagues Richard Madsen, William Sullivan, Anne Swidler, and Steven

Tipton are able to detail in the fieldwork and the attendant history that describe the American experience with liberal ideology. Bellah and his colleagues raise the central question of social ethics: How does the social world shape the character of the individual soul, and how do values, visions, and virtues become collective?[11]

Arguing that sociology is public philosophy and that social science is an open public conversation that is not only collective but historical, in *Habits of the Heart* Bellah explores the thesis that the relationship between *soulcraft*, the building of the good, moral self, and *statecraft*, the cultural building of a community, is a public virtue whose exercise could be encouraged in the specific American context. This requires a careful examination of the liberal language that describes this state.

For Bellah, the American state is organized around freedom, and the organizing question of the state is what institutions and virtues create freedom.[12] Bellah distinguishes two types of language and associated virtues that define the American social contract.[13] What distinguishes the two is the characterization of the relationship of the self to the other and the nature of social obligation. The biblical vision took the biblical narrative and its associated community as central, naming *ethical* relationships as defining. True freedom means freedom to make good, moral choices; true liberty exists in a covenantal relationship, to God and to others. Republican democracy is linked to this theme, and Thomas Jefferson's vision grounds this idiom, regarding equality as a universal principle that is "not always" applicable, and postulating the need for self-governance by relatively free equals.[14]

In contrast, the second and competing ideology, called utilitarian and expressive individualism by Bellah, is distinguished by an attachment to the freedom of the autonomous self. While the ideology and language of utilitarianism stress self-improvement, personal interests, and goals, the language of expressivism emphasizes the need for, and the power of, the free, expressive, independent self.[15]

Bellah postulates that the independent citizen, the entrepreneur, the manager, and the therapist have been models of the moral agents shaped by these languages.[16] Bellah describes this agency as developing in response to the demands of American culture, and its existence then further matured in the community thus created by such characters. The loss of communities of meaning, arising out of the biblical/republican ideology, and the substitution of lifestyle enclaves, arising out of the language of expressive individualism, represents, for Bellah, the loss of language that makes moral discourse in America possible.

In reflecting on the crisis of moral language caused by the loss of communities of meaning, Bellah invests a great deal of faith in the reclamation of a language of *citizenship*.[17] Bellah is optimistic about religion as a positive force in the creation of social communities of meaning. He argues that religious communities offer the possibility of intergenerational relationships, the maintenance of tradition, and the source of sustenance and vision. Here the tension between the withdrawal into the private, spiritual, personal sphere and the public life can be mediated. Language that is biblically rooted can be developed in common. Bellah argues for the development of a corresponding language of civic virtue, postulating that such civic virtue could mitigate the tension between conflicting solutions to economic and moral crises.

It is important when discussing Bellah's notion of community to understand his ideal of a national society. Bellah intends the development of a national American social community. His insight is that the language of *public good* is a construct demanded by this ideal of a national community. To support this insight he reflects on the language of historical source traditions—in the period of historic tension created by the Civil War, for example, when the discussion about how to achieve such a common language was framed by competing schematic answers that developed throughout the nineteenth and early twentieth centuries.[18] Bellah is skeptical of all schemes that were not founded in civic virtue and advocates a return to the Madisonian discourse of public good to create the language of political integration of the private moral life.

Bellah does not base his language of community on political economy or contract theory but postulates social coherence as the central theme. Coherence[19] is only possible in communities of meaning where silence, wholeness, God, and neighbor are primary. Civic virtue is public at its heart; conversational, and thus unfinished, by definition; and always linked to a larger shared goal.[20] The public discussion that emerges from this kind of attention creates the possibility of a meaningful moral discourse based on social solidarity and responsibility.[21] Bellah proposed that the term "community" include a larger sense of "settlement" and "cultivation." These two terms were to express the obligation of one generation for another not only as Rawls would have it, on behalf of a sense of fairness, but because it is through such obligation that our selves are created and re-created.

Beiner is similarly concerned with the language of liberalism and the call for a new moral vocabulary. Like Bellah, he frames his call as a language of "new republicanism" and a new language, and practice, of citizenship. In this call Beiner criticizes both the paucity of the language of liberal theories and the lack of a vision of a shared "discourse of public life." This discourse is central to Beiner's understanding of community and is prerequisite to the notion of a common good. Liberalism has so attenuated our very experiences that republican community is no longer possible. Indeed, a liberal state of this kind becomes barely intelligible.[22]

Beiner defines citizenship as a form of attachment to the political community itself. By this Beiner implies not only the theoretical justification of the act, but also the capacity to effect this attachment through various kinds of competent social, legal, and political praxis. But there are several cautionary notes about the language of community and citizenship, primarily that such language could come to be seen as a form of nationalism/xenophobia. Specifically, he notes that the language of community must be sensitive to the issues of gender, class, and racial particularity. He struggles with the notion of common allegiance itself— What meaning does this term have in a widely pluralist society?—and offers one specific answer to these issues: that as moderns we have been "socialized to be isolated and private, not to 'be good audiences.'" Beiner uses language that depends on the ability of a society to create a shared culture and sense of rooted-ness, seeing and acting on this shared culture rather than building institutions dependent on its absence.

•

The Nature of the Ideal Moral Agent

An overreaching and ultimately false autonomy is not the only problem of liberal-ism. In all of the liberal scenarios of justice there is an imagined agent behind the passive voice of the text; in classical Hellenism, the implied agent is male, a property holder, and a person who holds social power. At the very least, the implied moral agent is someone who understands the terms of the debate; at most, the agent is someone who has been specially trained as a philosophic expert to act as the identified public moral agent.

Even in the midst of the problems of social choice and social justice, the agent behind the passive voice is an individual, and his individualism is synonymous with autonomy. In fact, as autonomy is formulated in the Enlightenment text, the meaning of the language of the individual self takes a different shape and potency. The premise that an individual can exist independent of and willing to move through the world as such a free agent requires a vast and evolving set of social assumptions. Further, it implies a set of social roles and a universe made possible only by a certain stage of economic development. The ideological assumptions of a mercantile universe rely on a world peopled by consumers or workers who are essentially rootless, are concentrated in urban centers, and are able to follow the work without the pulls of rootedness.[23] In such a construct the enabling and the ends of production itself assume some life of their own.[24]

•

The Moral Agent in the Community

This language of human moral agency has been thoroughly challenged by theo-rists who insist that the moral agent stands not alone, but at the center of a responding and responsible community—embedded by necessity rather than au-tonomous. The issue of community is central to the practice of religious social ethics. Each act in the world is illuminated by the public reality of its context. Mutuality of language, commonality of history, and shared human space make the discipline of religious social ethics both possible and necessary. The ethical moment in systems of Jewish, Catholic, and Protestant thought can be placed only in the center of a responding and responsible world. For selected Christian ethicists this community is the main organizing principle, the empowerment that makes the ethical movement the most human of our acts. (The reflections of the Jewish tradition will be explored extensively in later chapters.)

To understand how religious theorists challenged liberalism and the Enlightenment project, consider the work of Stanley Hauerwas. No one in the Christian tradition of modern bioethics[25] is more closely associated with the necessity for community than Hauerwas, notable as a theologian, a communitarian theorist, and a bioethicist.[26] In framing a theory of ethics and rethinking the nature of moral agency, Hauerwas insists on the reclamation of both the language of Aristotelian virtue or character theory and the language of community. In framing the discourse of virtue as a modern necessity, Hauerwas uses the specific language of journey and frames the Christian task of responding to God's imperative as a pilgrimage of the character-in-process, as the mutable striving self embedded in a community of others. To form character, to be "marked" by choices made in the Aristotelian sense, means limiting a wide range of possibilities by choosing an order and setting a course for a journey through the choices, the journey imposing order on the self and on the world. For Hauerwas, there is no one "good" character; each journey will be uniquely good if it remains true to the larger tasks of participation in the believing community, by which he intends to describe his own Christian community.[27]

Hauerwas's method involves a self constructed with duration over time, consistent growth, and integrity and wholeness ("rondver" in Calvin's and "sincerity" in Edwards's terms). Wholeness is the goal of this process, a character that will be an example of the "already being, not yet" quality of Christian life.[28] The power of this language of virtue theory is that it reflects an essential felt reality: each act we make takes us, holds us, and shapes us subtly and irrevocably. It focuses attention on the agent in a way that was not anonymous, not abstracted as in the liberal term of an ideal self, removed from actual events. This self faces the concrete other with a narrative of concrete obligations. Additionally, the powerful metaphor of journey, growth, and unity of self gives an underlying optimism to this approach.

We need to be cautious, however, about the language of community used abstractly. The communitarians have observed that if history is constructed as not having an intrinsic thematic importance, an end, and a goal, then there is no shared notion of the meaning of goodness. Unlike a shared religious goal, such as the group project of Exodus, for example, the liberal goal threatens to be one of individual persons creating a fresh narrative as a project of their defining freedom. Hauerwas insists that calls for community do not avoid the problem of a struggle over a just end. He is skeptical of the uses of the languages of communitarianism, however, and troubled by the liberal assumptions embedded in the position itself. Further, Hauerwas is careful to make a distinction between the kind of community intended, a grouping of friends "bound by the love of one another and of God," and a neoconservative nostalgia for "small town America and the correlative 'family doctor' that no longer exists."[29]

Further, Hauerwas is wary that appeals for community that are linked to appeals to a superficial consensus mask the conflicts that exist between us, conflicts of values that are critical to reflect on and struggle with in a society in order to identify what goods we share in common. Hauerwas quotes Christopher Lasch in observing that it is the communitarian understanding that the goal of a state is not to protect the privacy rights of individuals that arise out of possession, but to protect praxis, skills, training, and practices that have become goods in common, a much wider claim for the state. The willingness to protect the work that is usually associated with private goals requires a view that freedom itself must be subject to exacting discipline, public discourse, and review. Medicine has offered the occasion for some of Hauerwas's most defining work because in medicine one can discover "what a substantive moral practice actually looks like."[30] Other theologians had also questioned the liberal language of unencumbered autonomous moral agency. For Bruce Birch and Larry Rasmussen, Protestant theologians writing collaboratively on the issues of the Bible and Christian ethics, community and moral agency were linked and central issues in ethics. Community was primary because it was the main shaping force of character/moral agency and made all demands and actions possible. We live in community because we are inherently social creatures. We live in many communities (communities of meaning), but each really moral, relevant community is one in which we can "be [construct] ourselves." Communities are the material ground of our moral lives.[31]

The role of the Bible is central for Birch and Rasmussen in the normative tasks of community. The language of community is not merely descriptive of the life they detail. Rather, two specific moral tasks are assumed by such a community. The first is to shape moral identity, to provide a context for the critical relationality of moral living. The second is to bear the shared tradition of the moral life, the narrative, and the placement of the story of each community next to the larger biblical narrative.

Community functions as a resource for moral development.[32] Community creates the context for ethics, the arena where morality, justice, and, ultimately, the discovery of conscience occur. Finally, community creates the accountability, the assessment of the moral act itself—acting as the self-correction to the moral agent. Further, once the community shapes its agents, it needs them. They set the vision, prove the history, and "stem the course" of the community. "Conscience is an expression of character, which is formed only in community."[33] This last point is of central importance. Like feminist theorists and others who criticize the liberal vision, Rasmussen and Birch make the link between the public and the private. The liberal sense that conscience is somehow removed from public moral attention, that it is the undiscovered country of the moral moment, is rejected by these theorists. It is the morally cognitive ability of the person that is shaped by life in the "called" community.[34]

The concept of the moral agent as formed by and responsible to the action of the community is certainly not the provenance of Protestants alone.[35] Theologians of the Catholic tradition argue that the historical experience of the early church ought to create a model for the language of community understood as *koinonia*.[36]

Koinonia describes the Paulist idea of a communal fellowship of God, allowing for the passive and active sharing of God's spirit, of meaning, and of blessing.[37] It is a *corporate* society, one in which all members are equal in fellowship and in which they contribute and share the gifts. John Mahoney, a Jesuit scholar, in describing the language of community, calls this a *matrix* of moral theology.

For Mahoney, God is by definition interpersonal. As Christ lived in community, so do we. Mahoney considers community the culmination of all of creation[38] and posits that in community all individuals could be the sharers of our "interpersonal being." *Koinonia* is at the heart of monastic discipline, but the ethics of *koinonia* can be described, argues Mahoney, as relationship/fellowship in general, fundamental to the *creation* itself, and hence constitutive of our human lives as lived, at best and most fully, in fellowship.

All these theologians vest authority, power, and vision in the act of *community*. While the parameters vary, the language is quite similar. Each speaks of the need for transcendence, for going beyond the self understood as an individual, in the practice of the moral act.[39]

Michael Sandel, writing from the secular communitarian position, also recognizes the centrality of relationship in the language of this account of moral agency. As moral agents, Sandel claims, we do not really construct or choose; nor can we claim deserts without a "thickly constituted self" capable of a "position of difference," with an identity tied to goals and journeys of growth, vulnerability, and achievement. To imagine a person free of attachments, according to Sandel, "is not to conceive of an ideally free and rational agent, but to imagine a person wholly without character, without moral depth. For to have character is to know that I move in a history I neither summon nor command, which carries consequences nonetheless for my choices and conduct."[40] Related to the self's capacity for knowing is the necessity for friendship. For Sandel, as for Aristotle, friendship is deeply a part of the moral experience. This means that self-knowledge ceases to be private; it involves the reflections of another, embeddedness in history, obligation, and the necessity for attachments and love.

A differently constructed agency is not the last problem with the language of liberal theory. Other theorists focus on the specific language of the rights, entitlement, and need.

•

The Language of Rights, Entitlement, and Need

The notion of rights and entitlement springs from the Lockean-Hobbesian sense of the term: a personal liberty with defined rights. The premise of Hobbesian autonomy implies that the self came into being, and into ontological being, as an isolated individual wary in a world that is not only unjust, but also treacherous. The world, quite literally, will consume the self unless bargains are struck.

> *Naturally every man has right to every thing.* And because the condition of
> man, as has been declared in the precedent chapter, is a condition of war
> of every one against every one—in which case everyone is governed by his
> own reason and there is nothing he can make use of that may not be a help
> unto him in preserving his life against his enemies—it follows that in such
> a condition every man has a right to everything, even to one another's body.
> And, therefore, as long as this natural right of every man to every thing
> endures, there can be no security to any man, how strong or wise soever he
> be, of living out the time which nature ordinarily allows men to live.[41]

These bargains, the social contract, are based on the language of the marketplace—deals made in terms of the possession of property and its associated physical boundaries that translate into the delineation of self. Thus is created a hypothetical, owned, private territory around each self and the things that each self can possess. The language of social contract is the language of the commodity. The self and the rights of the self could be negotiated and bartered in exchange for collective security. The implication is that everything is up for grabs (quite literally), that everything can be bought and sold, justified because the contract is made in a world of infinite possibility and infinite danger.[42] These two assumptions—that rights are commodified and as such can be bought and sold in a freely chosen social contract—create the premise that rights are relative not to necessity, but to desire and power.[43]

Nancy Hirshmann notes that the contract is not only made under conditions of fearfulness, but that the premise of consent itself is problematic on its own grounds. "Underneath the veneer of this exchange relationship is a relationship of power and dominations. Within the language of social contract and consent theory, one potentially puts oneself in another's power when one places oneself under an obligation by giving up part of one's freedom—one's essence—for something else. . . . The dangers inherent in this kind of relationship, this formalized connection are what requires the centrality of voluntarism as the legitimator of such a relationship."[44] The formal boundaries thus created must be carefully maintained even within the rights contract to constrain the empowered state from abuse of the power relationship that is inherent.

L. W. Sumner notes another problem with rights language itself: "Like the arms race the escalation of rights rhetoric is out of control. In the Liberal democracies of the West, and especially in the United States, public issues are now routinely phrased in the language of rights."[45] The language of rights is infinitely expansive. Used in public debate with finality, it is intrinsically limited in its ability to address conflicts because of this inflationary quality.

"Entitlement" is the term used in most modern liberal theories of justice to address the rationale for material possession of the goods needed for human flourishing. But basic entitlement, like rights, explains nothing about what to do in the face of competing entitlements or of actual scarcity. In fact, it is postulated on the premise that what is at issue in the discourse is the just distribution of shares and not primarily restoration or deserts.[46] The view of entitlements intended by libertarians but shared by other theorists as well is that entitlements have no relationship to deserts.[47]

Once the rules of justice were formulated in all classic liberal theories, then deservingness or undeservingness is secondary to legitimacy of expectations created by the freely chosen contractual relationship. For both Rawls and Nozick, the sense of community implied by the notion of deserts, the shared language of what the good life requires, is, by definition, absent.[48] How those in need come to be in need is irrelevant. What is at stake is the gravity of needs with respect to income, wealth, and other goods.[49]

•

Need, Provision, and Membership

How does language of "community" actually affect political responses to need in the real world? Michael Walzer's[50] insight is that the liberal language of the term "need" is used as an abstraction. He notes that need is always contextual: relative to political power, history, and culture. "Despite the inherent forcefulness of the word, needs are elusive. People don't just have needs, they have ideas about their needs; they have priorities, they have degrees of need; and these priorities and degrees are related not only to their human nature [sic] but also to their history and culture. Since resources are always scarce, hard choices have to be made. I suspect that these are and can only be political choices."[51] Walzer notes that need (like right) is not only elusive, but nearly infinitely expansive. Hence the limits on need, the social determination of priority, degree, or standard can only be politi-cally girded; there is no absolute priority that is given.

Walzer's language of justice rests on the perception that human societies are organized into different "spheres" or arenas. Each sphere creates different tem-plates and language for justice, and the construction of one unified field theory of justice diminishes critical differences in constructing appropriate schemes for adjudication of disputes and competing claims in different spheres. Member-ship in social community is necessary, complex, and interactive, argues Walzer. Walzer's analysis of membership and of what the system of redemption and indebtedness requires of us in the arena of social welfare is the most compelling for our purposes.

For Walzer membership in the community means the participation in the political, public arena of social needs and social exchange. This "sphere of se-curity and welfare" is marked by special obligations and relationships of exclusion and inclusion, much the way a family is marked. This division between member and stranger is constructed and maintained by provision, naming and defining what can be publicly offered to each in terms of security and welfare and what can be given up to create the community. " 'The process worked both ways,' notes Walzer, 'and that is perhaps its crucial feature. . . .' Mutual provision breeds mutuality. So the common life is simultaneously the prerequisite of provision and one of its products."[52] Communal provision is both general and specific to a given cultural and narrative location. What is common about communities of welfare and security is that public funds are spent to benefit all or most of the members, and goods are also actually handed over to individuals.

Thus, two levels of discourse on justice must take place. The first is the general discussion about the justice of common goods and needs; the second addresses the particular system of distribution to individuals based on some assessment of material principles. Walzer favors "need" even while noting the problems associ-ated with this criterion. Hence, for Walzer, distributive justice has a twofold meaning. It refers not only to how goods are distributed and on what basis, namely, the recognition of need, but also to the recognition of membership.[53]

Walzer's point is that no member can be said to have an individual right to any specific set of goods. All goods that are public are distributed as a result of some process that then marks the character of the particular political community. Members can claim two general things: (1) the right of membership itself and the right to a response to neediness and (2) some right to communal resources for the bare subsistence that makes life and, hence, membership possible to sustain. This second provision only exists as a result of some process of communal assessment and decision.[54] Walzer criticizes Rawls's language by pointing out its limited use in the actual world. "Fair shares of what?" Walzer queries the reader, cautioning that there is no comprehensive and universally approved list or method of justice that is formulaically applicable.

Interestingly enough for the purposes of my argument, he takes as his paradigm in explaining his alternate vision the example of the provision of public health. He notes, as I do in the next chapter, the strong communal provision of a public health that informs the historic Jewish communities of the Middle Ages and, after an examination of that example and a parallel one regarding education in the Hellenistic period, reflects on the provision of medical care in the modern period. He asks, "What do the citizens owe one another, given the community they actually inhabit?"[55]

Walzer resists a picture of "community" as a "mutual benefit club" and cautions the reader against ignoring the deepest moral bonds that underlie the obligation of provision.[56] Walzer's critical point is that arguments about communal provision are, at the deepest level, interpretations of the "union" and the definitions of membership in community itself. Such arguments are linked to the notion of the strategic assessment of both needs and the method and content that address the needs. Who is included in the conversation about the redistribution that of necessity precedes distribution will determine whether the rich or the poor or the powerful or the vulnerable bear the cost of community maintenance and community survival.[57]

Beiner raises the problem of rights language as the creation of rhetoric that occurs outside the context of the necessary ongoing discourse that is central to meaning.

> At a time when notions of individual rights have uniquely impressed themselves upon the political consciousness of my own polity, it can hardly be overlooked that much of contemporary political discourse is framed in the language of rights and entitlements. This forces us to reflect on the question of political rhetoric, that is to say, of the fundamental terms with which we address one another as members of a particular political community. This reflection suggests first, that the appeal to rights is not self-sufficing but depends logically upon the deeper moral considerations; and second, that the translation of this more primary moral language into rights discourse renders political relationships generally more adversarial than they would otherwise be.[58]

Beiner views the languages of rights and of values as not merely a semantic problem. Like Sandel, he considers the impulse to reconstruct the language as critical in constructing the possibility of a moral life.

Disputes over rights tend to be conducted in terms of absolutes, notes Beiner, and do not offer the possibility of negotiation and discourse. Positions are constructed, defended, and held much like territory. In challenging the view of Bruce

Ackerman, that liberal citizenship is equal to a minimal dialogue between citizens, Beiner proposes a definition that is the exact opposite: "Citizenship [ought to be] defined as participation in a dialogue that indeed weighs the substantive merit of competing conceptions of the good and that aims at transforming social arrangements in the direction of what is judged, in this active public dialogue, as the best possible (individual and collective) good."[59] Citizenship is public dialogue, argues Beiner. It is impossible without a community of discourse, a language that looks beyond the minimalist view of rights as borders and defenses, and a reflection on the problem of the good. But citizenship and its minimal requirements are not the most profound critique of liberal theory. Several challenges to the theory question the nature of the self as primarily "rational."

•

The Concept of Rationality

Kant, Locke, and Hobbes base the very possibility of justice on rationality. For them, it is the defining characteristic of human beings, critical for the entire postulate of ethics that is rooted in Aristotelian thought. "Laws of nature are to be obeyed because they come from God, not because of consent per se. But because God makes all men rational and coherent with the divine order, they will all naturally want to obey the laws of nature. For example, even if I am too dim or evil to see that the law of nature prohibiting waste is what God wants, I will at least be able to see that violating it is irrational, in that it wastes my labor."[60] The self, if it is to be truly autonomous, is a freely choosing self—importantly, not only a *freely* choosing self, but a freely *choosing* self.[61]

But language of rationality came into question even in the eighteenth century. David Hume noted in the 1700s that the human is also a creature of the subjective, or emotive, faculty.[62] Hume's insight was that the "sense of Justice" was an artifice, constructed out of the need for harmonious social relations under a fixed set of rules and out of a need for the absolute stability of property, and that such artifices were a part of what could be understood as constraints on less generous impulses. "Here then is a proposition, which I think, may be regarded as certain, *that it is only from the selfishness and confined generosity of man, along with the scanty provision nature has made for his wants that justice derives its origin.* The sense of justice . . . is not founded on our ideas but our impressions [and] *these impressions which give rise to this sense of justice are not natural to the mind of man but arise from artifice and human conventions.*"[63]

Rationality implies dominance over and control of the natural world and its attendant chaos. Hauerwas challenges these assumptions directly.[64] The problem here is the reification of human reason, and individual human reason, as a replacement for received wisdom or shared traditional narratives, which is correlative to the Enlightenment project of the liberation of the person. The rational person is free of all positions and communities other than those willfully chosen from a position of complete autonomy.

In this context, argues Hauerwas, suffering is absurd, because it is a threat to complete autonomy. Hence, the goals of medicine that emerge from a similar period are the elimination of the external threats to autonomy (as in germ theory) or the repair of the broken machine (as transplant surgeons use the metaphor of the Industrial Revolution). The goal is, in any case and at whatever cost, the restoration of lost freedom and independence, freedom from the necessity of the other.

Hauerwas follows Charles Taylor in pointing out that the language of "enlightenment" means far more than a new reliance on a quantitative cognitive and replicable scientific method. The language of science is based on an assumption that the dignity of a human life comes from mastery over the cause and effect relationship, that all of life is subject to causality and, therefore, to a disengaged, rational control. The central assumption of the Enlightenment was that everything that trespassed on autonomy—suffering, illness, and death—could be progressively eliminated. As God disappears from social explanations of events and as God is gradually eliminated as "superstition" and as an explanatory principle of science, then there is no sensible explanation for suffering. Thus emerges the new explanation for suffering that medicine hopes to address. In shifting the burden from reliance on God, a communal understanding of which will "place" suffering in context to the reliance on rational science, the belief in human understanding and power becomes utter. Then the goals of medicine became enlarged, and each occurrence of illness calls out not for a responding community, but for a progressively persuasive scientific, rational answer and cure.

Sickness, instead of being a call for the best possible community, becomes the worst problem an individual can face, a catastrophe both in body and in meaning, because we think of suffering as something we should be able to affect. Suffering challenges our most cherished presumption—not that we are alone, but that we can control everything. This is why we escalate the race and the passion for medical technology, Hauerwas reminds us. We think we do not need a community capable of caring for the sick; we need an "instrumental rationality made powerful by technological sophistication."[65]

Hence, all illness is pointless. The ill play no role; illness is a move out of a controllable narrative, a move further into isolation and absurdity, an abnormality. Nonrational, comatose, severely retarded, or severely mentally ill individuals are now hardly viewed as persons. The claim of those afflicted in these ways is only given tangential hearing by the state.[66] "The issue is not what we do, but rather who we ought to be in order to be capable of accepting all suffering as a necessary part of human existence. . . . The issue is not whether retarded children can serve a human good, but whether we should be the kind of people, the kind of parents, and community that can receive, even welcome them, into our midst in a manner that allows them to flourish."[67] Hauerwas defines the creaturely experience as the experience with limits (this is, he notes, after all, the point of the story of Eve) but suggests that this ought not to define our boundaries as human creatures. To fear limits or dependence on one another is to misunderstand the real promise of human freedom—not autonomy from the other, but the refusal to fear the other,[68] the ability to give as well as receive, and, as well, to give without using receiving or giving as a means to control the other.[69]

Feminist theorists take this critique of rationality further. Jane Flax focuses on how rationality is linked with control of the other. She argues that the philosophies of science and religion are based on the object relationship loss that creates a dual yearning for/fear of women and nature. Hence, divine perfection is posited as a realm apart from this primal tension. Western rational thought and Christian tradition are based on distancing the choosing self (the exemplar of the male ego-self) from the world of darkness and fecund disorganization. Fecundity is too close, claims Flax, to death, birth, blood, and relationships, and simply too reminiscent of the great loss of childhood.[70] Linked to the language of rights as control of the other, she notes, are the concepts of neutrality and universalism.

Objectivity in moral choice means moving from particularism to universalizability. This is the Kantian cornerstone of categorical imperative itself. True impartiality is linked to the rational observer's distance from the subject. The ideal observer stands removed from the world. Moreover, the observed world is peopled with moral agents that represent the universal and rational being rather than particular beings enmeshed in circumstance. Yet liberal theories of justice are not neutral about key concepts; they are passionate about them. The inherent commitment to the notion of progress, to technology, and to the marketplace as the means of maximizing consumer choices is hardly a neutral stand.[71]

Furthermore, the construction in liberal theory of a fact/value dichotomy sets in motion a conception of a stance where a particular description of reality is posited to be singularly true. This disembodied truth represents the given, fixed universe, the "is" of ethics, science, and social science, observed by the neutral describing self. This language places values apart from "facts." This is a linguistic and, therefore, framing choice. The construction of a "true" world separate from a world of values is more profound than the subsequent problem of the language that is to posit some choices as normative, logical, or natural and others as deviant.[72] This view holds that partisanship and particularity are divisive; passions, necessities, and yearnings of human life need to be apart from ethics, in this classic view, reserved for the separate discourse of politics.

The critique of the disembodied, neutral stand creates one of the strongest challenges to the liberal language of justice. Linked to this concept of the objective and neutral choosing will and the rational self is the notion of universalism. In all classical discussions of systems of justice, the approach is of both the objective and universal observer outside the human community and its particularism. The language of justice is meant to be transcendent language.

Beiner points out something paradoxical about the tension between universalism and diversity that characterizes the liberal tradition. The interior drive toward a universal notion of the good seems to enforce a monolithic culture that overcomes purely regional and particular perspectives in the name of a passionate defense of the dignity and unique worth of the individual.[73] Beiner's reflection on the problem of the universal assumption in the language of liberalism is linked to his insight that a discursive community is necessary to create a context for citizenship. It is his insight that the individual so defended by liberal texts was a construct of a particular social order. Worth and dignity, however, might also find their expression within the discursive citizenship for which Beiner argues.

•

Communicative Ethics

Beiner is not alone in his insight. One of the recent disciplines that uses the metaphor of community as central and places the self in the center of, and sequential to, a responding community is the postmodern philosophic school of communicative ethics. The communicative ethicists argue that the language of the discourse and the process that creates the language must be particular to location, to context, and to the conversation in which the language is located.[74]

The basic syntax of this work is Continental philosophy. Most prominent among its theorists are, in Europe, Karl-Otto Apel and Jurgen Habermas and, in America, Seyla Benhabib. The work of Benhabib, situated at the intersection of feminism and communicative ethics, is, I argue, most applicable to the problem of justice and community.[75]

Communicative ethics can be described as a "cognitive ethics of language," a type of cognition that, instead of stressing (factual or intuited) data, relies on insights garnered through participation in the exchange of a discourse community. The exchanges are actual, intersubjective, and reflective of the normative structure of language. This "linguistic turn" privileges a focus that is available to each speaker in a dialogue. Ethics from this perspective is not a matter of individual conscience but, rather, is created by "exchanges" based on the imperative of language itself, the premises upon which intelligibility is based. Persons are persons because we are linguistic beings, able to exchange meanings with one another. Ethics must presuppose this primary discourse, and ethical principles are only empirically valid if all participants in the discourse agree to, argue for, and participate in their premise.[76] Instead of the Kantian, private, thought experiment rooted in individual conscience,[77] the procedural model for communicative or discourse ethics is the argumentative praxis.[78] Benhabib suggests that an ethics of discourse captures the strongest aspects and the most truth about the moral world.[79]

> Instead of asking what I as a single rational moral agent can intend or will to be a universal maxim for all without contradiction, the communicative ethicist asks: what principles of action can we all recognize or agree to as being valid if we engage in practical discourse or a mutual search for justification? With this reformulation, universalizability is defined as an intersubjective procedure of argumentation, geared to attain communicative agreement. This reformulation brings with it several significant shifts: instead of thinking of universalizability as a test of noncontradiction, we think of universalizability as a test of communicative agreement.[80]

What is sought is not a logical unity but, rather, what is mutually acceptable to all agents in the discourse. Further, this model implies/asserts the *necessity* for the other. The intention of ethics is not to posit the single agent intuiting a specific outcome, but to direct an action of communication that is shared and mutual in a discursive community.

But how can the discourse be rescued from charges that it will be meaningless, trivial, and inconsistent? To address this problem, Benhabib frames three rules that she intends to toughen and specify the strong ethical standards of the discourse. First, she argues for *the principle of universal moral respect*, a recognition that all beings capable of speech and action have a right to be participants in the moral conversation. This principle is intended to address the need for inclusivity of discourse. Second, she argues for *the principle of egalitarian reciprocity*, whereby within such conversations each participant has symmetrical rights to various speech acts that initiate new topics and ask for reflection about the presuppositions of the conversation. This principle, argues Benhabib, demands an attention to power relationships between the participants in the discourse. Third, she "pleads for a *historically self-conscious universalism*,"[81] to emphasize the specificity of the implied language.

This model of discourse creates a moral community. The model of the postmodern moral community is one in which the boundaries and ontological limits of participants are challenged by the rules of inclusion and reciprocity. To be a participant is to engage in reversibility: to be able to "stand in" the moral location of the other. This quality of reversibility has the strongest implication both for civic virtue and for moral citizenship. All human communities, according to Benhabib, define some limited number of significant others in relation to which reversibility and reciprocity must be recognized. What is radically challenging about the ethics of discourse is that this community is coextensive with all beings capable of speech. It is the mutually binding and processional conversation that is the end point, the ongoing work of possibility that is the lifeworld of this moral community. The promise of contract consent is ephemeral. What is sought, rather, is open ended, a way of life in which normative practices, moral relationships, praxis, and word can flourish.

This conversation is not limited to the usual subjects of distributive justice. This discourse is intended to raise issues of the good life itself, thus addressing the concerns of the communitarians that a simple discourse of justice, as in Rawls, is a sterile replacement for the language of actual communities. This means that Benhabib intends ethical reflection of this sort to guide all areas of life. She argues for the necessity of a practical discourse in international relations, in banking, in fiscal policy, and in state security, all conducted under the constraints of the ideal speech situation.[82]

This idea challenges the actual power that all public speech references. In the current public dialogues, the arena of public policy is defined, and hence diminished, by a particular and accepted vocabulary, an officially recognized idiom. "Public dialogue," Benhabib quotes Nancy Fraser as pointing out, "is not external to, but constitutive of, power relations."[83] There are official words with which a claim can be pressed, a repertoire of available rhetorical devices and an included patterning that participants must put forward. To live in the correct grid of communication is to have one's speech sanctified over the speech of others, and it is this speech that is then reified as "public debate" to the exclusion of other speech, and of other actors.

It ought to come as no surprise, argues Benhabib, that the power that surrounds this speech derived its source from a particular conception of the self that is male and autonomous. This type of formal public speech is developed from the fictive model of the nineteenth-century agent, the self-made Man, the independent, rational agent of the Enlightenment vocabulary. The words and actions of women and children lie outside this discourse. The speech of women is defined as outside the wall, as hysterical (embedded in the body, the womb, the blood), and as enmeshed in the demands of children, by definition not public. It is, therefore, somewhat startling to think of members of this encumbered world as participating in the public discourse of real weight and substance.[84] Hence, we are used to conceptualizing all public discourse as being in the hands of experts, meaning, according to Benhabib, expert practitioners of the language.

But Benhabib urges us to think of the ideal conversational community not as a sanctified location, but as having the characteristics of ordinary moral discourse, of the sort with which we are all familiar—the discourse of raising children and of human relationships. By suggesting that ordinary moral conversations, not public forums or courts of appeal, be the model of moral community, the daily expertise that constitutes the actual world, as opposed to the privileged communication of a removed elite, becomes valued.

Knowing how to sustain an ongoing human relationship means to know what it means to be an "I" and a "me," to know that I am an "other" to you and that likewise, you are an "I" to yourself but an "other" to me. . . . Communicative actions are actions through which we practice the reversibility of perspectives implicit in adult human relationships. The development of this capacity for reversing perspectives and the development of the capacity to assume the moral point of view are intimately linked.[85]

In her most recent work, Benhabib continues her emphasis on the construction of gender and the construction of moral community.[86] She is careful to note that the subjects of the discourse of ethics are "finite, embodied and fragile creatures" rather than the usual abstract or disembodied cogitos of classic philosophic tradition. The human infant becomes a "self" only by participation in human community. Human community constructs a social self capable of speech and action and, hence, able to construct a narrative unity that integrates the moral voice— what one has been, what could come next, and what others expect of one. Such a self will always be in relationship to what Carol Gilligan has called the "concrete other," as opposed to the generalized other. Hence, the self will be able actually to experience in practice the power of reversibility that is the basis for the ethics of discourse and the sole process of the limited universalizability that could be claimed as valid. This multiplicity of perspectives then makes possible the creation of public space—a sphere that is "the crucial domain of interaction which mediates between the macropolitical institutions and of a democratic polity and the private sphere."[87] What a discourse or communicative view of the moral community attempts is a participatory restructuring of the civic conversation where difference is understood as necessary and legitimate. What is encouraged is not consensus or harmony,[88] but political agency and the sense that each one actually makes a difference in the participatory discourse itself. What is critical is that the widest-reaching democracy will result in the best civic polity, itself a processional community where the public venture can be realized. This is referred to as the discourse model of legitimacy.

•

Summary of Challenges to Liberal Theory

The model of moral agency that is constructed from the work we have just looked at differs entirely from the liberal model. It draws on the varied sources of the discourse of communitarianism, of feminism, of the new social and political science, and of religious reflection of the Christian tradition.[89] All of this language, in theory, should simply solve the much discussed crisis in liberal theory.

All these varied critiques call for a renewal of the language of justice. All struggle to re-create the moral in light of the good. All attempt to project a language of relationality and conversation. Yet the language heard thus far, while substantially useful in addressing the crisis of language that can be seen as correlative to the crisis of citizenship that the health care debate uncovers, is still incomplete. All of it has ultimately failed in the project of renewing a public model of a common good.

There is one discourse that is absent from these considerations. Its absence is scarcely noted in passing by some. In no work thus far cited is it central. In fact, many of the assumptions of even the secular language of the liberal tradition arise from uniquely Christian as well as Western postulates.

What is missing is the discourse of Jewish tradition, a rich and complex discussion that has actively considered the relationship of the individual to the collective responsibility for justice throughout the 4,000-year history of its existence. The next section of this book foregrounds the Jewish tradition with a radical claim: the choices that the Jewish community has made, the way that they are made, and the texts that drive that philosophic stand offer a central ethical norm. What they present, and what I argue for, is an ethics of encounter, an inescapable recognition of the completeness of the responsibility of the encounter in a world of scarcity.

The discourse of Jewish ethics was conducted in a parallel arena adjacent to the discourse of Western thought described here. As such, the Jewish tradition can be seen as standing in distinction and in tension with that tradition.[90] What the interior references were, and who the historical players were, remain distinctive. The issues that are addressed, however, must necessarily be the similar issues of justice: communal responsibilities in a time of terrible choice. These choices were a constant intellectual traveler in the Jewish community during long years of dispersal, exile, and return.

Jewish textual tradition is a dialogue, an argumentative exchange. It represents a tradition whose argumentation is not only substantively preoccupied with the ethical gesture of the daily life held in common, but whose methodology embodies the language and discipline of the radical encounter with the other across barriers of spatiality, temporality, and culture. Unlike a familiar rehearsal of debates about the liberal tradition, if we look at Jewish texts carefully, we can uncover new resources and largely unexplored terrain for the work of reconstructing language and meaning. This reconstruction can radically challenge what is seen possible in the relationship of the citizen-self to the other in the actual world.

•

PART TWO

THE TEXTS AND THE METHOD:
JEWISH ETHICS AS ENCOUNTER

•

•

CHAPTER SIX

THE DISCOURSE ITSELF
Method, Text, and Covenant

The first section of this book focuses on what have traditionally been the main points of debate in the field of distributive justice and on what some significant challengers to classic theories have noted about the debate. This debate provides the context for the ideology and the construction of the language that is public, political, and ultimately polemicized by the allocation of scarce resources in health care. Yet the language has not been entirely adequate to frame a solution to the problem of securing justice for the one amid appeals for justice for the many— it is language that has failed at the task of explaining social policy. And the language leaves inexplicable the radical solution of the Oregon community. Nothing we have seen so far fully explains how a responsibility for the stranger necessitates our attention. Why does justice require attention to the marginalized, or face-to-face dialogue with the disenfranchised? What is the logical next step in reflection on the encounter between the self and the other that stands at the center of justice debates? In the next three chapters I add yet another source tradition to the debate: the language of Judaism and its concomitant cultural response and faith tradition. Close attention to the text and history of Judaism gives precisely the vocabulary for renewed philosophy about justice, and scrutiny of its argumentative, multivocal, dialogic method yields a way to talk deeply and realistically about the difficulty of achieving justice in ordinary life and provides the vision we will need to pursue it.

Why Judaism? I introduce Judaism because it is my tradition, quite frankly; because I find there a method for the discourse of the justice for the vulnerable that informs my faith; and because, I argue, the faith commitment is precisely the idiom that millions of Americans speak in when they speak of justice. But in large part my exploration of this traditional method of analysis and debate offers a template for how to argue as well as what to argue about, a methodology as well as a specific vocabulary to reconstruct the (stilled) debate around health care reform. The Jewish tradition offers resources of method, text, and history for the recovery of a language of public values of community and the possibility for reconsidering the centrality of collective responsibility. The ethics of encounter demands a serious appreciation of the power of the stranger—*of the necessity of the stranger.* No other language explains the power of the stranger that is at the core of the Oregon experience. Careful, deliberate consideration of this distinctive theological perspective allows a shift in paradigm from reflection on the rights of the agent of moral action to the nature of moral agency itself—which is collective and which invokes the language of mutuality and interdependence. This shift creates the possibility for resolving questions of public policy and justice.

The question of what makes a right act right is a complex one. The discourse of response involves critiques not only of substantive issues, but also of procedural ones. Embedded in the problem are issues of context, causation, agency, norm, and assessment. Each of these issues must be addressed by whoever is describing whatever methodology of ethics they use, with the assumption that methodology in ethics involves not only a general theory of morality, authority, and value, but also "middle axioms," or the middle ground between general principles and the details of policy.[1] Methodology in any integral ethical system must address both the *why* and the *how* of a "right act" if the system is to have coherency and if it can be used in the human hands and heart of the world, and Jewish ethics is no exception. Jewish ethics presumes public choices; it assumes community, human sociability, and embodied dailiness, that ordinary human acts have a weight and meaning that ought to be the subject of urgent discourse.

What I do when I argue has some relevant moral meaning: the gesture of the discourse, the construction of what I call an ethics of encounter, and what others have described as conversational ethics can be critical to reframing a method of ethics. Further, such a method is of direct practical utility. This multivocity,[2] this face-to-face engagement must occur in the public arena that surrounds and informs every act of ethical reflection if we are to come to terms with ethical plumb lines in a society of such cacophonous cultural claims.

•

Responsibility and Relationship: Introduction and Starting Points

How do we analyze a system that is so distinctive in its method? Social ethics seeks not only to name the rules of the world, but to organize and judge the relationships between each of us as we jointly build that world. In ethics, as in all academic disciplines, this takes the form of a communal dialogue, and it is the sharing of language itself that defines the way that action and character are shaped, described, and judged.

We enter the discourse of religious social ethics in an academic and public arena that is theoretically deeply committed to pluralism and that attempts to name "the good" with a standard that can be jointly used. But this is in itself a paradox. Systems of ethics, especially religious ethics, may finally be true only to their own internal debate. What is central in one tradition may be unmeasurable in another. The tools of the trade, the plumb line and the level of religious ethical systems, fashioned by thousands of years of continual use, are worn by the particular hands that shape them and have a grain that is risen in them from good use— the history and social location of each particular people's story.[3] Given this and the intricacies of differences between religions, comparative measures can be used, nevertheless, in broad categories of thought. Moreover, descriptive ethics can be helpful in explaining how one particular tradition, Judaism, stands relative to Christian and secular ethical traditions. While simplistic analogies can be misleading, and complex ones arcane, if we are to organize the debate, we must seek some common ground and shared hermeneutics. One critical way to begin is to examine the methodology of disparate ethical traditions to distinguish structures and substructures before we attempt to reflect on the outcome. In this way we can offer parallels; starting points can be compared, and data can be clarified. We can understand the nature of the moral agent in each tradition and, from these beginnings, proceed to the world of human activity where we participate collectively. This effort is of particular importance among traditions that use the same text and share much common historical ground but arrive at pointedly dissimilar resolutions, such as the Jewish and the Christian traditions. Here distinctions can be seen in the methods that are the architecture of much of moral theology.

In this chapter, I use a standard ethical vocabulary as developed by ethicist Carol Robb to delineate the Jewish method in ethics and analyze the methodology with normative descriptive terms rather than the self-reflexive language of the Jewish tradition. This is an a priori and external standard, used deliberately so that readers who are not familiar with the intricacies of the Jewish tradition can organize the major points that I am making about comparative method. There is no parallel construction in traditional Jewish terms. While the Jewish discourse about ethics has well-developed debates on several of the topic areas that I address in the body of my work, I used Robb's terms self-consciously to create an organizational frame for the analysis. In this way, Jewish ethical thought can be both critically examined and placed with more clarity in the general discourse of ethical theory. My effort is not to demonstrate a fully developed comparative analysis of the whole of Jewish thought, but rather to clarify and give a typology for the method of ethics used in the tradition and to demonstrate how the method itself is constructed around a regard for community that radically challenges classical liberal theory and that renders an alternative language of ethics possible.

The effort is not, of course, exhaustive. I use only some of Robb's selected terms as follows: "starting point," "data," "analysis of the roots of oppression," "loyalties," "value," "source of claims," "motivation," and "the nature of the moral agent" to allow for a common comparative language in the dialogue.[4]

This chapter is devoted to some major structures of normative Jewish ethical thought. It delineates the methodological framework that underlies the moral philosophy suggested by this system. Because I take the position that the texts argue for an ontological as well as ethical choice, it is an inquiry into what I regard as foundational in Jewish ethics: a concern with community and the existence of the human person within community. I believe that respect for community is the organizing principle of Jewish ethical teaching, but as such it is not an inclusive framework. This chapter does not attempt to clarify the larger issues of Jewish theology or philosophy but to accomplish the more narrow task of considering normative relationships between people, the norms of social ethics as the covenantal community moves through history.

The notion of community is not a simple one. In the texts that I examine, the discussion is in large part one of ontology and of what is constitutive of self. Normative rabbinic Judaism understands a self as self-in-relationship, a relationship that is essential, obligatory, and constitutive of a human life. In rabbinic theology, the issue of the obligation of the collective to the individual and the individual to the collective is critical to the understanding of what is a right act, and what makes it right, a central question of method in ethics. Community is the organized collective being of the responsible self-in-relation and occurs only when all stand alert, listening both to the voice of the other person and to the command of God.

This direction was explored deeply, but not exclusively, by leading modern theologians Emmanuel Levinas, Joseph Soloveitchik, Abraham Joshua Heschel, and Martin Buber. Because each major theologian understood this relationship and the traditional sources of rabbinic Judaism uniquely, I discuss the particular response of each in some detail. Further, I use the work of contemporary commentators such as Judith Plaskow, Elliot Dorff, Michael Walzer, and David Hartman, each of whom has his or her own perspective on this topic, to reflect on some of the specific concerns that Robb raises. My concern here will be methodological rather than substantive, to explore how the deontological system of halakhah directs ethical choice. In the next two chapters, I look at the substantive justice claims that such a system proposes.

Jewish ethics is a system that was marked primarily by elegant and persistent argument and that used both deeply rooted textual and intertextual assumptions and the multigenerational simultaneous discourse. Hence, the argumentative nature of the text means that much of what I put forward as asserted by the text could be debated and disagreed with using alternate arguments from the texts themselves. There is no "Jewish view" on a topic, and all attempts to find one position are tempered by this methodological frame.

The discernment of right action itself reflects the substantive value of standing "face-to-face," in Levinas's words,[5] with the other in the discourse. To take on the tradition means to "enter the room" with this discourse. The central claim of Jewish ethics is that truth is found in the house of discursive study—the *bet midrash*.[6] Such a public discourse is created when we argue, face-to-face, about the meaning and relevance of the narrative, symbols, and referents. The conversation that seeks to explain Jewish ethics is not detached from the conversation about bioethics: Will we talk about principles; What will be mutable; What, if anything, can be regarded as a fixity; What texts will resist our efforts to finally know them?[7] Hence, the central definitional process will be a relationship that begins in a close examination of the claim of a particular thinker and widens to include the field.

•

A Framing Issue: Feminism

As with all social theories in all disciplines, the initial issue is linguistic inclusion. Whenever the discussion of community is begun, care must be taken to define boundaries. Hence before addressing the method of communal discourse, it is important to note that even this issue is a question of contention. Feminist theorists ask, Are women a part of community, or are women outsiders? Before I begin to describe the tradition in general terms that might gloss over this problem, we must explore the significant issues that feminist scholars have raised. Judith Plaskow has raised the issue of whether women are even seen as actual moral actors in this system.[8] Who was in the crowd, Plaskow asks, that was being exhorted to make daily justice with their own hands? (Who shaped the tools and whose prints were on the wood?) Plaskow argues that much of the tradition was written from the perspective of the male moral agent, and women's bodies and agency were "other," the strange terrain that was negotiated. More telling, Plaskow's work explores the ways that the tradition was silent: the voices of women were absent or lost.[9]

To understand how the system works requires the inclusion of both this critique and a working solution. While holding to the basic truth of the feminist insight (an insight that is true for all written religious traditions), the fundamental questions of any method remain: How does *anyone* know the right act? And does the way that women are spoken of negate the evidential claim for ethics? For while the existence of texts written by women are minimal, the stories of women's lives inside the Jewish tradition are not. The richness and complexity of the narrative must be judged, then, both extensive and insufficient.

For Judaism each act, at its heart, recalls that the world is unredeemed, broken, and more dark than light. This is constant, and the disconnection—the loss that Plaskow, Heschel, Ozick, and others show us—clearly is to be expected in a tradition that defines itself as incomplete. Hence, a modern critic can point to all the "silences" in the text. Not only is there an absence of women speaking as and for women, but also the views of the handicapped, for example, can startle the modern reader. The unredeemed world is finished in part by listening to ex-cluded voices. Ultimately, the judgment of the right act will address this question: How does this act move the Jew toward wholeness? To examine and focus on method is to look at the process and decisions along the way to that goal.

The world is fundamentally broken, in need of repair and healing, and, cen-trally, awaiting the yet-to-come Messiah. The people are in exile; that was "what was wrong with the world," to use ethicist Carol Robb's terms. This starting question contains a call to act: If the world is broken, how ought we to act to fix it? How ought a human community live in daily time and ordinary physical space in a just manner? Further, what does justice mean in a world that is acknowledged to have widely varying levels of resources, of access to goods and privilege?

•

Three Postulates: The Centrality of the Daily, the Necessity of Argument, and the Fundamentality of Exile

The relationship between daily justice and the sacred admits of two different, but related, features of the question of the right act and community. The daily tasks are not altogether priestly, although the details of anachronistic priestly duties remained in the Talmud long after the Temple was destroyed by the Roman conquest. Though the conquest rendered the performance of such tasks impossi-ble, they persist as issues that are carefully debated in the halakhic literature. The divine daily act makes ethics a concern for each Jew, and each relational encoun-ter is mediated by the spiritual call to come to the other "with full hands" and with complete presentness. The daily lives of Jews—rearing children and cooking food—are what construct a world of sociability and human continuity. This focus on the holiness of the daily characterizes an essential democratic thrust of the tradition. This is key because it means there is a clear and prominent role for women, children, and men within the family context. Many of the central obser-vances are to be carried out in the home with the assumption of full participation. Two examples are the Passover seder, a reenactment of the central drama of Judaism, and the building of the *Succah*, the frail harvest booth constructed by each family to re-create the experience of wilderness exile. Kashrut, the daily preparation of food that was important to the maintenance of distinction as community, is a home ritual.

> In this dialogue God speaks to every man through the life which he gives
> him again and again. Therefore man can only answer God with the whole
> of life—with the way in which he lives this given life. The Jewish teaching
> of the wholeness of life is the other side of the Jewish teaching of the unity
> of God. Because God bestows not only spirit on man, but the whole of his

existence, from its "lowest" to its "highest" levels as well, man can fulfill the obligation of his partnership with God by no spiritual attitude, by no worship, on no sacred upper story; the whole of life is required, every one of its areas and every one of its circumstances. There is no true human share of holiness without the hallowing of the everyday.[10]

The stress on home responsibility, the assumption that every adult would be responsible for the rearing and teaching of children, was striking in light of other religious systems that did not deal centrally with this sphere.[11] It was a central and substantive claim of justice that the ethical relationships of the daily were the measure of the ethical claims of the entire system.

•

Embodiment as an Organizing Principle

The method of Jewish ethics is rooted in the power of this listening, reading, and then interpreting community, both contemporarily and historically. Because Jewish ethics is based on text, it creates normative guides for basic behavior, standards that can be coherent guides for daily life. Since its method is inherently dialogic, fellowship is required, and response and accountability are part of the method itself. It takes into account the real circumstances of being human in the world, with an attention to detail and daily human life that is extraordinary. As such, every moment of human life, of the polis as well as the life of the most intimate human sphere, is addressed and mediated. Each moment of the day is examined, holy, and accountable to the community norms. Inherent in the method is deeply mutual responsibility for both the past and the future. Nothing is completely disregarded—no little story, minority opinion, or tangential point. All is recorded; attention is due. The method at its best is flexible; because it is casuistic, it is by nature so. It assumes human moral agency as a given and the assessment of consequences as a requirement.

Despite the categorization of Jewish method as hyperlegalism even by significant and loved ethicists (for example, Niebuhr), it is informed with the essential discursive spirit of halakhah itself. The method dictates that human life is essential, that human flourishing is rooted not simply in justice, but in love and mutuality, and that righteousness (*tzedek*) and loving kindness (*hesed*) are at the heart of human survival.

The concept of justice in the traditional liberal ethical models that emerge from the Aristotelian tradition usually mean "treating similar cases similarly." Judaism posits a radically different assumption. At issue here is the recognition that the world is unjust in its manifestations, and therefore the problem of justice is how to treat not only equals with equal fairness, but how to act in such a way that the marginalized are treated with compassion and hence made whole. The tradition insists on this, and the calls to include and differentially favor the stranger, the widow, and the orphan are everywhere in the text.

To live faithfully, argued Levinas, is to know also that nothing is of greater importance than the approach made toward one's neighbor, the concern with the fate of the "widow and the orphan, the stranger and the poor man," and that no approach made with empty hands can count as an approach. The adventure of the Spirit also unfolds on earth among people. The traumatization of one's enslavement in Egypt constitutes one's very humanity, that which draws one closer to the problems of the wretched of the earth and to all persecuted people. It was as if I were praying in my suffering as a slave, said Levinas, but with a pre-oratorical prayer, as if the love of the stranger were already given to me in my actual heart. My very uniqueness, argued Levinas, lay in my responsibility for the other; nobody could relieve me of this, just as nobody could replace me at the moment of my death.[12] The preoccupation with justice, defined in this way, is a singular mark not only of the ideas, but of the method itself. Thus, the foundational questions are How does one make justice in the unjust world, and How does one act justly even in the face of a society that is not always in one's control?

The rabbinic understanding of the prophetic call is to enact the justice of the disempowered, which is substantially different from performing the just acts of an individual person. People in a disempowered community draw their meaning from one another. Indeed, throughout most of Jewish exilic history the community was the unit of survivability, and the just relationship of the entire community was the justice necessary for survival in the fundamentally hostile and uncontrollable gentile world.[13] The theme of justice returns us to Levinas's idea of the community as a group of listeners. The listening people must hear in the voice of the commanding God the voice of the other as well. The right act is right only if it is imbued with this call.

•

Procedural Questions: How One Walks the Way in a World of Exile

Judaism is both a casuistic and a deontological system, rooted in rules, duties, and normative conduct and concerned with motive and process. But it is unlike a purely deontological system because the real world and the context and outcome of each case count in their assessment. Consequences, once enacted, are re-examined and debated: hence a modified deontology. Human reason is needed both to negotiate the system and to interpret intelligently the sensory natural world. Talmudic methodology is argument structured by text, history, and community. These three elements and the use of reason to decipher them modify the deontologic method of Jewish ethics. It is *deontological* because it assumes Torah law as motivational, central, and binding, and *casuistic* because it is also inductive and case (context) modified.[14]

Such a method raises the problem of how to achieve good ends in a non-teleological system. How are the norms in a modified deontological system evaluated and enforced over time if neither classic consequentialist nor classic deontological ethics are part of the tradition? Judaism answers this in a way that is the unique hallmark of the method. The basic procedure for the evaluation of norms of justice is the mode of argumentation, commentary, debate, and discussion.[15] Essentially casuistic, the halakhic system uses the encounter with the Torah text and the encounter with the other's encounter with the text to create a continuous discursive community. Cases are raised to illustrate points of law and then to illustrate alternate interpretations of the law. Narratives, in a variety of literary forms (metaphor, allegory, historical reference, and intertextual mirroring) called *aggadah*, are embedded in the text. While the details of the aggadah did not create binding laws, the form was used to grapple with and embellish the discussion of the details of the halakhah. The casuistic account attempts to decipher the particular and specific human ways the principle has been or could be, even theoretically, applied.[16]

In Jewish thought, the crucial text is that of the Torah. Here, in the scriptural source, analysis begins.[17] Since the Torah text itself is laconic, elliptic, and contradictory, with much unsaid, the commentaries on the text are numerous, spanning the 2,000 years of the Oral Law.[18] The Talmud, which is the written compilation of Jewish Oral Law, is divided into two areas: the Mishnah, which contains aphoristic delineation and exposition on the Torah text, and the Gemara, which contains recorded historic comments and debates on virtually every phrase of the Mishnah by rabbinic scholars (*Hazal*, or the sages, or the rabbinic commentators).

The Talmud is not arranged systematically. It is the multivocal, multitemporal record of a long and often rambling discourse. Scattered throughout are ethical considerations, stories, and legal discourses. Talmudic disputes are often left unresolved. At times the section of the debate will end with the expression *tayku*, which means, in effect, "the question stands."[19]

Within the Talmudic text there are tensions as well between the weight of the old and the importance of the new, between the pull of the majority and the rights of the minority. If even a minority position can be found among the Talmudic debates, or if a later commentator has furthered a minor point, these data can be considered relevant proof text for an ethical argument. An ethical argument cannot be made, however, within the horizontal and vertical community of Judaism without a commentary or proof text that was scripturally or Talmudically based.

The Present Continuous

The commentaries are a kind of long argument, often focusing on the struggle to clarify the literal interpretation of the text (*pshat*) with a homiletic one (*midrash*). It is centrally important for the methodology itself to note that all discussion takes place in a "continuous present." In this Talmudic time, rabbis, separated from one another by hundreds of years, communicate as though all were in the same room (face-to-face). The reader of the text, at any historical time, is also assumed to be in that room. There is an assumption of reversibility in the text, a recollection of a concrete moment of human gesture that creates an internal logic based on the effort to identify the hearer of the story or midrash with the players in the narrative. The story makes sense of the textual quote that itself is a sign of the argument about the original query in its context. The text, the example, and the explanatory narrative create a tension that places the hearer of the argument in the position of the subject, and thus the hearer is given the opportunity for reflexive analysis. Often, the problems, the narrative, and the textual fragment exist at different historical moments, thus allowing the contemporary account the same privilege as earlier commentary. The text is reversible in that it ought to apply, given this logic, to a variety of circumstances, each slightly unlike the other, linked by an analogy that places index and subject against context. The logic is not linear, but convoluted, conversational, and vague; the categories evolve around types of moral gestures, a sort of fuzzy set theory.[20]

The authority and the premise of the Oral Law are that God gave it to Moses along with the written Torah (the Pentateuch) at Mount Sinai. This means that not only did the writings of the prophets and the other canonized texts have divine authority, but so did the arguments of the Talmud and the decisions of the rabbis. Thus, the commentary of the Talmud, the Tannaim, the later medievalists, and all the responsa (the analysis of the body of case law that was debated and decided after the redaction of the Talmud) that follow and "enter" the text, and the person engaged at any moment in the act of study, are in this way connected to the event of revelation and to the entire responding community.

Bounded by the system of legal behavior that is called halakhah, the individual Jew, once past the age of thirteen, is responsible for the performance of mitzvot, or divine commandments. (There are 613 such commandments in the traditional reckoning, a metaphorical number that stands for the completeness of obligation.)[21] Many are concerned with the daily details of life that grace the smallest moments. Some authoritative rabbinic commentators do not see these worklife commands as "ethical commandments." They consider as ethical commands only those mitzvot that address the broadest social relationships, such as the injunction against murder or commandments to "do justice" and to make peace.

However, the whole of the law is commanded and the whole fabric lives as a piece. If the world is not straight, then the task is to make it right. The concept of *tzedakah*, or righteousness, is expressed by the word that also means charity; the term for the fitness of food, *kasher*, is also the term for a person of high character.[22] To be concerned with the ideal is to be concerned with the ordinary. The idea that rules and laws form the base of the system can be agreed on, yet the methodology of argumentation creates nuances of interpretation.[23] The central procedural question stands in tension with the praxis. The dilemma of the achievement of justice within certain parameters is *not* resolved, and the quest itself will serve to "open" the method.

Exclusivity and the Discourse

The method of Jewish ethics is rooted in the exegesis, interpretation, and argument of halakhah. Hence, at issue is whether there is an ethics that is apart from halakhah itself. Commentators have long disagreed.

Marvin Fox, writing in *Modern Jewish Ethics*, one of the central works in English in the modern period on this topic, noted that the first essential procedural question concerns the conflict between the commitment to following the mitzvot and "intrinsic ethical values," as in Kant's categorical imperative. The question of whether there is an ethics apart from halakhah is implied in this debate. Both contradictory views exist in Jewish sources:

> Ethics as an intrinsic value is indubitably an atheistic category. . . . The Torah does not recognize ethical commandments whose source is in the recognitions of natural reality or the recognition of man's obligation to man; it recognizes only *mitzvot*. The Torah and the prophets never appeal to a man's conscience, for such appeal is always suspect as a possible expression of idolatry. In fact, the term *conscience* is not to be found in the Hebrew Bible.[24]

> On the other hand, the covenantal pole emphasizes that halakhah is not only a formal system concerned with the rules of procedure but also an expressive system grounded in the love relationship symbolized by God's invitation to Israel to become his covenantal community. The understanding of halakhah as a covenantal relational experience guards against the mistaken notion that a dynamic living relationship with God can be structured exclusively by fixed and permanent rules.[25]

At issue is not only whether Judaism does admit extra-halakhic norms, but whether halakhah itself subsumes these norms within its general stance.[26] As Abraham Joshua Heschel wrote in support of the first position, "The goal is to live beyond the dictates of the law; to fulfill the eternal suddenly; to create goodness out of nothing, as it were."[27] Louis Jacobs explicates the latter contention: "The statutes and ordinances are not recommended because they are in the law but, so it is suggested: they are in the law because they are 'righteous.' "[28]

Life in community holds both views in tension as necessity. The categorical imperative, in Levinas's view, constitutes the very ground of being. To be a human is to assume responsibility for the other. The laws exist as given to *this* people but are only possible if acted upon by the person who is both self and other, if people are mutually responsible for one another's commandments (i.e., responsible for the other's responsibility).

Aaron Lichtenstein, responding in the same volume to the problem posed by Marvin Fox, addressed the legal basis for halakhah and posed the central question in this way: Was there an ethic independent of halakhah? His argument was a qualified yes. Lichtenstein struggled with the issue of inclusiveness and breadth: How much of halakhah was meant by the term itself? How were non-halakhic choices made in a modified deontological system?

Lichtenstein began his assessment with a discussion of all the ways halakhah admits of a legal system that was outside halakhah. He first noted the discussion in Eruvin: "Rabbi Yohanan stated, 'If the Torah had not been given, we would have learnt modesty from the cat, [aversion] to robbery from the ant, chastity from the dove, sexual ethics from the cock.' "[29] This text was quoted throughout the tradition in debates that seek to establish a version of Jewish natural law theory. (It is, of course, disputed just as thoroughly.)[30]

Further, he noted the concept of *derekh eretz* (correct behavior), as described in the Mishnah ("Without Torah, there is no *derekh eretz*, without *derekh eretz* there is no Torah").[31] He mentioned the description of Abraham's argument with God about justice, as though there was a divine standard beyond the (as yet ungiven) Torah to which even God was accountable. He also noted that natural morality establishes a standard, the basic minimal standard of the Noahic laws, below which the demands of revelation could not possibly fall.

> Thus in proving that the killing of a gentile constitutes proscribed murder (although the Torah at one point speaks of a man killing "his fellow" [Exod. 21:14], i.e., a Jew), the *Mekhilta* explains: Issi b. Akiba states: Prior to the giving of the Torah, we were enjoined with respect to bloodshed. After the giving of the Torah, instead of [our obligations] becoming more rigorous [is it conceivable] that it became less so? Moreover, this limit does not just reflect a general attitude but constitutes a definitive legal principle to be applied to specific situations.[32]

If such a basic standard existed for the gentile, the rabbinic texts argue, surely such a minimum standard also existed for the Jew. Thus natural morality assumes a justice and a peace to which, "as it were, God Himself is bound."[33]

However, Lichtenstein noted that the notion of an "independent natural law" was not simply described in rabbinic thought, and he delineated points to support his theory of the inclusiveness of the halakhic system. Lichtenstein first noted the phrase from Shabbat 135b: "Torah has been given and *halakhah* innovated." This means, argued Lichtenstein, that "although the substance of natural morality may have been incorporated as a floor for a *halakhic* ethic, it has nevertheless, as a sanction, been effectively superseded." Lichtenstein argued that Maimonides, the great twelfth-century philosopher and legal scholar, noted that Sinaitic law superseded all that preceded it (e.g., we circumcised not because Abraham did, but because the command was given at Sinai).[34]

Second, Lichtenstein argued that there was a complete association between the religious and the ethical: "They are inextricably interwoven; and what holds true of religious knowledge holds equally true of religious, that is *halakhic*, action. This fusion is central to the whole religious tradition."[35] He cited Jeremiah as proof text. In this text, the ethical moment was constitutive of God. ("But let him that glorieth glory in this, that he understand and know Me, for I am the Lord who exercises mercy, justice, and righteousness in the earth—this I desire.")[36] To know God was to know that God was an entity that both performed and was ethical choice itself, defined here as mercy, justice, and righteousness.[37]

Third, Lichtenstein noted that it was not a violation of the system to go beyond the rules of the system or to violate them in certain circumstances. Tradition was both "elastic and historical." He introduced two classic rabbinic concepts to explain this argument further. *Lifnim mishurat hadin* (to go beyond the letter of the law) and *midat Sodom* (the trait of Sodom) were terms that described the ability of halakhah to adapt in the way Lichtenstein argued was fundamental. For Lichtenstein and others, the language of justice itself contained an explanation of this paradox. *Din*, the word for legal justice, was not the same as *tzedek*, the word for justice-in-the-sense-of-righteousness.

Lichtenstein retold the story of an incident in the Gemara in which Rabba, son of Rav Huna, had hired some laborers to transport barrels of wine for him. In the course of their work, they broke a barrel of wine, apparently due to their own negligence:

The strict letter of the law would have held them liable for the damage; and since they had been remiss in performing their assigned task, it would have allowed them no pay. By way of guaranteeing restitution, Rabba held on to their clothes—which had apparently been left in his possession—as surety. Whereupon they came to Rav [who in turn] told him, "Return their clothes to them." "Is this the *din*?" he asked. "Yes," he [Rav] answered, "That thou mayest walk in the way of good men." He then returned their clothes, whereupon they said to him, "We are poor, we have labored all day, and now we are hungry and left with nothing!" [So Rav] said to him, "Go and pay their wages!" "Is this the *din*?" [Rabba] asked. "Yes," [Rav] answered, "And keep the path of the righteous."[38]

In this struggle of both law and meaning between Rav and Rabba, the point emerged that the moral obligation toward the other exceeded the requirement of *din*, which, because it was limited, was necessarily "unrighteous." *Lifnim mishurat hadin* was contextual, requiring the discursive community to interpret and define the language of its use.

In describing *lifnim mishurat hadin*, Lichtenstein first noted that the essential organizing principle repeated in the Torah was "You shall be holy." This phrase implied adherence not just to the letter, but to the spirit of the law. This and the general rule "You shall be right and good" were a kind of categorical imperative. Lichtenstein argued that to the medieval rabbinic commentator Nahmanides and others in the responsa literature, halakhah was multidimensional, inclusive of both legal and superlegal actions.[39] Thus, *lifnim mishurat hadin* was a part of the legal system itself.

The Talmud spoke of *midat Sodom* to explain that the Sodomic error was excessive rights language: What was mine was mine, what was yours was yours. It was immoral, argued Lichtenstein, because it reflected "obsession with one's private preserve and the consequent erection of excessive legal and psychological barriers between person and person."[40] It also reflected a broader ethical call within the system itself.

Halakhah allowed for supererogatory acts as part of the system as well; technicalities could be disregarded and exemptions not taken advantage of. Rabbis extended the law to normalize consequences and make them consistent, and this could be done even in regular cases. Of course, in all instances of life and death and urgency, all but three laws (adultery, idolatry, and murder) could be voided.

Lichtenstein noted that halakhah allowed for filling in the lacunae in the text (by the use of midrash), adding "aspirations" that were non-obligatory but approved. In this interpretation, following the interpretation of Rav Huna, halakhah was not just *din* (law) but, because of *lifnim mishurat hadin*, was meant to include all the legal and extralegal fictions and interpretations as well.

Nahum Rabinovitch, responding to the same question that Lichtenstein posed, argued that halakhah was "equal to a moral code." It was a narrower set of rules used to judge how one should act in particular contexts. Torah was the plane of ethics and the ultimate reality. Rabinovitch thought that because we did not understand the theory completely, we could not know if the moral code was complete. He stated that since people/society were temporally and historically based, moral codes (halakhah) change, and therefore the system was open ended. He added that individual responsibility to the halakhah was the organizing principle of Jewish ethics and that part of the halakhic method itself was the intellectual study and the training in both argument and rational discernment. In cases of urgency, however, if no one else was around, the individual student was urged to study, examine his or her own motives, and determine the proper course of action. Even a transgression might be acceptable in this type of case, argued Rabinovitch, noting that it could be considered "great" if done for the "sake of God."

Rabinovitch contended that the rabbis saw all of reality as polarity, as a dialectic relationship between *din* (the law) and *rahamin* (mercy), and he urged halakhah as the "middle way." Hence, he believed what was required by halakhah was not obedience, but struggle, which made it a spiritual and not a secular or purely legal experience.

Rabinovitch argued that he stood with Maimonides in believing that halakhah leaves some areas undefined. At these points, the method employed was to use the categorical imperative of the Torah, the principle of justice, the urgency to do the good and the right and be holy as paramount. He gave much attention to the moral actor—a user of halakhah was versed in law but confident of his ability to interpret it.

Rabinovitch argued that this moral reflection can only happen with surety in community, and he urged the reader to see how the assumption of *kehillah*, community, was critical to the resolution of the key procedural question. The Oral Tradition itself cannot stand as a soliloquy. The premise requires response. The method assumed the voices of many in discourse and in discord with one another. It assumed that the view of the minority will be heard, respected, and answered, and that the majority had inescapable responsibilities for actual leadership from a real base. The discord was very important. It was central to my claim that this discursive community can be used as a model for policy debate and that the sharpness of the debate in the Jewish tradition was honored and expected. The method of ethics is rooted in genuine questions that arise from the praxis of an actual world and a specific moral, material location.

•

Text, History, and Allies: Source of Claims

Not only the starting questions, but their authority distinguishes the Jewish ethical method. Jews are called by God to live by the halakhic path. God's call to the people, and their responsive listening, is the source of the ethical claim, not the people's assertion that they understand or are able to rationalize the claim; rabbinical authorities tell us that one cannot and ought not to do this.[41] Jews ought to live under the "yoke of the kingdom of heaven." The people have made a *brit*, a bargain/covenant that they accepted before they heard its terms. Elliot Dorff, a leading scholar of the modern Conservative movement, argues that this basic and prior covenant is a characteristic of the ethical system and is critical in distinguishing Judaism from American democratic theory. "Rules are instituted to secure rights; American individualism can only be set aside by American pragmatism, in this case being the practical need to ensure that all can enjoy what is theirs by right. The source of authority of the law is the consent of the governed, who presumably see the practical need for imposing a law which restricts freedom. For Judaism, the author of the commandments is God, not the governed."[42]

If Torah, halakhah, and responsa are the main interpretive sources of the claims on human action, there is another manifestation in community praxis, called *minhag* or custom. For Lichtenstein, *derekh eretz* referred to the natural morality that was accessible and observable in the world of nature. Yet the term has another important meaning. Nonbinding yet restraining, *derekh eretz* also meant the "proper way" in which ritual and ethical behaviors were customarily done in specific communities. The collective, historical practice that followed from this shared and accepted veracity gave the weight of tradition to custom. (In fact, many modern Jews will be unsure about the actual source of *minhagic* customs and think they are halakhic in origin.) Reason and habit, rather than received textual tradition, were the source of these customary ethical behaviors.

Can Jewish ethical method admit to other disciplines and to such things as reasonableness of custom as sources of truth in the sense that Robb intended? As in the extended procedural discussion above about whether an ethics could exist outside halakhah, there are two conflicting traditional responses in the texts. Marvin Fox argued that the halakhic system itself includes an accountability to a variety of sources. His insight is that the basic method incorporates science, philosophy, and natural reality into the traditional texts. The rabbis used exegesis and interpretation as the most important device to reconcile the basic and sacred text with the reality of exile, change, and science. In Fox's view, "fundamentalism"[43] poses the main danger to the method, freezing it in a static position when its essence is adaptability.

Fox further noted that the incorporation of "external to Sinaitic" sources was always a part of the discourse. Fox described Judah HaNasi's confession that, in some arguments, the gentile sages "vanquished the sages of Israel." This was cited in the tradition as a case of how best evidence and best argument from whatever source ought to prevail. (That even this point was disagreed with was noted by Fox.)[44] Saadya Gaon made this point, according to Fox, even more forcefully by insisting that reason existed both prior to and after Sinai. Further, Fox noted that interpretation has always varied widely, even at the heart of basic texts (such as the Moses story, the Ruth story, the view of the Nazarite vow, and the problem of creation itself). Additionally, he pointed to the flexibility of the aggadah as indicative of the freedom at the heart of Jewish method itself. He reminded us that tradition has each Jew at Sinai now and for eternal generations and noted the rabbinic midrash that says each Jew hears the revelation through his or her own body and experience.

> Even at Sinai the divine voice went forth to all Israel and was assimilated by each person in accordance with his particular capacity—the elders in their own way, the youth in their own way, the children in their own way, the sucklings in their own way, the women in their own way, and also Moses in his own way. . . . For this reason it is written, "the voice of the Lord is according to *the* strength" and not "according to *His* strength" to teach us that each one grasps His message according to his own particular power and capacity.[45]

Since the tradition further assumes that the call from Sinai goes out every day, each Jew must continually hear the call in his or her particular way. Fox argued that Maimonides developed a line of reasoning that claimed and accepted external sources and assumed that math, astronomy, and "speculative realities" were better known by the Arabic world than by the rabbinic sages. Jews need to "accept truth from any source," claimed Maimonides. Because of his authority in the tradition, his idea became the majority viewpoint and has been followed by most scholars in the modern period.[46] Acquiring the Greek truths of medicine, he contended, was an ethically proper response because the Torah was a vehicle of truth. If science can prove miracles by clear explanation (tides that would make a Red Sea into dry land, for example), then we ought to act on and understand these truths.

Rabbi Joseph Soloveitchik, the leading contemporary halakhist, developed an analogous position more fully.[47] He remarked that physics and the theory of relativity teach us that truth can be viewed from many perspectives, and that the universe was not a Newtonian machine, but a complex of related happenings. One's perspective, then, will determine the "true" view of the object.[48] Further, Soloveitchik understood that human perception is a function of the truth that each person perceives, as each individually views the "real" from the perspective of a particular and chosen order. What is seen as actual is a chosen fact pattern based on a system of value and belief. He posited the notion that to be religious or to be scientific, while they may be radically different worldviews, was not only to value the world differently, but to experience and to see the phenomena of the world differently as well. That notion was entirely consistent with the concept of truth understood as "plural truth" and explained how specific events could be seen either as miracles or as functions of the events of the causative natural world.[49]

•

Text and Data

Ethical systems admit certain data as relevant; other data are excluded. This question of action in the actual world is the question of all ethical systems. As religious systems, however, both Judaism and Christianity ask additional framing questions in this discourse: What is our relationship and, hence, our responsibility to God? What are we, as religious thinkers, commanded to do by the divine voice we hear in this world? When the voice of God is heard as having its source in history as well as in text, as it was for Jewish theologians, the response will be made in a manner different from that of Christian theologies that have their source in gospel alone. For Jewish theologians Torah, Sinai, rabbinics, and lived experience are the critical data that distinguish the tradition of ethics.

The Torah text begins as an account of human history. While this text is part of the shared testament of both Jews and Christians, the fundamental light of the respective traditions illuminates the text in ways that are strikingly different, and the difference begins with Bereshit (Genesis). Consider the Jewish discourse relative to the exit from *Gan Eden*. Notably, this exit was not seen in rabbinic thought as entirely negative but, rather, as the entrance into history itself. History, procreation, and the passion of sexuality and reproduction are made possible by the entrance into history, time, and human struggle. While this history was often tragic, paradoxical, and frustrating, it was necessary for the relationship of God to human being. Eve's role, while causative, was not degraded or irresolvable, and the call from God to Adam ("Where are you?") would be repeated over and over until the Abramic *hineni* ("I am here") was unquestionably established.[50] Bereshit was the prehistory of the call and response, and rabbinic midrash pictured the God of Bereshit as a "king without his retinue,"[51] found in the desert by Abraham. This not only pictured a God in search of a relationship with human persons, but a God in a relationship of mutual obligation, in the midst of a history that was intentional.

Contrast this with the narrative accounts of Christianity: the expulsion from the garden was a fall. In the Christian tradition this acted, in a sense, as a proof text of the human depravity that "stopped" history. Thus, Augustine, as well as Luther, and Niebuhr were able to see all that followed as fundamentally born into the human condition. For Christians, the Fall was ahistorically inescapable: the event was concurrent, present, and essential to humanity.[52]

For both Christian and Jewish theologians, the revelation at Sinai was a key organizing event. In Jewish theology, at Sinai the Hebrews became a chosen people rather than a promised tribe. The Sinaitic experience was directly linked to the very historical, political struggle of Exodus. The event must be preceded by the historical act of speaking truth to power, of liberation from actual historical oppression, and of the physical participation in the liberation. It cannot be separated from the events of the historical moment.

For Christians, however, the Sinaitic covenant was an instant of command with a specific focus. Like all Torah text, it was read "forward," as a predictor of the coming of Jesus and an anticipation of the New Testament. The command at Sinai was "free but not freed" from the passion story, and "true but not complete" in that it was placed not at the center of the Torah, but in the context of the New Testament.

The texts of the prophetic books are another point of divergence for the two traditions. The prophetic calls to Israel are specific and historical; they meant for Jewish theologians that history as promised was in question. Real enemies, wars, and dissolution threatened and had to be addressed and reconciled with the historical mission of the people. Jeremiah and Isaiah dealt with the condition of exile and dispersion; how could this have occurred, and what ought we to do as actors in history? The call of the prophets was heard in the Jewish tradition both as ethics and as political theory.

For Christian theologians, the ought (ethical call) of the prophets was both a challenge to political order and a promise of Christ's coming. The New Testament itself was proven by the promise of the prophets, lifted from the historical reality of Babylon to the metaphor of Babylon.

History was also central to rabbinic texts. In a way that was fully explored only by Jewish theologians, rabbinic theology was completely understood only in light of the Talmudic discourse relative to the historical destruction of the Temple and the exile of the Jewish people. The exile from the land of Israel and the destruction of the Second Temple by the Romans, so utter and devastating in light of the promise of the Lord, was the "other" proof text of Jewish theology. The survival and struggle of the people in history was the issue at the heart of the work of Philo, Saadya Gaon, Judah HaLevi, and Maimonides, as well as the rabbinic commentators. Like the prophets, the rabbis and later theologians had to make theological decisions that were also ethical and political. The actual questions of ethics— What was human flourishing? What was the relationship of soulcraft to statecraft? What was the right action of human persons relative to one another?—were different depending on the relative power a people had and what kind of access to the means of production its members possessed. Rabbinic theology is deeply cognizant of this. In Marxist terms, the production of history was itself human creation, and, hence, the ability to act in history was both the text and template of the Jewish answer to ethical questions.

Data that were central to the system of ethics were also the particular experiences of the Jewish people. The history and geography of the Jews was the particular terrain upon which the drama of the ethical quest was played out; there was no claim to use a universalist concept of the history of the world's peoples as the ground of ethics. Case law evolves out of specific historical circumstances—for example, the problem of the legal status for the Jewish widows of the First World War when there were no witnesses to the deaths of their husbands.[53] In this way, a deontological system admitted history into its considerations. As Hartman states, "Halachic norms are grounded in shared historical moments."[54]

The resultant case law framed this last source of data. This was the most important way in which ideas of science and mathematics, insights of psychology and sociology, and similar secular disciplines were admitted into the tradition and its text.[55] The responsa literature was the written record of the systematic attempt of the leading rabbinic authorities in a particular location to answer questions that arose for their community. The law was interpreted through the context of particular cases and commentary. This responsa tradition continues in the modern period, in some form, in all three branches of Judaism. And here again, we find the insistence of community and continuity. The particularity of casuistic argument revealed in this literature can seem startling, even queer, to a reader outside the world that is addressed. As the real was admitted into the terrain of the metaphysical, we see the events of the world taken into the small circle of the rabbis to be turned over and over, then returned to the community for more discourse, and then taken inside the debate once again. Because there was no central authority, the wisdom of the collective will hold even over the *bat kol*, the voice from heaven.

In the clearest move to strengthen the value of community-based discourse as the arbiter of the true norm, the rabbinic story was told:

> On a certain occasion R. Eliezer used all possible arguments to substantiate his opinion, but the Rabbis did not accept it. He said, "If I am right, may this carob tree move a hundred yards from its place." It did so. . . . They said, "From a tree no proof can be brought." Then he said, "May the canal prove it." The water of the canal flowed backwards. They said, "Water cannot prove anything." Then he said, "May the walls of this House of Study prove it." Then the walls of the house bent inward, as if they were about to fall. R. Joshua rebuked the walls, and said to them, "If the learned dispute about the *Halakhah* (the rule, the Law), what has that to do with you?" So, to honor R. Joshua, the walls did not fall down, but to honor R. Eliezer, they did not become quite straight again. Then R. Eliezer said, "If I am right, let the heavens prove it." Then a heavenly voice said, "What have you against R. Eliezer? The *Halakhah* is always with him (his view is always right)." Then R. Joshua got up and said, "It is not in heaven" (Deut. xx, 12). What did he mean by this? R. Jeremiah said, "The Law was given us from Sinai. We pay no attention to a heavenly

voice. For already from Sinai the Law said, 'By a majority you are to decide.'" (Exod. xxiii, 2 as homiletically interpreted). R. Nathan met Elijah and asked him what God did in that hour. Elijah replied, "He laughed and said, 'My children have conquered me.'"[56]

The text records a dispute among the authoritative rabbinic figures of the period. At issue is the way that meaning will be interpreted and transmitted. The text argues for the interpretation of the majority of the scholars to stand, rather than the "logocentric" school of Rabbi Eliezer, who, despite having the halakhah always with him, did not represent the understanding of the majority. Meaning itself was determined by the understandings of the community. As Daniel Boyarin describes the process, "Meaning is not in heaven, not in a voice behind the text, but in the house of *midrash*, in the voices in front of the text. . . . [Further,] the majority of the community which holds cultural hegemony controls interpretation. To put it another way: correctness of interpretation is a function of the ideology of the interpretive community."[57] History, context, and community culture all reinterpret textual veracity. There is no unmediated "truth," no vantage that is not particular to this history.

The data of the tradition and how it was used and applied can best be understood by looking at the work of Maimonides, the major philosopher of the twelfth century whose works are still considered pivotal in the modern period. The admission of the critical data of revelation, of history, and of the centrality of the rabbinic response are central to his philosophy. Maimonides, like other Jewish theologians to follow, took historical responsibility for ethical choices in the political world.[58] He was a leader in the diaspora community of North Africa that was buffeted by *galut* (exile); he wrote about the ethical and political response to this difficult exile, and his writings were not only theoretical but became normative throughout the *galut*. Because the Jews were stateless, Maimonides argued for the primacy of family and community. His epistles to the Jewish community of Yemen frame his theology. He stressed to them that it mattered how they lived daily life—not only the daily work, which was the response to Sinai in the observance of mitzvot, but also how the community would survive in the world. The acts of mitzvot were to be understood as both large and intimate; to live the ethical life was not merely to be cognizant of the parameters of creatureliness, but to act in the real life of the community—caretaking, *tzedakah* (charity), and "teaching your neighbor to fish." By making the smallest human acts sacred, Maimonides sanctified counterhistory itself; the action includes the people on the banks, not just the flow of the river.

For Maimonides, the Torah's central organizing event was the revelation.[59] The historical event at Sinai was true and historical and must be believed. This was one of his critical premises. Just as critical—and he insisted on this in an age where he was surrounded by doubt and challenge—was the Oral Tradition of the rabbis (*Hazal*). The actual rabbinic reflections, the halakhic details, were to be trusted. They were based in real human history, space, and time. Maimonides also argued that the aggadic details of rabbinic thought were true, necessary, and relevant. Maimonides believed that the rabbis, like the prophets (and as a continuous part of the prophetic tradition), spoke paradoxically so that their truths could both be heard in their historical era and be relevant to contemporary history.[60]

Maimonides insisted on staying with the rabbinic tradition of Jewish thought. He did not reject the praxis or the theory of the rabbis. He polemicized against the Karaites, his contemporaries who rejected the Oral Law. Because of his inclusion of the whole of Talmudic thought, and not simply the Torah, he made rabbinic interpretation, on its own terms, imperative for the entire tradition that followed.

In the *Guide of the Perplexed* and *Mishnah Torah*, two very different works, Maimonides shaped his theology by writing about the actual historical situation of his community and particular individuals within it. *Mishnah Torah* was normative. It described how one ought to respond to the command of God and what the details were of such a response. This text was readily accessible then as it is now, completely available to the laypersons that follow halakhic tradition. In this text one notes how specific praxis in real human hands is the concern: it would both shape and be shaped by Maimonides' text.

Maimonides considered *teshuvah* (return, understood as repentance, even radical change) central to theology and ethics. Repentance, human action for human choice, was always possible and was linked to human redemption. The two mountains lie before Jews always—which choice will it be? Ethics was possible within halakhah because human beings were both creaturely and capable of *teshuvah*.

This brings us to an insight central to Maimonides and the final way in which his work is an example of how Jewish ethics used historical data, in Robb's terms, to inform and develop the tradition. Living in the twelfth century C.E., Maimonides was faced with the enormous pull toward the intellectual life of Athens. While insisting on the primacy of Jerusalem and the specifics of the Jewish story and the Torah text, Maimonides acknowledged and used key Aristotelian notions in his work. The *Guide* was a major attempt at synthesizing Aristotle and Judaism. Rationality and the necessity for activity of the soul in light of considerations of virtue were seen as central concerns of the just person. Additionally, Maimonides had a notion that justice must take account of the situation of human beings in a world where goods are both abundant and contested. He understood justice as having to do with the actual public distribution of goods in a polis. For Maimonides, like Aristotle, relationality (friendship) was a subject of ethical discourse. And, as did Aristotle, the historical choices he discussed were made in the context of actual family and city life.

The *Guide*, written to "one [gifted] student" rather than to ordinary Jews, nevertheless dealt with ethical themes similar to those addressed by the *Mishnah Torah*: how to act well in light of tradition (Jewish history) and the history of the general society—including the work of Aristotle and contemporary Arab philosophers (rooted in Hellenistic thought). This challenge was specific and historical. According to Israeli philosopher David Hartman, Maimonides refused to "split" his theology—that is, he did not have a historical, scientific understanding of Aristotle and an intellectually separate faith commitment to Judaism. Maimonides created a textual world in which both Aristotle and the rabbis were present. Hence, he remained placed in the world of both sensory, physical, mathematical, and philosophical empiricism and rabbinic discourse.

Maimonides argued that all rational thought and empirical wisdom were, however, given and understood in the light of the Torah. This attachment to text shaped even the strongly historical conditions that Maimonides addressed. As would later theologians, Maimonides grappled with the notion that God's textual command must make sense to a human community struggling within the perplexities of a world in which they are isolated and endangered. History shaped texts that were given as bedrock, but all texts would be taken with the community on the journey through a history that was consciously chosen by theology.

•

Analysis of the Roots of Oppression

As discussed earlier, there is a basic notion at the heart of Judaism that the world is broken and essentially unredeemed. The embodiment of this concept is both the central story of the Jewish people and the organizing principle of Judaism's ethical method: the exodus-to-exile journey. In paradigmatic form, this notion suggests the struggle that is part of the ongoing hermeneutic; the communal exodus was referred to as both method and as telos.

Exile was the real state of being in the world; God was in exile along with the Jews.[61] The Messiah had not yet come, according to Jewish thought, and Calvary had not occurred in any redemptive sense. Hence, the narrative history of exile and of return and deeper exile was the reality and the language that surrounded the location of the Jewish ethical method.

For Jews, the task was *tikkun olam*, the modern meaning of which is "to repair the world."[62] Since Jews were God's partners in this task, it must be in some way meaningful that they were in exile.[63] Each prophet had made the claim that the exile deepened when Jewish communal action went awry. This referred not merely to observance of rituals and ritual mitzvot, but most particularly to the mitzvot of social justice, to the stewardship of the needy, to the care of the land, and to the seeking and making of peace.

But such choices were not always freely available to the Jewish community. The relationship of the people to power and production varied considerably as the circumstances of their exile changed. Michael Walzer, in *Exodus and Revolution*, notes that Exodus is the story of political triumph and victory by both human struggle and divine intervention.[64] To understand fully the roots of oppression and the liberatory framing of Jewish ethics requires an attention to this organizing principle. Walzer was concerned with how the Exodus story places the Jews in history ("We are always and everywhere to remember and act as if we were recently freed slaves"). This principle would have peoplehood shaped by the whole story (not just Sinai)—oppression, slavery, disbelief, struggle, liberation, exodus, rebellion, wandering, conquest, genocide, and promise.

Walzer noted that exilic history was more normative than the history of the land; the people were outside the land more than they were inside it. In the Exodus story the land remained the Promised Land. Walzer, however, suggested that return shaped history. While attached to the normative power that Walzer claimed (that we remember slavery and redemption as constitutive of the Jewish people), he also insisted on the reality that Jewish community life continued *without* absolute victory as a nation.[65] Walzer viewed the Exodus story as inherently revolutionary, to be evoked as a radical snap in history.

The Jewish tradition focuses in a way that Greek tradition does not, on the position of the most vulnerable and most powerless in both the social and the political world. Thus, while the Exodus story is central and explanatory in these two ways, it does not speak as thoroughly as the Greek sources do to the dilemma of the achievement of power for the community. Walzer's work emphasizes, first, that it was the textual and historical responsibility of Jews to account for the full range of human capacity in history. The most vulnerable, the most wretched, and the most lost must be redeemed. God acts in history not on the side of the pharaoh, but on the side of the slave. Hope was the central stance of the human condition, and community (not single disparate individuals) the central moral agent in history. Second, Walzer reminds us that ethics was historical as well as based in community and dependency relationships. We were going somewhere, yet we were not there; the community was freed, but not home. Solutions in ethics would be partial, historical, and limited by actual time and place.

Loyalties

The analysis of the roots of oppression is critical to the understanding of ethical method, but it is only half of the description of the context for ethical theory. Ethical vantage positions are also defined by who was in alliance with the tradition. Loyalty, solidarity with a particular group that the method identifies as allies, is one of the key notions of any partisan ethical theory.[66] The method asks with whom do you stand as well as who stands against you.

Jews view the Jewish community as central and the "faithful remnant" as the locus of the ethical debate. This explains, in part, why there has not been a vocal application of Jewish texts to modern secular public policy. There is, to be sure, a strong universalist element in Judaism. (One need only look at the prophets Isaiah and Jonah to see this.) But it is not self-evident that such universalism is the dominant trend in the tradition. In a long and well-researched look at the concept of "neighbor" in the phrase "And thou shall love thy neighbor as thyself," Ernst Simon and Harold Fisch debated whether Judaism intends the term *re'ah*, neighbor, to refer only to Jews.[67]

The texts of Judaism differed sharply throughout history on this point. Yet all agreed that fellow creatures were creatures of God and worthy of infinite respect and communal obligation, even if not love. Despite this, the mitzvot were commands for Jews alone. Non-Jews had a different set of responsibilities. They were expected to be committed to the seven Noahic commandments. The mandate of Judaism for the Jewish people was to be a "light unto the Nations," to make the living action of the whole of the community an exemplar for all peoples.

Jewish ethical thought, however, reflected the basic insight, cited above from Walzer, that the Exodus story, imbued with the sensibility of the slave experience in Egypt, informed all the actions of Judaism. The prophetic voice of Judaism insisted that there could be no spiritual ritual observance without attention to ethical social justice. The Torah text, drawing on the Exodus paradigm, reminds us that Jews "were strangers in the land of Egypt, therefore [they] know the heart of the stranger." Jews were specifically bidden to act accordingly, standing with the excluded and the enslaved against oppression and injustice. This accounts for the social location of this system of justice; Jews were always and everywhere a community of freed slaves, posited Walzer.[68] This loyalty to oppressed peoples had pervasive contemporary effects, contended Walzer and others. Even when Jews in the twentieth century achieved financial success and objectively changed class position, as a group they continued to "vote poor." In other words, they continued to vote and behave politically as though the slave experience, the exile, the shared history of Eastern Europe, and most of all, the Holocaust were an ever present danger.

This last agony of Jewish history, taken with the subsequent founding of the State of Israel, had methodological implications for contemporary theorists, themselves the first post-Holocaust generation of ethicists. The nightmare of powerlessness and the difficulty of the administration of power have shaped the community. Jews reside in the world as historical and social beings, exquisitely aware of this history. A familiar methodological claim in contemporary Jewish ethics is that one must remember and learn directly from the Holocaust history when making an ethical assessment of a current dilemma. Central to this claim is the importance of the community itself, the simultaneous fragility of the community, and the tenacity of the communal relationship.

•

The Centrality of Community

In her analysis of methods, Robb asked for the central values of an ethical method as a way of describing it more fully. What did the centrality of community mean for the assessment of value in the method of Jewish ethics? I argue that it meant that value was placed on the collective good rather than on the competing claims of individuals. Acts were assessed as valuable when they fostered a community life. Acts were problematic when they destroyed community endeavors. David Hartman explained, "Religion is often regarded as essentially an activity of the individual. The movement of the 'alone to the Alone' or 'what one does with one's aloneness' are plausible definitions insofar as they focus on the common belief that ultimately the religious experience is personal and individual. Such definitions, however, are inaccurate when applied to Judaism. The covenant is made between God and the people of Israel."[69] Hartman added that the primacy of community accounted for the "democratization of the spiritual."[70] Numerous halakhot and stories supported this thesis. Perhaps the most telling indicator was the level of difficulty that surrounded a choice to live in isolation. Jews needed a minyan, a group of ten adult people (men in the Orthodox tradition), to pray, for prayer itself was a collective act. Prayer was not spontaneous but traditionally was the ritualized resaying of a set order of invocations. The individual Jew, therefore, was in community, as it were, with all Jews who prayed before and with all who will follow; they have said and will say the same words.

When Jews came to a new place, the community first built a *mikvah*, or ritual bath, for the enactment of the laws of ritual purification. Then they established a center for learning. As David Hartman made clear, the practice of the commanded life itself demanded community:

> The significance given to practice within Judaism not only makes the creation of a shared language a logical possibility, but also provides the sense of urgency to make that attempt. *Mitzvah* illuminates the *centrality of community* within Judaism. Halakhah is a way of life of a community, and serves to develop a collective consciousness within the individual Jew. Systems of thought in which the individual is dominant cannot do justice to a world view where law, which is vital to community, plays a central role.[71]

When speaking of values and the relative weights given to principles it must be also stressed that halakhah serves to develop collective conscience as well as consciousness.

•

Postmodern Reconfiguration(s)

The issue of community was central to the work, the *doing* of social ethics. Each act in the world was illuminated by the public reality of human action. Shared language, shared history, and shared human space made social ethics both possible and necessary. The ethical moment in systems of Jewish thought could only be placed in the center of a responding and responsible world.

For Emmanuel Levinas community was the main organizing principle, the location of empowerment that makes the ethical moment the most human of our acts. Levinas's work represents both a radical break with the secular assumptions of liberal tradition and an innovative reappraisal of Jewish thought. Levinas remained firmly within the rabbinic tradition, yet his creative critique of the tradition enabled an altered reflection and use of the basic texts.

Levinas's work on community must be understood in the context of his philosophy in general. He argued that ethics was primary to and preceded any ontological discussion in philosophy. What made this extraordinarily demanding construct imperative was the radical encounter with the "naked face of the other," an encounter that "broke into being" itself. The vulnerability of the face imposed its own demands. What was at stake at all times, argued Levinas, was the potential for violence suggested by such a vulnerability. One could always kill the other, insisted Levinas, so essentially defenseless and so ultimately distinct in its otherness before you. But the vulnerability recalled the command not to kill, and alterity recalled the respect for difference.[72] In this way, the Torah is the essential frame for relationship, the assertion of the responsibility that is the most human and the most transcendent of gestures. Levinas postulated that we live in the epoch of "totality." Totality is the tendency of human reason, made binding by Western tradition, philosophy, and science, to create orders and systems that can be rationalized. Seeking unity and totality has created a seamless functionality for persons to fit into. One's life and being are to be part of a rationally understood process, an order that is static, rigid, and boring. It is the life of the dis-*inter*-ested person—of anomie, homelessness, and ultimately loss of self.

Everyone totalizes the world. However, a radical transcendence of the human position in the totalized chain of science and reason is possible. One could, on occasion, leap out of an individual ego, out of totality, and into "infinity" and restore the possibility of true individuality and human freedom.

The ethical moment is the moment that creates this break with totality. In the ethical moment, one has to stop reducing the other (person) to an object in the universe and to really see him or her. This essential act is liberatory, one that makes self possible, as well as an act of community and fellowship; but it is risky, unguarded, and utterly complex. "Justice . . . means we are responsible beyond our commitments."[73]

When the other is truly seen as a person and truly recognized in all his or her separations, then he or she is also seen, paradoxically, as the same as the self—a real self, inspired by God (breath of life, as in Genesis).[74] The other can then refute our objectification of him or her and create his or her own meaning; he or she can accept or reject our approach. Yet this authentic encounter is the whole of ethics for Levinas. The other comes to us as each alone can bring himself or herself—naked, without the clothes and baggage of totality, place, and hierarchy. Like the widow and orphan of the Torah, the other person needs us. And if we allow ourselves to acknowledge this need fully, that is the fundamental act of basic justice, *tzedakah*. That is the act that sets the world right and takes us, for that moment, out of totality.

Levinas described the moment in the biblical text when Jacob put on the clothes of his brother, Esau. This midrash, Levinas claimed, was a metaphor for radical responsibility. Levinas used a Hebrew wordplay, based on the similarity between the sound of the word for clothes, *begadav*, and the sound of the word for rebels, *bogedav*, to open his discourse on accountability.

> How does one preserve oneself from evil? By each taking on himself the responsibilities of the others. Men are not only and in their ultimate essence "for self" but "for others," and this "for others" must be probed deeply. . . . Nothing is more foreign to me than the other; nothing is more intimate to me than myself. Israel would teach that the greatest intimacy of me to myself consists in being at every moment responsible for the others. *I can be responsible for that which I did not do and take upon myself a distress which is not mine.* . . . The scent of Paradise is Jacob bearing the weight of all that he will not do and all that others will do. For the human world to be possible—justice, the Sanhedrin—at each moment there must be someone who can be responsible for the others. Responsible! The famous finite liberty of the philosophers is responsibility for that which I have not done. Condition of the creature. Responsibility that Job, searching in his own impeccable past, could not find. "Where were you when I created the World?" the Holy One asks him. You are a self, certainly. Beginning, freedom, certainly. But even if you are free, you are not the absolute beginning. You come after many things and many people. You are not just free; you are also bound to others beyond your freedom. You are responsible for all. Your liberty is also fraternity.[75]

This is a complex point. Jacob, the younger brother, deceived his father by dressing in Esau's clothes (*begadav*). In putting on Esau's clothes he took on his being, Esau's self as well as Esau's future, Esau's responsibility, and Esau's rebellion (*bogedav*). Hence, this rebellion of Esau (rebellion that was put on like clothes) was carried forward on all the embodied generations of Jacob's kin. Levinas meant us to understand, by way of this midrash, that one was responsible for the responsibility of the other; one had taken on the responsibility of the other, no matter where that may lead, and even if such a relationship was taken on in deceit. And if a relationship taken on in deceit was so utterly formative, Levinas argued, how much more so the one taken on in full consciousness?[76]

For Levinas, then, the major ethical event was "hospitality"—a call to the other to share your whole world. You must take responsibility not only for the other, but for his or her responsibility (commanded life) as well. This creates a community of fellowship that is beyond language, transcendent and existing completely, unreliant on a particular and separated self. "Justice . . . means we are responsible beyond our commitments."[77]

The value of community was embedded in justice. It was the meaning of the phrase "Love your neighbor as yourself." The encounter was so total that it involved the substitution of self in the place of the neighbor.[78]

In discussing the relationship of Adam to Eve as "one human head with two faces," as the two "sides," Levinas wrote:

> To be under the sleepless gaze of God is, precisely, in one's unity, to be the bearer of *another* subject—bearer and supporter—to be responsible for the other, as if the face of this other, although invisible, continued my own face and kept me awake by its very invisibility, by the unpredictability that it threatens.[79]

> Humanity is defined not as liberty . . . but by a responsibility prior to all initiative. Man answers for more than his freely chosen acts. He is the hostage of all the universe. Extraordinary dignity. Unlimited responsibility.[80]

This intense fellowship admitted of no compromise. Levinas was making an innovation here; this was not the normative stand, but it was strongly textually supported. He declared that outside this relationship with the other there was no possibility of an encounter with God, because a "Jew was never alone with God; it's always a threesome"—the Jew, the other, and God, with God revealing Himself only through the other.[81] "[This] thing is the worst, worse than the enthusiasm for idolatry. Isolation within Judaism, a *no* uttered to the community. To be outside a synagogue filled with people, that is the extreme apostasy; to say 'that does not concern me. . . . Here is the condemnation that is beyond recall.' "[82] For Levinas, isolation from relationship makes the self impossible.

Levinas teaches both secular philosophy and Talmud. The encounter with the other happens in the context of a specific community—for him, the Jewish community. Here the ethical gesture is expressed in the terms of the halakhah: "The Law essentially dwells in the fragile human conscience, which protects it badly and where it runs every risk."[83] His insistence on community is linked to this radical recognition that it is a *specific* community in which one must locate each act. Community is not a comfortable abstraction; it must be based on each actual encounter with each other real self. Direct, unmediated, and as discomforting as it is liberating, this encounter is the initial basis for ethics, law, and praxis among the generations of Adam.

In discussing the gesture of Abraham toward the three strangers in the desert, Levinas wrote:

> The heirs of Abraham—men to whom their ancestors bequeathed a difficult tradition of duties toward the other man, one which is never done with, an order in which one is never free. In this order, above all else, duty takes the form of obligations toward the body, the obligation of feeding and sheltering.[84]

> But here is where the logical integrity of subjectivity leads: the direct relation with the true, excluding the prior examination of its terms, its idea—that is, the reception of Revelation—can only be the relation with a person, with another. The Torah is given in the Light of a face. The epiphany of the other person is *ipso facto* my responsibility toward him: seeing the other is already an obligation toward him. A direct optics— without the mediation of any idea—can only be accomplished as ethics. Integral knowledge or Revelation (the receiving of the Torah) is ethical behavior.[85]

The question of religion and ethics in the modern world was, for Levinas, of necessity both tentative and tenacious. It was tentative because of the realistic appraisal of the situation of modernity and because of the fragility of faith in a world of limits, condition, violence, despair, cruelty, and loss. Yet it was tenacious, a tough and persistent surviving question that was tangible, compelling, and human and spoken in a distinctively human voice. "To hear a voice speaking to you is *ipso facto* to accept obligation toward the one speaking. . . . Consciousness is the urgency of a destination leading to the other person and not an eternal return to the self."[86]

Levinas believed that "intelligibility" is prior to any human enterprise and "protects this enterprise like the cloud" that follows the tribe of Israelites in the desert. This intelligibility was also spoken of as a prior innocence, "an absolute uprightness which is also absolute self criticism, read in the eyes of the one who is the goal of my uprightness and whose look calls me into question. It is a move-ment toward the other which does not come back to its point of origin the way diversion comes back, incapable as it is of transcendence—a movement beyond anxiety and stronger than death."[87] And language itself is not disinterested or instrumental. Language is ethical. "The original function of speech consists not in designating an object in order to communicate with the other in a game with no consequences but in assuming toward someone a responsibility on behalf of someone else. To speak is to engage the interests of men. Responsibility would be the essence of language."[88] This task of human community is at once the most difficult and the most essentially human of acts. "Our text teaches us that not everything can be bought and not everything sold. The freedom to negotiate has limits which impose themselves in the name of freedom itself."[89]

The discussion is, then, about the issue of humanism, which Levinas defined thus: "The man whose rights have to be defended is in the first place the other man, it is not initially myself. It is not the concept 'man' that is at the basis of this humanity, it is the other man. The other man's right is practically an infinite right."[90] Levinas was alert to the fragile nature of this value, not only as protected by the vulnerable human self, but as historically placed against real and tangible evil. "Evil surpasses human responsibility and leaves not a corner intact where reason could collect itself. But perhaps this thesis is precisely a call to man's infinite responsibility, to an untiring wakefulness, to a total insomnia."[91] For Levinas, the responsibility that was total necessitated the community of others. One could only encounter the infinitely expansive being of the other in a world governed and directed by such encounters.[92]

This point was also made vividly by Levinas in an essay on the giving of the Law.[93] Levinas described the occasion of the giving of the mitzvot to the com-manded community, the "Listeners." In the rabbinic telling, the Law was given three times to the people assembled as community: first, at Sinai (described in Exodus); second, on the plain of Moab (in the Deuteronomic retelling); and third, in the ritual described for the people to do when they enter the Land ("I have set before you two choices"), as they assembled on the mountains of Gerizim and Ebal (described in Joshua and discussed in the Mishnah 7:1; Balvi Sotah 37a–b).

Levinas was struck by the wholeness of the staging of the event described in this Mishnah. "The words of the Levites will reach everyone's ears: each person here is in the presence of all the others. Each person shall say: 'Amen.' The pact con-cluded, then, is an authentic one, made in the presence of all the people, mem-bers of a society in which—I continue to emphasize the point—everyone can ob-serve everyone else."[94] Levinas was struck by the fact that all were present and none excluded, not even the "stranger, or children, or women."[95] But more re-markable was the ceremony itself, where everyone saw everyone else in the face-to-face receiving of the Law, in "full view" of one another's reception of the Law.

One was responsible, then, not only for everyone else, but for the *responsibility* of everyone else. In classic rabbinic hermeneutics, the number of times events occurred in the narrative was of critical importance. This attention to the numerical detail was an additional hermeneutic device for understanding the meaning of the text. The number of times the listening community heard the commandments (in complex rabbinic calculations this was forty-eight times) must be multiplied by 603,550 (the number of people who were assembled), and the product multiplied again by 603,550 (because each one hears the other's hearing of the commandment). Each person heard the command not only as an expression of personal revelation; each heard the other's hearing and saw the face of the other as he or she received the command. Each heard the other's responsibility, and each one's hearing and hearing of the other's hearing was named and honored by this numerical calculation. This point was extremely important because it insisted that in the act of personal accountability (personal hearing of God's commands) a central and inseparable role was played by the recognition of the other. "To such an extent that I offer myself as a guarantee of the other, of his [*sic*] adherence and fidelity to the law, his concern was my concern."[96]

The description, while graphic, was not simple. What seemed to be going on at the moment of the choice between Good and Evil was the recognition that the choice was not merely personal, that the human choice for justice was fundamentally public, made in full view of the next and the next. To be in the community meant not only to be a listener, but a watcher, standing with and witness to each other's listening.

Levinas argued that the recognition of the other, in the community as a context and location for the recognition, was the central moment in Jewish ethics. It was the commitment to this moment of attention and radical encounter that was constitutive of self. Human life, ethical choice, and society could not exist prior to this recognition.

Inherent in the methodology was the emphasis on focused and sustained learning. Literacy was expected in this tradition. How else could one pray from a written text? How else could one argue and engage in discourse?[97] Since the great covenant between God and the people was based on the complex text of the Torah, as opposed to a single act or a specific miracle, then to interpret this text carefully was the first goal of religiosity. Levinas explained how the relationship between teacher and student was integral to the revelation of the Law itself. Once again, he argued that the ethical tradition assumed and counted on each moral agent taking responsibility for the one beside him or her at Gerizim and Ebal: "In the four last books of the Pentateuch, there is a verse which constantly reappears: 'Speak to the Children of Israel *le'mor* ("thus").' . . . In my own reading of this verse, *le'mor* would mean 'in order to say.' This gives us: 'Speak to the children of

Israel in order that they speak' [and] teach them so profoundly that they themselves begin to speak, let them listen until they reach the point of speaking."[98] Teaching enabled the democratization of the tradition. The expectation was that the language itself needed to be made intelligible. In part, this explains the tremendous emphasis on textual analysis. Every word had to be understood, taught, and debated. This means (theoretically) that anyone could be a participant in the discursive community, because the text was given to all.[99] The issue that emerged at this point was complex. What was the relationship between the values described and the necessity to enact them? The next category of ideas described by Robb's analytic terms suggests an answer.

•

Motivation

Judaism rests its motivational justification on clear textual statements that the world works and is held together by the collective power of right conduct, by the attention to the deeds that are done in accordance with a divine command. But does this scheme work by itself? How can such a system be regulated, since many of the 613 mitzvot are enacted in the small and private daily moments of a human life?

It is interesting that this question, asked with some degrees of speculative curiosity in earlier historical periods, assumed full voice after the Enlightenment in Europe. The question of living a "life outside the law" was seriously raised and acted upon. The rabbis were skeptical of such a life. They felt that the yoke of the kingdom of heaven was lifted at one's own peril. And yet, in many Talmudic discussions, it was made clear that it was not lack of attention to halakhic detail that was said to have caused the worst catastrophe in Jewish history, the destruction of the Temple in Jerusalem and the final exile from the land of Israel, but "baseless hatred" of one Jew for another. In the text of Job we clearly have a strong rebuttal to the theory of immediate cause and effect. Job's friends were wrong: Job's actions were not to blame for his tragedy. The argument, of course, continued throughout the textual tradition. Dorff cited several motivational reasons that were given in the tradition. "The Bible delineates several reasons to obey God's laws. These include: to avoid divine punishment and/or receive divine reward; to fulfill the promises of our ancestors and abide by the Covenant, promises to which we, too, are subject; to have a special relationship with God, thereby becoming a holy people; and to express our love for God. None of these aims, however, is to secure rights."[100] It was not securing rights, but establishing obligation to covenant that was critical in securing motivational adherence. But there was another motivational factor. To follow the mitzvot was to be part of a motivational *community*, and for most people relationality, shining in the light of each other's eyes, was a very powerful incentive. The community was "in full view of one another," Levinas would remind us.

To live outside the gaze of the neighbor is a condition of exile itself. How much harder to compound the unchosen historical exile with a self-imposed one. At the heart of Judaism is this nagging mandate: Do not be satisfied with the unredeemed world as it is; act to change it, criticize it, show up the injustice of your society, expose the falsity that Jeremiah knows and the pretension that Isaiah sees. This edict is expressed by Hannah Arendt's notion that Jews must be pariahs, outsiders with necessary vision. Yet the performance of this task needs the solidarity of the exiled people. The ordered method of Jewish thought, even when the mitzvot are challenged and struggled over by deep internal debate, creates a community to live in, a place from which to start and to which to return.[101]

Mitzvot are tempered with compassion, with *hesed*. Thus, the praxis emerged from an empathy with an exiled and endangered people (it was sensitive to social location) and from a God and a lawgiver who could be called to task by God's prophets for the same requirements of justice and mercy that guided human action. Jews are urged by the rabbis to find the most compassionate way to solve the dilemmas of ethics, for the "Torah is to live by and not to die by." Formative compassion is built into many of the mitzvot themselves. The requirement that "one cannot stand idly by" the blood of his or her fellow is a call not only to *tikkun olam* and not only for justice, but also for direct and human caring. The mitzvot provide ample source texts for the mandate to heal. Jews are obliged by the halakhic method to give charity when they feel generous and when they do not, to offer hospitality without judgment, and to live in ways of selected care not because they want to, but because the world in some way will fall apart if Jews do not walk on this path.

This mandated rising to goodness means specific things for the individual. Fundamentally, the commanded life is one of urgency, that language of necessity about which Levinas spoke. It calls on each one to follow the rules as heard because humans are interconnected in mutuality, not merely out of concern for their own fate. As Hartman argues, "In contrast to certain Greek notions of self-sufficiency, the revelation at Sinai proclaims that perfection is to be realized in relationships. The covenant God of the Bible chose interaction with men [*sic*]. The Lord of history as opposed to an impersonal ground of being, pronounces that interdependency is the ultimate datum of reality. History and community, therefore, are central to a tradition where perfection is grounded in relationship."[102] The perfect, complete person is incomplete unless he or she is with another. The notion that human beings are bound to one another, that human fate is tied to others, is strongly suggested by the texts themselves. One of the difficulties in understanding a deontological mode in a consequentialist world is a certain inability in language to discover the necessity of this collective meaning.[103]

Of all the categories that I have addressed, however, none is as important for understanding and differentiating the language and the resultant ethical methodology of Judaism than the radical difference in the traditional view of the moral agent. The view of community and the language of self are integrally connected. This view of moral agency offers the strongest challenge to the methodology of the classic, liberal secular, and Christian tradition.

•

The Nature of the Moral Agent

Each ethical method must come to terms with the person who will enact the deeds of the system. It is striking that the ethical language of the liberal tradition of Locke, Mill, and Kant, which positioned individual autonomy as a central goal, depicts the moral agent as a single male actor. Choices are made that maximize the liberty of this moral agent, who is often portrayed by this language as performing on the stage of a solitary drama, acting for the right, frequently on behalf of others who are voiceless or powerless. The ethical man is seen as potent, reasonable, resolved, and objective. Ethical language is depicted as universally applicable, neutral, rational, and consistent.

While there are some sources in Judaism that firmly support that anthropology, there is strong evidence to support an alternative view. As Plaskow pointed out, even when gender-biased sources predominate (and they are by far the majority of all sources), to understand that a fuller anthropology could be realized by the tradition, we must "listen to the silences" as well as the voices that are textually recorded.[104] I contend that not only the silences, but the methodological, legal, and ethical structure along with the history of oppression have radically altered the portrayal of the male agent, endowed with rights, as the ideal. The Jewish moral actor is seen mostly, but not entirely, as male; indeed as Daniel Boyarin has claimed, the texts often portray this agent as a feminized male.[105] While the Torah text reflects the life stories of female figures who are locked in their own limited historical veracities (how could it be otherwise, given who recorded history and who nurtured the children?), the textual accounts of Genesis and of Judges contain narratives that suggest women who occupied the central stage of the ethical relationship by either overt or covert demonstrations of power relative to the male actor in the account.[106] Further, the midrashim, which in part explore what is missing from the text and in part challenge the text itself, often focus on women's narratives. As such, midrashic texts often reveal women's motives and women's differing perspectives of the textual account in the Torah, offering another traditional source of language about the ethical action of the moral agent in Jewish life.

As noted before, in numerous texts the actions of each Jew were expected to be made contextually, rooted in community. This was true when discussing moral agency as well. The moral agent acted in the present as a part of a community at large, in the context of a history that shaped him or her, and in the consciousness of a future to which he or she was responsible. The human life, as conceived by Judaism, had no resonance without this rootedness in community.

The moral agent was a limited self with a transcendent task: he or she was called upon to change the world.[107] Hence, the task of ethical reflection was required also to involve ethical practice, and that practice was not merely the small series of acts that could circle an individual human life, but the largest of human goals and plans. Martin Buber and Abraham Joshua Heschel, whose writing about moral agency figured notably in the modern understanding of the Jewish view of the self as self-in-relationship, offer further considerations on how the necessity for relationship is implied in the description of the moral agent.[108]

•

Martin Buber and Revelation: The Call of God in the World

Levinas was not the only Jewish theologian to write of relationship as constitutive of personhood. Martin Buber was the modern theologian most associated with the description of the moral agent as a person in an encounter or meeting with God and with the other. Buber, like Levinas, who also wrote in a world shadowed by the worst horrors of the twentieth century, was a European Jew conversant with both the Hasidic tradition of Orthodox Judaism and secular philosophy. Of all contemporary Jewish theologians, he was a critical "bridge" figure, the Jewish theologian most centrally read by Christian theologians in the modern era. Buber wrote from a particularly Jewish perspective, focusing on aspects of the tradition infrequently encountered and clearly fascinating to a number of his Christian contemporaries.

Buber stated the central question in Jewish thought as "What is our relationship to God?" Buber's answer was "to be in dialogue with God's presence." Buber's view of God stemmed from his basic philosophy of the I-Thou relationship. All selves, all beings, were defined in relationship. One was either in an I-It encounter, which was instrumental, cognitive, practical, and objectified, or in an I-Thou encounter, in which both beings were fully present to each other and where a true encounter was made.[109]

Buber insisted, moreover, that the encounter with God as the Eternal Thou (one that cannot ever be made into an It) is a central moment of faith, but not the whole of religion. Religion itself encompasses the whole of our everyday lives.

Religion is not a revelatory moment extracted from our "real" lives, broken into and illuminated; religion is the daily illumination of our lives. The core of Hasidic teaching, Buber believed, is that the holy could be found in the everyday and that humans could best approach God by becoming what we were created to be—human. This unity of life is the other side of the monotheistic unity of God.

The question of revelation involves the nature of God's call to us. This call, Buber believed, comes daily and in every interaction. We cannot control the call or manage it; we can only risk an openness to it and live in the moment, the situation of presentness to the call of God. All things, situations, and people address us without overt words or gesture. They make a claim on us simply by their being. A dialogic encounter with them is a response of our whole, open being, a risk-taking response to the Thou that addresses us.

According to Buber, living means being called by an intimate, indwelling God. The signs are everywhere and happen without respite. In revelation God gives this "presentness" and "direction" more importantly than dogma or rule. Buber did not stress the specifics of mitzvot but, rather, the need to be answerable to the revelation itself. In revelation, God is transcendent yet constantly very near to human beings. What is given is not a verbal command but an ultimate value, a Thou that cannot be objectified. The call in the ongoing dialogue is the revelation. Revelation helps to turn one toward the mystery of God by enabling a person to live his or her life in response, which is the true nature of human responsibility and human nature itself.[110]

For Buber as well as Levinas, the call that is heard from the Other/other is the beginning of a process of human response. The critical next step is to understand the response itself. For Buber, this call was addressed to us in the concrete world of creation. The questions in the actual world are not only "What is the way of faithful ethical response?" but also "What is the nature of the human person?" and, finally, "What is sin?"

Human beings stand in creation—which is Buber's name for the concrete reality entrusted to human beings in which the "signs of address" are given. We are in creation and, of necessity, in a world that is peopled and therefore shared. The journey is joint; God is not responded to by the exclusion of other peoples, but only with and by means of relationship to others. In this way, humans are in partnership with God's creation. This notion of partnership is central to Buber's thought; creation is unfinished, and human beings are needed to complete the work. Ethics, the work of response, is specific to the actual work of the moment: encounter. It is not universal, detached from creation, but specific to the concreteness of the world.

For Buber, the Torah was the record of creation, of the encounter with God. It taught the real history of the world, which was a narrative. Creation was the beginning, redemption the goal, and revelation the midpoint event.

The nature of the human person, according to Buber, is to have a variety of relationships. Some relationships are, of necessity, I-It; work and being in the world would be impossible without I-It relationships. Humans will be "its" to one another—each person will experience himself or herself as an it at moments and then move ahead. Yet the faithful response will be to try for encounter in each daily act. This gives human life possibility and transcendence.

Sin, then, Buber understood as the turning away from the possibility of an I-Thou encounter. For all Jews, it is *het*, the act of "missing the mark." To miss the mark is to lose unity and direction, to compartmentalize, and to pull away from encounter with the other and with God.

Responsibility is the proper answer to God's calls in creation. It implies both answerability, the ability to hear and respond, and the sense of recognition of the assertive claim of the address. While Buber was nonspecific about the action of the response, he was clear about its nature. One must wholly encounter the other. Encounter does not mean emptying oneself into the other, however. Each thou remained distinct, separate, and worthy in the concrete world of creation. (The self is also the other, and so cannot be instrumentalized either.) The central encounter is an equal meeting rather than a sacrifice, an empathy toward, or a selfless encounter with the neighbor.

Redemption, for Buber, is the goal of human history. Like creation, this goal provides meaning and surrounds the decision for the encounter. Buber argued that Judaism teaches that this power works to redeem the world, and in that work humans are partners in creation.[111]

Redemption is, for Buber, the ultimate fulfillment of creation. It is implied in the religious tie to the concrete, which does not detach the spirit from the physical and finds redemption of the latter in the fulfillment of the former. Redemption is God's action in the encounter with the human. Humans respond in a way that is capricious, and God answers deeds in ways that are unexpected and unpredictable. For Buber, redemption is not possible outside community, where relationships of true encounter are shaped and experienced and where redemptive action is to be expected.

For Buber, community is living with, not merely alongside, other people. Community presupposes mutual responsibility, self-reflection, and mutual recognition of others' essential otherness. Community confirms and strengthens personal existence in a life lived toward the other based on selfhood and dialogue. Buber called community the "basic structure of otherness." A human being cannot live only by answering God's call to him or her without answering for his or her neighbors as well.[112] True community cannot be manufactured; it arises naturally from an unselected reality. The Eternal Thou is the true center of all real community, and the relationship to God defines a legitimate obligation to the group.

For Buber, the Jewish people exemplified this kind of community. Jews were not an abstract grouping, but a continuing and historical band, a natural group that attempted to realize an ideal because of the covenant—the essential acceptance of God. This community was directly ruled by God, and the fact that it had no sovereign, argued Buber, gave it a special role in the world. The community was an example of the truth that humans had a purpose in the world.

Israel was elected to fulfill this role in redemption. Israel created the possibility for the perfection of the world and the ultimate unity of humankind. The whole community heard the charge of revelation and, ideally, acted out lives of unity and justice as a commitment to redemption. This was done in dialogue, encounter, and recognition of the other *in* community. In the realization of real community with its own natural life in a different kind of nationhood—one of justice and righteousness, not mere political striving—the Jewish community could realize the ideal goal of relationship to God, a covenant and a dialogue.[113] It was Buber's insight that the moral agent in the Jewish ethical system was not the individual actor, but the Jew within this whole community.[114] Thus, Buber's work is critical to my argument.[115]

•

The Issue of Autonomy and the Liberal Social Contract

The principle of personal autonomy so constitutes ethics in the dominant liberal secular tradition that it deserves discussion in greater detail. The notion that self-rule and personal intentionality (the good will) were major components of deontology depended on a self that was existentially alone. Levinas, Plaskow, Buber, and Heschel understood that this type of self was not the model of the Jewish person. One reason that this is such a difficult concept for modernity to grapple with is that all post-Enlightenment thought rested on the notion of the discovery of an autonomous self. It is difficult to postulate the meaning of human freedom without freedom from covenantal responsibility, yet this is precisely what Judaism asks, conceiving of human freedom within the commanded life.

In an American context, as Elliot Dorff has noted, living freely within the covenant is particularly difficult.

> If rights are the primary reality of my being, the burden of proof rests upon anyone who wants to deprive me of those rights or restrict them. Since other people are born with the same rights, there are times when my rights are legitimately restricted, and even times when I have a positive duty to others. In each case, however, the duty arises out of a consideration of the other person's rights. If, on the other hand, the prime fact of my being is that I have obligations, as it is in Judaism, then the burden of proof rests upon me to demonstrate that I have a right against the other person as a

result of his or her duties to me. My rights exists only to the extent that others have obligation to me, not as an innate characteristic of my being.[116]

Rights are not innate or constitutive of self. Autonomy, which figures as the central organizing principle of liberal consent theories and their attendant ethical systems, is neither a presupposition nor a goal of Judaism. The rabbinic conceptualization of the body as lent by God for limited temporal use, rather than "owned" by the "self," as it is in the language of liberal theory, is useful in understanding this fundamental difference. The human person is a created being made in the image of God, with a self (body and soul are one entity in this system) that is essentially on loan from God and will return to God at the time of death. By no traditional accounts is a person "entitled" to act in complete freedom; he or she is required to act in community, in covenant with God, and in accordance with halakhah.

At issue here is not what feels right to the individual, guided by an individual heart, but "What does it take to live an honest life within this particular community?" Hence, a number of actions may be argued for, but all ought to be directed toward the community interest, not only the self.

Dorff notes the constitutive frame of collectivity, and quotes Milton Konvitz to illustrate his point: "The traditional Jew is no detached, rugged individual. . . . He *is* an individual but one whose essence is determined by the fact that he is a brother, *a fellow Jew.* His prayers are, therefore, communal and not private, integrative and not isolative, holistic and not separate. . . . Although an integral part of an organic whole, from which he cannot be separated, except at the cost of his moral and spiritual life, let each man [*sic*] say with Hillel, 'If I am here, then everyone is here.' "[117] Even the inner world of prayer is to be experienced in terms of the collective. This is in stark contrast to modern constructions of the goal of the autonomous self in an era when the consideration for the social and ethical is nearly eclipsed by considerations of inner emotional states of feeling.

It should be further noted, when discussing the issue of autonomy, that adult Jews are expected by Jewish sources to live not only in community, but in family, which is the embodiment, quite literally, of the obligatory, nonvoluntary human relationship.[118] "Membership in the group (the Jewish people) is not voluntary and cannot be terminated at will; it is a metaphysical fact over which those born Jews have no control. This indissoluble linkage between the individual and the group means that each individual is responsible for every other and that virtually everything that one does is everyone's business."[119] As discussed previously, the expectation of this methodology is that all adults have partners, parents, and children. Dorff's insight is that this is only the first level of nonvoluntary relationship. The obligatory character extends to the larger circle. Here he quotes the Talmud: "Whoever is able to protest against the wrongdoing of his family and fails to do so is punished for the family's wrongdoings. Whoever is able to protest against the wrongdoings of his fellow citizens and does not do so is punished for the wrongdoings of the people of his city. Whoever is able to protest against the wrongdoings of the world and does not do so is punished for the wrongdoings of the world."[120] The notion that one is in a family and hence in a specific relationship is textually related to the generalized situation of the human person. The Torah's first story tells us that the essence of creatureliness is partnership and relationship. Whether Adam and Eve are co-created (Gen. 1), or fashioned from each other's bone and flesh (Gen. 2), the imperative to committed companionship is clear in Judaism; this is not necessarily true of other traditions. Sexuality and procreation are part of the right way to stand with the world. This creates some powerful assumptions that cannot be overlooked about women as part and parcel of the human self (a notion that was actually rare in systems developed at the same period; it was not structured into Hellenistic thought, for example), and about the obligation to relationships that are distinctive.[121]

Basing the search for both the collective language of justice and its application in the methodology and the text allows for the richest meanings. Additionally, it allows us to see the whole tradition as the basis for the discourse and opens the system of halakhah to the most, yet traditional, ethical meanings and directions. It reminds us of the largeness that is possible in this particular ethical system and permits us to use the relationality inherent in the language as proof text for the contemporary issues of choice in a world of scarcity, of doing justice and right action in an unrighted, limited world.

Finally, the analysis of method, the pulling out and lifting up, the taking into the light of these tools we use daily and giving them critical examination, has a goal. Only by this lifting to the light and honoring what is unique can we see what is given in company with other ethical traditions. Then the task of listening, we can say, is not yet enough, and the task of developing shared language that expresses the collective is not yet enough. Then the task of acting together can begin. How the Jewish tradition applies this method, and how the method itself can be used in direct application to the problems of distributive justice in health care, is the subject of the next chapters.

With this limited review of the methodological assumptions of the tradition, placed in the context of the discipline of social ethics as described by Robb, in this chapter I have set in place the fundamental terrain of the larger Jewish discourse on which the debate about the details of distributive justice occurs. In the next chapter I discuss the major halakhic sources that are classically used within the halakhic system as proof texts for the arguments about distributive justice.

CHAPTER SEVEN

LIMITS, LANGUAGE, AND TRADITION

Jewish Textual Sources, Casuistry, and the Details of the Discourse

The debate about allocation of scarce medical resources seems radical, even startling, in the American social discourse, since we have grown accustomed to a medical enterprise powered by unlimited expansion and supported by a corresponding ideology and text of autonomy. However, within Jewish tradition, text, and historical circumstance, evidence abounds of both the problem of scarcity and the discourse of rationing and distributive justice. In Jewish tradition the issue of allocating scarce resources has shaped the language of the very measure of obligation between persons both in normal situations of obligation and in crisis.

Jewish ethical reasoning cannot be fully separated from the religious legal system of halakhah. What this means in practice and in text is that reflection and analysis in regard to ethical questions is based in case, narrative, and context. Arguments about principles are made analogically from precedential cases. Further, the end result of any discourse on a question is precisely that, a discourse. The question raised and the case review examined can and do span generations of respondents, and the process of the argument is closely preserved. It is the dispute within the faith community rather than a set of rules applicable to specific dilemmas that is preserved. This is why I took care in the previous chapter to make clear that there is no one Jewish truth about a rule of conduct, that any author reflects on views held in tension, on majority and minority viewpoints, and on counterhistorical and intertextual meanings in a tradition that values nuance in text and, above all, the transhistorical argument.

It is part of my premise that this tradition is more than an interesting historical artifact and is indeed exactly the public policy model we need for contemporary debate on social goods. Only through face-to-face dispute and discourse, the actual case story and/or the actual face of the other, can policy be resolved. The discursive relationship, here expressed by the textual interdynamics, creates the template for this moral discourse. This chapter analyzes the traditional sources of teachings on questions of justice and reviews critically their content, their language, and the justification employed by each as they use the method of halakhah to construct both a social world and a moral meaning for the dilemmas they seek to resolve.

•

A Flask in the Desert: Who Shall Live When Not All Can Live?

When searching for texts to support a judgment about the question of micro-allocation (e.g., in the debates that surrounded the first kidney dialysis machines), most modern Jewish commentators in medical ethics turn to a single classic text in the Talmud,[1] as modern Jewish theorists still readily do. It has become the standard for initial discourse in the discussions of the subject. Although micro-allocation is the focus of this text, the language of larger social problems of macroallocation is, in part, developed out of this specificity of detail at the individual level. While the issue of the microallocation of a scarce medical resource is not directly addressed by the rabbis of the Tannaitic period, the matter of scarcity of life-saving technology or objects is addressed.

The Talmud recounts a dispute involving two travelers in the desert with only enough life-saving water for one of them.

> Two people were walking along the way, and in the hand of one of them was a flask of water. If both of them drink, they die, but if one of them drinks, he reaches civilization. Ben Petura expounded: it is better that both of them should drink and die and let not one of them see the death of his fellow. Until Rabbi Akiba came and taught: "That your brother may live with you"—your life takes precedence over the life of your fellow. (Bava Metzia 62a)[2]

The situation is as follows: If both drink from the flask, both will inevitably die. If one drinks, he will be able to reach the next city and live, but his comrade will surely die. The text asks, "What is the just course of action?"

An extensive literature follows this startling text. At its heart is the problem of the phrase from Ben Petura, "it is better that." This is taken to mean that there is a tension between the prophetic and the practical: it is a supererogatory gesture to offer water that you possess to a fellow traveler and expect a miracle, but it is not necessary either to offer the water or to live expecting miraculous rescue—it is not the *din*. In fact, the premise of *pikuah nefesh* (the necessity to preserve life) must be remembered; it is critical to save as many lives as possible (in this case, one).

Immanuel Jakobowitz, David Bliech, Fred Rosner, and other commentators in the field of Jewish medical ethics have pointed to this text as definitively addressing the problem of rationing. The dispute in the text is resolved in favor of Rabbi Akiba, the great Tannaitic sage of the fourth generation. In the event of scarcity, saving one life takes precedence over the moral gesture of equality. And the life saved is not random; it is that of the owner of the life-saving resource.[3] Rosner would have us focus on the issue of ownership as critical. Yet a responsa literature surrounding this text seems to alter the analysis of the text; it details cases that might result in agreement with Ben Petura and provides a different basis on which to analyze the meaning of Rabbi Akiba's commentary. The very starkness and brevity of the textual language lends itself to the analysis of each moment of the story. This is the basis for the rich responsa literature that follows this text.

•

Reconstruction of the Argument

What is occurring here? First, the context for this *baraita* is a section of the Talmud that begins with a discussion of the rules and obligations involved in lending money and charging interest. The discussion of the marketplace, of charging interest, brackets the text. In fact, the Talmudic argument about interest could be presented seemingly seamlessly if the text on the flask in the desert were excised.[4] Why is this text, then, placed as it is?

Distinctions are being made: How far must one go to assist another in a monetary transaction? Is lending with interest similar to actually "shedding the blood of the neighbor"? Can restitution be made for the damage that may result from charging interest? If not, how can the obligations of society be continued? How is it that "your brother may live with you," and what are we to make of this verse? Suddenly, a story of two travelers, our text, is told. What are we to make of this narrative? What is at stake here? How does the context comment on our narrative and our narrative explicate the larger discussion of obligation?

Two People Were Walking along the Way

The two are alone on the road. Crisis emerges. Friendship, ownership, and necessity are in contention, and the stakes are the highest. The issue is forced choice; short of a miracle, no help will arrive. In the actual world, no help will come in the desert, and choices, finally, must be made.

Civilization, meaning social choices, order, and abundance, cannot be found in the midst of this moment of heightened peril. It is the compelling nature of the stark choice that places this text at the heart of the rationing debate, even if the details vary. The language must be carefully examined. Is what is at stake the necessity of self-preservation, the rights of ownership, or the methodology of response to competing claims? At issue is *language*. What are we to make of the verse in question: "Let him live by your side: do not exact from him advance or accrued interest, but fear your God. Let him live by your side as your kinsman" (Lev. 25:36)?

Interestingly, for the purposes of this discussion, the verse in question in Leviticus comes in the middle of a section of the Torah devoted to the obligation not of strangers or even of friends, but of those who are to be regarded as kinsmen who fall into poverty (the verb in Hebrew is *mwkh*, meaning "to collapse").[5] The entire section follows the discussion of the Laws of the Jubilee, the radical mandatory redistribution of land and property that occurs every fifty years to undo all the injustice inherent in the free marketplace, the system of inheritance, and the problems of a labor-agricultural system with all its natural caprice. The point of the Jubilee is to realign the given world of property, what is experienced as "real" and fixed in human relationships, to the justice of a theological law, the "original position" directed at Sinai that is based on equal shares of the land. But what if this breaks down in the generation that waits for the Jubilee? What if the call for equality cannot be reasonably answered in the actual world?[6] Then the obligation of the kinsman is to become a "redeemer" to the person in need, in fact, to treat the person by his side *as* a kinsman. It is a powerful charge. Being responsible is not adequate; even being conscious of the humanity of the person in need is not enough; in this text, even being neighborly is not enough. What is called for is kinship, brotherhood. From this moment in the text of Leviticus comes not only our text in Bava Metzia but also the text that forms the halakhah for the Ruth story, the textual context for the story itself, which is examined in the next chapter.[7] In its entirety, the quote from Leviticus (25:35) that Rabbi Akiba uses as a proof text to explain his position reads as follows: "If your kinsman, being in straits, comes under your authority, and you hold him as though a resident alien, let him live by your side: do not exact from him advance or accrued interest, but fear your God. Let him live by your side as your kinsman. Do not lend him money at advance interest, or give him your food at accrued interest. I am the Lord your God, who brought you out of the land of Egypt, to give you the land of Canaan, to be your God."[8] To live as a commanded Jew according to the dictates of the Torah text, argues Rabbi Akiba, means modeling one's behavior on the behavior of God. If a man falls into poverty, his life is your responsibility, in a sense. One ought not to take advantage of his poverty, and one ought to remember that strangers (*gerim*, or resident aliens) are to be allowed to live under the same consideration as a family member, "by your side." Thus we are enjoined by the direct command in this verse to support resident aliens just as we would support a fellow Jew.

But the verse is curious; it sounds as if the converse ought to be true: "Let him live by your side" could support the argument of Ben Petura! The text did not put a limit on the amount of support. Rabbi Akiba is drawing the inference, from other sources in the Talmud, that one ought to support him only if one is able to live oneself while enabling him to live. But why is it that one's life takes precedence over the life of one's fellow? Is this precedence descriptive or directive?

According to Moshe Sokel, at issue is the conflict over how to divide a scarce resource.[9] (Indivisible resources are a different sort of conceptual problem; whether we properly focus on problems of indivisible or divisible resources and which the issue of health care is best modeled after is addressed later.) Ought saving as many lives as possible (in this case, one life) be the principle of justice upon which rationing is based, or ought extending each life as long as possible be the goal of just distribution?

This text has at least two different interpretations (Sokel named an additional four, but they are not directly relevant to this discussion). The first follows nineteenth-century commentators Naftali Zvi Yehuda Berlin (known as the Ne'tziv) and Rabbi Abraham Karlitz, popularly known as the Hazon Ish, and has been described by Sokel thus:

> Rabbi Akiba, in this explanation, is of the view that it is better to permanently preserve one life, even at the expense of the other, and thus only one should drink. Ben Petura is of the view that it is better to temporarily extend the lives of both and therefore both souls drink. In the words of the Ne'tziv, explaining Ben Petura, "if both drink, at least they will both live another day or two . . . and perhaps then water will be found." As formulated, the logic of the argument is such that it makes no difference whether A, B, or such third party, C, is in possession of the water: Rabbi Akiba's reasoning, that only one should drink, would apply no matter who had possession of the water, as would Ben Petura's reasoning, that both should have a temporary extension of life. Possession is relevant only in determining *which of the two should drink*; were Ben Petura to agree with Rabbi Akiba's basic logic, that only one should drink, then he too might well agree that it should be the owner of the water that does the drinking. At issue between them is whether one drinks or two drink, *not* whether the owner drinks or they both drink.[10]

Here are not one, but two issues, one of possession and one of quality versus quantity of life. Sokel explains the Ne'tziv's comments as intending to focus the reader on the justification of the second argument, whether only one or both should drink. Leaving possession aside, Ben Petura comments on the quality of faith and the importance of social solidarity, which for Ben Petura exists prior to rights. If a third party had to decide the fate of the two travelers, he or she would still have to confront the issue: Ought two to live longer and in comradeship, or ought one to be selected to live? In this interpretation, the issue is not possession, for the logic holds in either case.

Sokel, thinking that saving a life is a consequentialist goal, counters with the more normative Jewish system of deontological goals to hear the claim of each equally and address the need of each equally. For this reason, Sokel claims, later commentators considered this text useful if a third party is rationing the resource; the issue is the competing moral appeals, the nature of the resource (divisible), and how best to establish a response, not rights or entitlements, in this case, to ownership of property.

And in the Hand of One of Them Was a Flask of Water

A second interpretation addresses the consequentialist problem—that the scenario will end with two dead travelers on the road, if Ben Petura's argument is accepted. Rabbis Chaim Ozer Grodinski, an early twentieth-century commentator; Eliezer Walenburg, a modern Israeli commentator, upon whose authoritative work much of the interpretation of Jewish bioethics rests; and Samuel Edels, a sixteenth-century commentator, focused on ownership as key. In other words, certain things about the situation itself might be critical, property rights being foremost among them. If both travelers were partners in ownership, that would be the basis for a split of the resource. What is at stake is the moral relevance of ownership, not outcome, with Ben Petura holding for a world in which ownership is of no moral weight and Akiba solving the problem, as it were, in a world of property and possession. Here the "it is better that" voice speaks for the moral equality of each traveler. In the previous interpretation, the "it is better that" voice speaks to the possibility of miracle and the justice of the process itself.

In the case of the usual context for the application of this text, the distribution of a divisible resource (e.g., medication, state funding, or the resources of a limited institution), neither party could be said to own the resource in a personal way. Hence, most commentators would argue, the resource ought to be divided equally, on the basis of the second interpretation of the text.[11]

What is striking about this response of perfect equality is that if the divisible resource is to be divided equally, despite the consequences, it does not matter what the status or need of the two parties is. If the resource can be split, it ought to be, even if one party is "more worthy" than the other, according to this interpretation. Thus, in this interpretation of the text, the claim of justice and the deontological appeal are prior to the outcome. After a systematic review of the history of the responsa literature in different rabbinic and medieval periods, Sokel notes that three deontological principles can be derived from this and other texts of allocation: first, a *principle of equal respect*, that all human beings must be treated with respect for their equal value; second, *the maximize life principle*, that one ought always to act so as to extend the sum total of human life; and, third, the *nonarbitrariness principle*, that reason and law ought to govern choices in life and

death situations. The claims of each traveler must be taken with equal seriousness; the principle of life extension can be met partially, and the nonarbitrariness
principle can be satisfied.

Because this text has been subject to such utterly contradictory uses, it might be
helpful to suggest another possible application. Rather than using it as a normative example for distributive principles of justice in any situation at any level of
scarcity, we can take this case as an outward parameter, the point of extremity
when a person is in danger of losing his or her life, where no other options exist
(no "civilization" can be reached), and where anything less than a desperate
choice for survival is untenable. A clue to the intention of the rabbis lies in the
very language of the example, in the starkness of the metaphor, in the harshness
of desert travel itself. Surely, those familiar with the ancient Near East would not
need the elaboration necessary for the contemporary reader, but the rabbinic
theme is clarified by the assumption of the systematic removal of *all* hope of other
human options. Were one able to count on any social response, the ethical
response would be immediately different. This text may stand, then, to give us an
ultimate bottom line: If there is no choice possible that preserves both human life
and human relationality, *only then* can individual life take precedence. And,
given this, the bluntness of Rabbi Akiba might hold: self-preservation is at the
bottom of any justice theory.

It is interesting to note that a parallel text occurs in the Stoic literature; and,
indeed, our text can be read as a counterdiscourse to the Stoic one, which has
been encapsulated by one scholar as follows:

> A second-century Stoic by the name of Hecaton purportedly posed a
> question which appears to be identical to a classic case in rabbinic
> literature which was alluded to earlier. It reads: "or like two people in a
> waterless desert. One of them has in his possession an amount of water
> sufficient to sustain himself, but not enough for both of them. Under such
> circumstances it is proper that the water be assigned to the one more
> useful to mankind." The Stoic solves the problem on the basis of *utilitas*,
> giving preference to the individual whose life is of greater value.[12]

In the Stoic view, the issue is not one of comradeship; the issue is one of prioritization. What, the Stoics asked, is the material principle upon which the water ought
to be divided? It is the principle of utility, of worth. The assumption of the text is
that one traveler will of course be given the water. The issue is which traveler?
The morally relevant thing about the two is not their essential humanity or need
for equal respect, but their relationship to the production of a society.

For the Jewish commentators, the relative value of each traveler is not a consideration. (The next set of texts that I will discuss does address this issue, but it is not

the issue of this particular text.) Value of persons is not a solution to the problem of the travelers in the desert; it is the subject of another discourse.

Of further note is the fact that none of the rabbinic commentators suggested martyrdom in this instance. After all, it might occur that one could give up his or her claim on the flask to save another. While a dominant theme in Christian texts, the limits of martyrdom were narrowly prescribed in the earliest Jewish source: only if being forced to commit murder, idolatry, or adultery was it permissible to allow oneself to be killed. Since the travelers' situation did not meet any of these three criteria, no commentators ultimately suggested that they take such a path, and, of course, neither Ben Petura nor Akiba implied that martyrdom would be a possibility.

What of a resource that is not divisible, however? Ought different rules of justice apply if there could be no temporizing option or if ultimately only one claim can be addressed? This is often the question that confronts us in medical situations. The resource is a physical entity that cannot be divided, a procedure that cannot be "half given," or an intervention that is ineffective (would not keep either party alive for any length of time) if given below a certain basic standard. Perhaps the theory of justice suggested by texts dealing with indivisible resources, and not the travelers' text, is the casuistry that ought to be used in delineating theories of distributive justice.

•

One by One: The Ranking of Salvation

A second set of texts concerns the issues of treatment priorities. These are a series of texts that are contemporary to the traveler text, Mishnaic in origin, and, as in the traveler textual tradition, quoted widely in literature intended for use in the field of bioethics. Abraham Abraham, writing the chapter on priorities in medicine in Rosner's most recent edition of *Medicine and Jewish Law*, quoted the Mishnah. He stated that the order of priorities ought ideally to be followed in a medical situation, but later he cited Moshe Feinstein, who wrote that it would be "difficult" to apply them in practice without "great deliberation."[13] Moshe Feinstein was the dominant *posek* (rabbinic decision maker who is an expert in the halakhah) of the current generation in this field. By citing the difficulty of application, he was noting his understanding of the actual medical situation. In the context of emergent care, the Mishnaic categories of ranking seem particularly indefensible. Abraham and Feinstein were both referring to the following Mishnah, which is the classical source of all such discussions: "Mishnah. A man takes precedence over a woman in matters concerning the saving of life and the restoration of lost property, and a woman takes precedence over a man in respect of clothing and ransom from captivity. When both are exposed to immoral degradation in their captivity, the man's ransom takes precedence over that of the woman."[14]

Here, in contrast to the radical equality of Ben Petura, is a complex taxonomy of rescue when only one can be saved. The paradigmatic example is rescue from a river, but the texts suggest other examples for prioritization—redemption from captivity and ships passing along a dangerous and narrow river. The subsequent section from the Mishnah and Talmudic discussion further illustrates the hierarchy: "MISHNAH. A Cohen takes precedence over a Levite, a Levite over an Israelite, an Israelite over a bastard, a bastard over a nathin, a nathin over a proselyte, and a proselyte over an emancipated slave. This order of precedence applies only when all these were in other respects equal. If the bastard, however, was a scholar and the high priest an ignoramus, the learned bastard takes precedence over the ignorant high priest."[15] This text explains that the status into which one was born took precedence if all else were equal, but that learning negated these set categories. The learned person of the lowest status outranked even one similarly educated of the highest possible social standing.

In reflecting on these types of ranking texts, Sokel delineated five types of categories that are relevant. These are the "material principles" discussed in Chapter 4 in another context. Of note here for our purposes is that while the categories themselves sound abhorrent to the postmodern reader, the notion that one can rank rescue and define priorities on the basis of some sort of social evaluation is certainly at the heart of these texts. Sokel's five categories are as follows:

1. *Yihus*. If all other things are equal, this tells us that simple clan status must be considered. Of course, in the Mishnaic period this was more closely watched than in the modern period, but it provides the first division that is permissible.

2. *Social need*. Sokel meant here the usefulness of the person to society. Kings, military officers, and persons that are useful in periods of crisis are considered next. Sokel noted that this is not developed, but that the existence of this as category is clear.

3. *Capacity for mitzvot*. This is how Sokel and most other commentators (charitably) interpreted the precedence of any man over any woman. One might argue for the explanation of this text by pure misogyny, or that in political economic terms women are really of less value to rabbinic society than men. Significantly enough, when discussing these texts, Sokel placed this ranking by gender as his third category. Yet the actual text places this as the first category of relevance. I submit that the text is more to the point: all else being equal, any man is to be saved before any woman. Further, anyone else whose capacity for the performance of mitzvot is impaired, usually understood to mean the handicapped, is also of lower value.[16] Not to note this and honestly confront the oppression

embedded in such an ordering is to gloss over what is at the disturbing core of all such ranking systems based on social worth.

4. *Talmid Hakham*. Torah learning, which is, after all, the relationship to production that shapes the consciousness of the writers of our text, is, not so unexpectedly, a critical determination for ranking rescue. Remarkable for its candor, the Pharisaic insistence on the ability of even a bastard to trump the high priest stands as an equalizing moment in our text, a counter-hierarchical challenge embedded in the text of hierarchy. Sokel noted that this ought to be read in light of the Pharisaic critique of the corruption of the Sadducean priesthood. Its impact on the discourse of justice in subsequent centuries was considerable. In fact, this point is so determinedly made in subsequent texts that providing clothes for the wife of the scholar takes precedence over the life of the ignorant.

5. *Relative degree of need*. In the Mishnah quoted, the text is concerned with both the likelihood and the nature of rape. It was likely that a female would be raped; but in the case of males, the rape is homosexual, and the text assumes it is more demeaning and more painful.[17] In these ranking texts, in siege texts, and in the *rodef* texts (which will be discussed later), the Talmud assumes that there are worst-case scenarios for rape (e.g., capital rape). In the case of the male, the virgin, and the child, the rape is to be judged more strictly than the rape or threatened rape of the already sexually active, married woman. The Mishnah seems to be saying, according to Sokel, that using the criterion of relative degree of danger is mandated. This is apparently true even if the issue is not death, but the mental anguish associated with rape. Rabbi Meiri commented on the Talmudic mandate to allow a loaded ship to reach port first, passing an unloaded one in the harbor. From this, Sokel noted that prioritization can be done both on the basis of need and of danger.

6. Finally, Sokel identified a category of *relationship to rescuer*. This ranking derives from texts about the rank ordering of need in cases where charity is allocated. In contrast to other teachings that suggest that charity pennies be given equally to each, as noted above, deriving the principle from Ben Petura, these ranking texts suggest the opposite. The following text is from Bava Metzia, the same section of the Talmud that we addressed earlier in the travelers text. Here the text discusses an opinion from Rav Yoseph about resource allocation properly ranked by proximity. "Rav Yoseph taught: 'If you lend money to any of my people that is poor among you.' My people or a non-Jew—my people comes first. The poor or the wealthy—the poor comes first. Your poor or the poor of your city— your poor comes first. The poor of your city or the poor of another city—the poor of your city comes first."[18] In considering allocation, relationality is of significance. If one's first duty is to self, as in the previously discussed (and related) travelers text,[19] then one's next duty is to family first, then to nearby strangers, and

finally to more distant strangers. This ability to rank by relationship adds an interesting nuance to the debate. The relationships are subtle: note that two issues are being addressed by this text.

First is the ordering of allocation by relationship ties, with the strongest obligation being the one that is the most inescapably intimate. The second issue is the placement of the needs of the nonfamilial, non-Jewish poor over the needs of the wealthy. If we interpret the text as describing a concentric prioritization of resources, it would appear that one attends to one's family first, then to the Jewish community, then to the poor of one's city, then to the poor of other cities, and then to the wealthy. At issue is the lending of money, so it would be odd if the needs of the Jewish wealthy were placed before the needs of any poor. There are several possible explanations. Perhaps the category "my people" and poor are synonymous, and perhaps the author of this text did not experience any Jews to be wealthy in the way that he experienced non-Jews to be wealthy. Much more likely we are simply meant to interpret the list as a series of ranking decisions, unrelated choice pairs, which are not intended to be in any lexical order. In this case, all poor are to be helped before any wealthy.[20]

Sokel noted that the categories that he described remain relatively fixed until the period of early modernity. In this later period categories were expanded and altered. Commentators became skeptical that scholarly endeavors trumped legitimate claims on life and health by the less well educated. Yacob Emden considered dropping the entire category of *yihus*: "The superiority of the priesthood and leviteship have declined in these generations."[21] The texts began to discuss women both as having the capacity for learning and as having worth outside that associated with reproduction. Further, linked to the capacity to reproduce, in Emden's work, was the "capacity to maximize life," a new category innovated by his ranking system.

In more recent times, the authoritative American commentator Moshe Feinstein added a ranking order based on queuing as morally significant. Sokel commented on what he considered a "general reluctance" by Feinstein to use the classical source texts of ranking for prioritization systems. Feinstein's queuing or chronological prioritization, according to Sokel, stood as a significant rabbinic innovation. It was an interesting innovation to trace through the texts, since it clearly showed how the method of halakhah itself was based on argument and reconsideration. What could be said, however, was that ranking was a category of thought that was not external to Jewish law; in fact, given the evolution in the categories in the discourse across time and generations about what was the proper way to allocate resources, it quite literally was a textual reflection of the pressing social discourse. Since prioritization was always necessary for Jewish survival, the legal discourse then struggled with how this ought to be done most justly.

The texts of ranking had their most prominent use when they referred to the parallel texts of the Mishnaic period and the responsa literature of the Middle Ages. Here the ranking gained specificity and passion; it was not a theoretical construct. The siege texts I will next discuss raised further questions that must be confronted in describing systems of distributive justice: not only which one would be saved, but what was the nature of a society's obligation in general to the endangered and vulnerable? To what extent ought a society to endanger or impoverish itself to rescue?

•

The Texts of Siege

Elliot Dorff has suggested that neither the travelers text nor the texts of ranking are appropriate to use in problems of macroallocation. He suggested, instead, that the siege texts found throughout Jewish history should be used as an alternative source for this sort of justice deliberation. Dorff's insight was to address the actual historical circumstance faced by the community rather than relying on thought experiments that were speculative. Dorff pointed to the siege texts as potentially useful in allowing the discussion of rationing to proceed as it did historically in Jewish communities faced with such decisions and in extrapolating from that experience to the medical context.

Dorff suggested that we conceptualize a given society as a group under siege from the Angel of Death and that in such cases rules about the limits of redemption and the responsibility of the community toward the threatened person ought to apply. Dorff comments, "Recent statistics on American health care clearly indicate that comparing our medical situation to a siege is not stretching matters much at all."[22]

There are a series of such texts of siege that range from questions in the Talmud about the proper response when a caravan is attacked by brigands, to medieval questions about the siege of walled cities, to horrific halakhic questions about the sacrifice of the one to protect the many when Nazis hunted for Jews in the ghettoes of eastern Poland. (There is a depressing similarity among such texts, preserved over four centuries, but that is the subject of another discussion.)

In 1620, Joel Sirkes, the new rabbi of Cracow, Poland, was confronted by a question from the leadership of the Jewish community of Kalish. A Jew was accused of stealing the host (or possibly a Christ icon) and was arrested by the authorities. A large crowd, Jews and non-Jews, gathered to watch, amidst them the father- and brother-in-law of the accused. The accused man handed his things over to his father-in-law, who functioned in that town as the *shamash*, Jewish representative to the gentile community and a person of stature and importance. Shortly thereafter, officials of the royal court handed down the following verdict: The stolen host might have been contained in the things handed over to the *shamash*; hence, the elders of the town were responsible for surrendering the *shamash* to the Wojewoda, the Polish authorities. The *shamash* fled and was hidden by a fellow Jew, who was aware that the charges were both unfair and inescapable. Should they not surrender him, the elders of the community would suffer the penalty handed down by the court. These elders had reason to believe that these punishments would involve tortures and finally death, a judgment beyond what even the Polish court allowed, since the very request for the community to stand trial was already in violation of Polish judicial procedure. What, they asked, is the ruling regarding this man? Is it or is it not permissible to surrender him to stand trial?[23]

The responsum delivered by Rabbi Sirkes is emblematic of the medieval response to the problem. (A responsum is an official reply to an official query by a leading rabbinic interpreter of halakhic texts [*posek*]). Couched in the classical language of the halakhah, it illustrates the issue we confront in our discourse: How far does a community extend itself to protect the hapless innocent from death? This responsum was carefully translated and analyzed by Elijah Schochet (all translations that follow are his).

Sirkes's response was that an individual has a responsibility to act in such a way that he does not endanger himself, but if he does, he is "guilty," must suffer the consequences, and cannot expect the community to protect him at cost to themselves. If he is not guilty of such behavior, then he cannot be surrendered. (In the case of the elders of Kalish in 1620, the *shamash* was not guilty; hence, the elders paid a large sum yearly as ransom to keep him free.) For our discourse, however, the texts themselves, uncovered by this responsum, are applicable as a source for the language of community and conscience.

The first text is the discussion in the Jerusalem Talmud. What might be described as the *principle of deserts* is what is at stake. If the victim of the kidnap in some way has contributed to his plight, perhaps his moral appeal is weakened.

> *Jerusalem Talmud: Terumot*: Caravans of men are walking down a road, and they are accosted by non-Jews who say to them: "give us one of your number from among you that we may kill him, otherwise we will kill you all." Though all may be killed, they may not hand over a single soul of Israel. However, if the demand is for a specified individual like Sheba son of Bichri, they should surrender him rather than be killed. Resh Lakish stated: "[He may be surrendered] only if he is deserving of death as Sheba son of Bichri." Rabbi Yohanan said: "even if he is not deserving of death as Sheba son of Bichri."[24]

The text says that if the brigands want to kidnap a random individual, it cannot be permitted. There is no justification for such a choice. If the brigands specify a person, however, then the Talmud considers it acceptable to surrender him. Resh

Lakish disagrees. He would advocate the sacrifice of the one on behalf of the many only when the one named is guilty of a capital crime.

Resh Lakish's point is critical. His argument is that you ought not to surrender to the enemy even if it means endangering the community—except in a case that is like the case of Sheba son of Bichri. But our text does not tell us *in what respect* like this Sheba. Is it that one can surrender the specific victim on the basis of his being *named*? Rabbi Yohanan supports this majority view. Naming a specific individual makes the rationing, as it were, of the resource of safety permissible for him, because the death that follows is arbitrary, or at least chosen out of the control of the community. But what ought to be the characteristics of the named person? If, as Resh Lakish suggests, specification is not enough, is culpability?[25] Is it enough that he is guilty of any crime, or only a capital crime? Sheba son of Bichri was involved in a number of actions. Can one hand over the victim who is guilty of rebellion, the victim who rebels against kingship, or the victim who is guilty of seeking the overthrow of a Jewish king? Is the mere act of specificity enough? Is the power in the naming or in the choosing?

Note that the texts themselves differ on the intent of the language and whether the language holds in all cases.

> *Genesis Rabbah* 94: It was taught . . . when Nebuchadnezzar went up to subjugate Jehoikim, he went up and sat in Daphne of Antioch. The Great Sanhedrin went down to greet him and asked him, "Has the time come for the Temple to be destroyed?" "No," he replied, "but Jehoikim king of Judah has rebelled against me. Surrender him to me and I will depart." So they returned and told Jehoikim, "Nebuchadnezzar demands your surrender." "And is it right to act thusly?" he exclaimed, "can you push aside a soul for a soul? Is it not written, 'Thou shalt not deliver a fugitive slave unto his master'" (Deuteronomy 23:16)? "Did not your old one do so to Sheba son of Bichri," they replied, [when they said to Joab] "Behold, his head shall be thrown to thee over the wall." As he would not listen to them, they arose, seized him, and lowered him down over the wall and he cut him in pieces.

This text recounts a teaching about both the concrete application of the text and the power relationships described within the text itself. The Babylonian king Nebuchadnezzar is besieging the Jewish kingdom of Judah. He waits in Antioch, and the religious leaders approach to negotiate. For them the issue is the continuance of the Second Temple, center of Jewish spiritual life. The Temple will be spared, and I will leave your world intact, Nebuchadnezzar tells the leaders, but you must surrender the Jewish head of state, Jehoikim. Jehoikim is approached by the rabbinic leaders, and he is horrified at the suggestion that he turn himself over to be slain. He resists with texts: You cannot push aside a soul for a soul; you cannot deliver a fugitive slave to its master. The argument is to no avail. The rabbis cite text of their own: It is the story of Sheba son of Bichri. They argue that Jehoikim fits the relevant categories: He is a man who has rebelled against a king (even an enemy king), he is specified, and he is indeed guilty of a capital offense in the law of the accusers. They can turn him over to save the community. And when language will not persuade, they seize him and lower him to his violent and hideous death.

The following text raises a new question: Is the extent of responsibility that a community assumes dependent not on the guilt or innocence of the victim, but on the level of risk to the community? The following text suggests that it might be the latter case, based on a *principle of actual need*. In a walled community, the invaders outside the wall stand a reduced chance of capturing the victim. But within a walled ghetto the chances that all could be killed are greater; moreover, the fleeing captive could hide out only with another Jew. As in the case of the elders of Kalish, all would know where he was hiding. Thus, if the threat is real, inevitable, and ominous, then the text suggests the victim may be sacrificed.

> *Tosefta*: Rabbi Judah said: "When are these words intended to apply, when he (the individual in question) is inside and they (the Non-Jews) are outside. But if he is inside and they are inside, since he would be slain and they would be slain, let them surrender him so that all of them will not be slain."

If the brigands were outside the walled city, perhaps the community had a chance of resistance. If they were inside, both the victim and perhaps all of the community would be killed. To protect many from great harm, a harm to the one could be allowed.

Yet another look at the texts of siege suggests that the relationship of the endangered individual to the community is tempered by the *problem of precedent*. In the cases that the texts discuss, the issue is the encouragement of the hostage takers: If you accede this one time, they will repeat their demands, a real threat in the cases at hand. For our discourse this has interesting implications. To what extent might the language of these texts allow us to reflect on precedent in setting up the exception in rescue? The suggestion of a category of argument is made: What is done in any particular case will affect the future cases of many to whom we also have obligation. This, too, sets a limit on what a community is obligated to do to redeem.

> *MISHNAH*: *Gitin (divorces) Chapter 4, Mishnah 6*: They should not redeem captives for more than their worth, for the benefit of the world, and they should not cause captives to escape, for the benefit of the world. Rabbi Shimon ben Gamiel says, "for the benefit of captives."

> *Gemara*: *Gitin 45a*: They asked them, "is this for the benefit of the world," is it because of the pressure on the community or perhaps because they (the hostage takers) should not be encouraged to take others?

Come and hear: Levi ben Darga freed his daughter for thirteen thousand golden dinarii. Said Abaye, "And who told us he did so according to the will of the sages? Perhaps he did so against the will of the sages."

"They should not cause captives to escape, for the benefit of the world. Rabbi Shimon ben Gamiel says, 'for the benefit of captives.' " What is the difference between them (the first sage and Rabbi Shimon)? The difference between them is when there is only one captive.

What is at stake in this story? The Mishnah begins with the statement that it is critically important not to pay ransom to kidnappers beyond the usual price for kidnapped persons, because such a course of action would have negative consequences for the continuance of a unified community. Shimon ben Gamiel adds that it is not acceptable to pay exorbitant ransom for one captive, because such an action might have negative consequences for the other captives who had been taken at the same time.

The Gemara asks for more detail: Is this ransom denied because individual Jewish communities would be quickly driven into poverty and it is not just to ask them to sacrifice as a whole to rescue one person, or is ransom denied because the kidnappers would, sensing a profitable business, simply take more and more townsfolk away? And what of the case of the wealthy man Levi, who ransomed *his* daughter for an exorbitant amount?[26] Abaye then points out that this could be an unauthorized private action, "against the will of the sages." Perhaps this exception had something to do with the initial dispute? The text leaves the question open to our speculation. The words of Shimon ben Gamiel are then reviewed. If it is not permissible to redeem captives for exorbitant amounts, perhaps it is impermissible not because of the effect this action would have on the society at large, but because of the fear of consequences on other captives. This is the interpretation of Rabbi Shimon. If this is so, he argues, then perhaps it is permissible if there is only one captive? (Presumably this is the case of the daughter of Levi ben Darga).

Rashi, the great French Talmudic commentator, interpreted these text as follows:

"Because of pressure on the community": We should not press the community and bring it to poverty because of these.

"or perhaps": The idol worshippers should not exert themselves to capture others, for they sell them at a high price. And the practical difference is, if he has a rich father or other relative who wished to redeem him for much money and that will not fall on the community.

"for thirteen thousand dinarii": we see it was because of pressure on the community.

"when there is only one": captive. The first sage is concerned with the benefit of the entire world, lest they jump on other captives in the future, and put them in chains, and Rabbi Shimon is only concerned with the other captives with him, lest they jump on them and torture them.[27]

At issue here is the recognition that each captive rescued has a direct effect on the others in the same plight. Note that Rashi's first premise was that limits can be set: A human life does not necessarily take precedence over the collective life of the commonweal. The impoverishment of the community is a real factor, and it must be considered even when a life is at stake. The project of the community as a whole must be affected by the plight of the one, according to Rashi, but there are limits on obligation. Note, however, the proviso for the supererogatory gesture of parents.[28]

This proviso leads us to suspect another principle: *the role of the exception*. In another text it is mentioned that a spouse has an obligation to redeem his wife even above any community obligation and even if it would encourage the brigands. This is explained because of the existence of the *ketubah*, or marriage contract. In this interpretation, the obligation of contract trumps social and public policy.[29]

Later texts continue the discourse. But what if a family cannot redeem? And what if the hostage is of exceptional value? Should merit count?

Talmud: Gitin 58: The rabbis taught: an incident with Rabbi Yehoshua ben Hannayah, who went to the great city in Rome. They said to him there is a certain boy in the prison who has beautiful eyes, and a good appearance, and his curly hair is beautifully arranged in locks. He went and stood by the door of the prison and said "Who gave Jacob for a spoil, and Israel to the robbers?" (Isaiah 42:24). The boy spoke up and answered, "Is it not the Lord, against whom we have sinned, and in whose ways they did not want to walk and neither did they listen to his teaching?" (Isaiah 42:24). He said, "I am sure about him that he will be one who shows the way in Israel. By the Temple sacrifices, I shall not budge from here until I redeem him for all the money that they ask." They said that he did not budge from there until he had redeemed him for much money, and it was not many days before he showed the way in Israel. And who was he? Rabbi Ishmael ben Elisha.

Tosafot on Gitin 58a: "All the money that they ask": And when there is danger to life, do we redeem captives for more than their worth? . . . Certainly here, where there is danger of killing, or else because this one was eminently wise.

Tosafot on Gitin 45a: "That they not be encouraged to take others": . . . And Rabbi Yehoshua ben Hannayah who freed that boy for much money, that was because he was eminently wise, or else because at the time of the destruction of the Temple, it was not relevant "that they not be encouraged to take others."

The Tosafot is the major school of Talmudic commentators that followed Rashi. Their commentary is included alongside the written text of the Talmud in all standard editions. They are arguing about the issue of the exceptional hostage. Clearly Levi ben Darga was not the only case of the inapplicability of the rule. Why was this exception made, and why was it justified by a prominent sage? The commentators disagree. Perhaps it was allowed because of the extraordinary worth of this boy (who turned out in the story to be a gifted Talmudic scholar), and, hence, perhaps relative worth ought to matter. Perhaps the exception was made because of the danger to his life, not simply his freedom. Or perhaps, the text goes on, because the social chaos of the period was so extreme that the normative rules did not apply. What is important is how this text differs from the original, in which the parental gesture may be unauthorized, the act of a desperate rich father, and this text, which involves key rabbinic authorities.

This raises a further problem. How does a community set the worth of a hostage? What is a fair share of the community resource, the fair price for a person held hostage, and what is an exorbitant amount? The question was raised in a fifteenth-century text written in Egypt by Rabbi David ben Shlomo Abu Zimra.

Responsum #40: You asked of me to let you know my opinion about what we learnt in a Mishnah that they do not redeem captives for more than their worth, if their worth is calculated as a slave in the market, or at the rate at which idol-worshippers buy their captives.

Responsum: All Israel is long accustomed to redeem captives for more than their worth if sold in the market, for an old man or a child is not worth more than twenty dinarii in the market, and they redeem him for one hundred or more. And the reason for this custom is that we have established that the reason is lest they be encouraged to exert themselves to take others, and we see at this time that the kidnappers do not go out on purpose for Jews, but for whomever they find, therefore even if they redeem them for more than the [other] idol worshippers do. . . . But they should not redeem them for more than the captives of other languages, it is not proper, for now we must worry lest they, since we pay a higher price than other captives, will go out looking for Jews . . . and there is also pressure on the community.

And if you will ask, we see that they redeem them for more than the worth of other captives, and this is an everyday occurrence, and whoever does more to be involved in this *mitzvah*, that it is praiseworthy, the answer is that they rely on one of three or four reasons:

> One, some idol-worshippers redeem their captives at the value that we redeem Jews, even though this one is strong and that one is weak, this uses his own money and that uses the money of others, still the kidnappers will not go after Jews in particular, but after anyone who will fetch a high price. . . .

> Or else, there might be among them a sage, who should be redeemed for whatever price, or even if he is not now a sage, he might be ready to become one. . . .

> Or else, there might be among them children, and they will make them transgress against their faith, and we do not redeem so much as the faith, and in general they force them to break Shabbat and festivals, and torture them with torture worse than death. . . .[30]

The text struggles with the rule and the exceptions. There is concern about the systematic impoverishment of the community and about the issue of Jews becoming targets if generous ransoms are paid. Yet there is the persistent exception, clearly an everyday occurrence. The texts admit several problems that strain the rule. There are the forces of the marketplace, the enormous importance given to hostages who were intellectually gifted,[31] and the special exception made for children.

There is clearly tension in the tradition between the concept of the sanctity of any one life and the arithmetic logic of saving as many lives as possible. Schochet traced this dispute with care. The ruling of Rabbah in the Talmud that the blood of one person is no "redder" than the blood of another, and hence one is forbidden to kill an innocent third party in order to save one's own life, is not evoked in the siege texts. It forms the basis for the general restriction on both martyrdom and opportunistic killing, but it was not a Talmudic response to the problem of resource allocation.

Later commentators did address this problem, however. Moses ha Cohen of Lunel, a twelfth-century contemporary of Maimonides, was the first to introduce an arithmetic solution into the discourse. These commentators were concerned about the problem of justifying a public policy that led to all being killed, the innocent individual accused as well as the crowd of innocent community members, on the basis of a philosophical principle. (It must always be remembered that these debates were, for twelfth-century Jews, not abstract theory, but actual questions that arose out of desperate circumstances.) This position is found throughout the centuries of the Crusades, noted Schochet, but becomes less prominent in the literature. Maimonides himself had suggested the principle of protection from the community was absolute for the innocently accused. The debate continued among twentieth-century commentators:

It is therefore most interesting to note a twentieth-century commentary by Abraham Isaiah Karlitz, known as Hazon Ish, wherein a purely arithmetical measure is once again applied to the saving of lives. The case concerns an arrow speeding through the air towards a group of people. If unobstructed in its course of flight it will surely endanger their lives. The author rules that the arrow may be deflected from its course unto another direction so that only one person will be killed, rather than the many. This deflection is viewed as an act of "saving life" rather than "taking life" because of the reduction in casualties thereby achieved.[32]

Rabbi Kook, writing in the twentieth century as chief rabbi of Palestine, raised another important issue, a reframing that focused the reader on the *obligation of the specified*. Does any one individual have an obligation to sacrifice his own life to save many? In reflecting on the texts, Kook did not find a rule that is binding: "For the inner worth of a man is hidden from the eye. One single human being can be the equivalent to a multitude of six hundred thousand, and even if he, himself, may not seem to be worthy, it is possible that his descendants will be the spiritual equivalent of multitudes."[33]

L. E. Goodman, writing on justice, sought to use this issue to shape a theory of justice. In writing on the problem of deserts, he turned to the text of Sanhedrin 4:5 that argues for the irreplaceability of each human individual, "for each human individual has the uniqueness of a people, a kind, a world."

> That uniqueness, which rests in its highest phases on the fact of subjecthood, is the mark of inestimable worth as persons. Our primal existential deserts are due no greater or lesser weighting than those of other persons and may not be bargained away, since to forfeit them would be to forfeit the irreplaceable subject that we are. Here, in the givens of our own being, not in any compact or theory of what we might find rational, lies the inalienability of our fundamental deserts—our freedom to consent or withhold consent, our right not to be tortured or toyed with, even when we merit punishment.[34]

Of course, then Goodman had to address the tension that such a suggestion placed on the discourse of distributive justice. If all are a world, it does no good to note this and defend the one while the many are also at risk. Goodman resolved the tension with an appeal to community: "The life of the Law is through community, through generosity, consideration, recognition of personhood in self and others. Refusal of such recognition is morally unsustainable and pragmatically unwise."[35] Goodman surveyed the sources for community and found, as in our previous chapter, that the Torah legislature was the "locus of an alternative paradigm" to the metaphor of the marketplace and contractual obligation, acting as a restricting text to the power of ownership, the use of the poor, and the use of the land itself. Hence, all of the tension in the dialogue was about the necessity to set public policy in a way that was both consequentialist in some aspects and respectful of the individual exception in others.

One way this tension was addressed was by the relationship of the duty of the individual relative to the community. The text that follows suggests the methodology of such an interaction. It was critical because it takes as central the voice of the individual that is specified. The entrance of this voice into the discourse allows a radical redefining of the problem of covenantal citizenship.

This text was written by Rabbi Shlomo ben Yehiel Luria, a Polish contemporary of Rabbi Zimra. It was from *Yam Shel Shlomo*, the Sea of Solomon, a sixteenth-century halakhic work. It concerned the most famous case of the redemption of captives, that of Rabbi Meir ben Barukh of Rothenburg (1215–93). This text sets authoritative limits on redemption because they were established by the great sage of the generation from "within" the captive experience.

> *Gitin 66:* . . . I have heard about Maharam MeRotenberg [Rabbi Meir ben Barukh of Rothenburg], may his memory be for a blessing, that he was taken prisoner in the tower of Eigesheim for several years and the prince demanded a great sum from the communities, and the communities wanted to redeem him, and he did not permit it, for he said, "they should not redeem captives for more than their worth." I am astonished, since he was an eminent sage, and there was not another like him in his generation in Torah and piety, and it is [therefore] permitted to redeem him with all the money in the world; and if, in his humility, he did not want to hold himself as an eminent sage, he should have at least considered the waste of Torah, as he himself wrote that he was sitting in the dark shadow of death, without Torah or light, and he lamented that he did not have the books of the decisors of Jewish law and the Tosafot, and how did he not concern himself with the sin of wasting Torah since many needed him.
>
> Certainly, his opinion was that if they would redeem him, there would be grounds for concern that all the princes would do that to eminent sages because of the great amount of money, until all the money of the [communities of] exile would not suffice to redeem them, and the Torah would be forgotten from Israel.
>
> Therefore, the pious one said that it is better to lose a small part of the extra wisdom of Israel than to lose the basic knowledge of the Torah, and that this is the sign, for then that ended the plague and destruction of taking the sages of the exile.

This text suggests two things. First, an individual himself may, though not bound by a Mishnaic rule, reflect on the use of his life relative to the life of the whole and act accordingly. This opinion is linked to the siege texts, which suggest that a medieval Jew has a responsibility to act in such a way that he is at all times acting "in public," as it were, aware of the effect his behavior has on the fragile whole. Second, this text suggests that merit, even Torah learning, a category of ranking outlined in the Talmud, may not trump community in the actual world of survival.

If these texts suggest that exemption for the learned person ought not to hold in some circumstances (not, one must note, for reasons of justice, but for practical reasons of community survival), what of the person of marginal social worth? Are some people, by virtue of their status, physical health, or behavior, *less* likely to be saved by the rescuing community?

The answer is a highly nuanced "yes." Schochet reluctantly called this the category of expendability. For our discussion it might be more accurate to call it *the principle of differential risk*. It is the relationship of this self to the community that is at stake. The following texts suggest that a person in a liminal state has a reduced moral claim on the resources held in common. Who are these expendable persons? According to some authorities, this category includes the already defiled woman (whether this is a professional prostitute, a woman suspected of casual sexual habits, or merely a nonvirgin is not clear) in cases of surrendering a woman to enemies who will rape her.[36] The text seems to assume that a woman who has had multiple sexual partners will be less at risk for severe emotional harm following a rape than will a virgin.[37]

There is also a discussion in the texts about categories of men who are expendable. A recurrent problem in the siege text genre was the forced conscription of Jews for the armies of assorted rulers in Europe and Russia. Community leaders, in a long series of queries to their rabbis, asked if it was permissible either to protect the leadership, the scholars, or the wealthy from the draft or to offer to the authorities community undesirables, rebels, and "immorals." Rabbi Samuel Landau followed the classic pattern: If an individual is already specified, it is wrong to rescue him, as this would surely mean that another would go in his place. He cited the issue of the equivalent redness of each man's blood.[38] What is important for the discourse is the admission into it of the *category* of thought that describes a differential risk spectrum.

A category also exists in rabbinic thought for the person who is already condemned to death. Dorff, who noted the importance of this category in the work of Daniel B. Sinclair, found it of importance in the problem of both discontinuation of treatment and allocation of the scarce resource.

> The term, *gavra ketila*, occurs four times in the Babylonian Talmud. According to Sanhedrin 71a, once a person has been sentenced to death, he is immediately a *gavra ketila*, a killed person. Because of that, Sanhedrin 81a deals with the possibility that one might think a person

sentenced to one of the more lenient forms of execution, since immediately presumed dead, could not be subsequently sentenced to a harsher form of execution for another crime. It rejects that conclusion, but in the meantime reaffirms the description of a doomed person as a dead one. Sanhedrin 85a adds the consideration that one sentenced to death, since considered an already killed person, is no longer "abiding among your people" in the terms of Exodus 22:27. And, perhaps the most relevant for our purposes, Pesahim 110b says that a person who drinks more than 16 cups of wine is a *gavra ketila*. There it is medical, rather than judicial, factors which make the person thought of as dead.[39]

Dorff linked to this another category of person—the *terefah*, a person with an incurable, fatal organic disease. This category emerges in Talmudic texts to describe both persons and animals who have a fatal organic defect or have been diagnosed with an illness thought to lead to death in twelve months. Dorff noted that since the death of a *terefah* is by definition inevitable, the rabbis allow for the deserted wife of a *terefah* to remarry and the killer of a *terefah* to be exempt from the death penalty. The intentional killer of such a person is still subject to divine punishment and moral sanctions, but the legal status of the *terefah* is analogous to that of a dead person.[40]

Dorff discussed confusion on the boundaries of this nuanced state. Clearly, it is a category different from that of the *goses*, the clearly dying person, the person on his or her deathbed who is to be treated, all agree, with the complete status of person. Why this confusion? According to Dorff, it is because the definition of the dying process and the appropriate response are complex issues. The view of this critical liminal state involves a definition of the period at the end of life and a highly nuanced view of personhood. The *goses* is not "more alive" than the *terefah*. The terms are, rather, different linguistic attempts at characterizing the process of dying. This is extremely difficult to understand, in part, because of the modern attachment to the "moment of death." It is important in clinical medicine to have such a moment, because it is at that moment that everything about the person as patient changes. The language of rabbinic ethics reflects a sensitivity to death as process, with the person retaining certain aspects of personhood even beyond the cessation of cardio-respiratory function, and losing other aspects of personhood prior to clinical death. The rabbis struggled to define these states, just as we do today, and used different vocabularies in an attempt to describe with accuracy a difficult and essentially mysterious boundary of human life. Alan Weisbard, in an early article on this concept, explained the terms as follows: "It is also difficult to understand because the English rendering of both terms is 'moribund' or 'in a dying condition.' The operational criteria and the legal status attaching to the two concepts are different in significant respects. . . .

The death of the *trefah* is regarded as ultimately more certain, although perhaps less imminent, than that of a *goses*. As the *goses*, unlike the *trefah*, is regarded as having at least the theoretical potential to return to health, the *goses*, unlike the *trefah*, is not regarded as 'a man slain.' "[41]

A parallel in rabbinic categorization exists, Dorff explained, in the case of the beginning of personhood and the debate that surrounds abortion. Here too, Jewish law suggests a liminal status for the fetus and, exempt from the death penalty, its destruction. Hence, given these thought categories, the discussion emerges in light of the siege texts:

> It is as if all of us are besieged by the Angel of Death, who calls specific ones of us (those who already have irreversible, terminal illnesses) to be sacrificed for all the rest of us. Since terminally ill people are already under a "sentence of death" (albeit a medical one, not a legal one), it is permissible, although often heartrending, to suspend our efforts to prolong their lives in order to preserve the lives and health of others.[42]

> What if the designated person was a *terefah*? R. Menachem Meiri says: "It goes without saying that in the case of a group of travelers, if one of them was a *terefah*, he may be surrendered in order to save the lives of the rest, since the killer of a *terefah* is exempt from the death penalty." Meiri specifically does not extend this to a *goses*. This is surprising, for a *goses* is typically closer to death than is a person who has just been diagnosed as having an incurable illness. Nevertheless, one can understand R. Meiri's reasoning: the *goses*, after all, is a living person in all respects, and hence any complicity in his/her death would be tantamount to murder. The *terefah*, on the other hand, is, as it were, already dead, and hence killing a *terefah* does not entail capital punishment. These facts mean, for R. Meiri, that in a case in which many lives might be saved as a result of the death of a *terefah*, the latter's life does not possess the same value as that of the other viable persons.

The siege texts, then, are complex and varied and difficult to summarize as a source for the language of justice. Yet, taken as a whole, they offer a rich assortment of Jewish responses to the discourse. The siege texts have a haunting urgency. They again and again pose the most difficult question of justice: the forced choice between the individual and the whole, the nature of innocence and desert, and a world without justice in which a community struggles to make rational the irrational and unfair. Nowhere is this choice more catastrophic and the chaos of injustice more utter than in the texts of justice that emerge from the Holocaust. These texts serve as yet another halakhic source for the discourse on distributive justice.

•

The Texts of the Holocaust

The texts of the Holocaust are unique in their power and their contemporary urgency and, as such, can be seen as related to the siege texts but distinct from them in important ways.

Responsa of Rav. Shimon Efrati of Warsaw
This is a question to make one's hair stand on end. In a bunker lived a large group of Jews hiding out so that the cruel, defiled, accursed oppressors, may their names be blotted out, would not find them. It was certain that if they would be found they would be killed. Once when the wicked ones were conducting a search for those unfortunate people, an infant among those hidden burst out crying. It was impossible to quiet him. If his voice was heard outside, they would all be seized and taken out to be killed. The question arose: is it permitted to place a pillow over the baby's mouth to stifle him? If they did this there is fear that the child might suffocate. Meanwhile, one man drew near and placed the pillow over the baby's mouth. After the accursed wicked ones had passed, they removed the pillow and saw to their horror that the baby had suffocated.[43]

This question was addressed to Rabbi Shimon Efrati of Bessarabia years after the event that occurred in the bunker. The after-the-fact quality of this text is extremely relevant. In a sense, the survivors were asking for the halakhic language that would again order the chaos of such a choice. And the rabbi carefully responded in the language and method of the classic halakhah.

The case is compared to the siege texts, and the verdict of Maimonides is again raised: it is impermissible to hand over a "single soul of Israel" unless the victim is a capital criminal specified by the enemy. Yet Efrati argued that even if a victim is specified, it is forbidden to surrender him unless it is certain that he will be put to death in any event. Since it is clear that, in this case, all would die if discovered, including the victim, it is permitted to sacrifice the baby. The child is, in a sense, *terefah*, already under a sentence of death.

The child also fell under another category of rabbinic thought: the *rodef*, or pursuer. If, by his being, this child endangered the life of another, can he be considered a *rodef*, and thus was it permissible to kill him to save the life of another? In this case, the child's pursuer status was involuntary; hence killing him was not mandatory but was permitted. Nonetheless, it was the doomed status of the child that decided the issue at last.

Can one ration the chance at survival so as to benefit the whole community? In this text, as in the other siege texts, the answer is a guarded yes: if it will not encourage further hostage taking, if it will not lead to systematic killing of the weakest, and if the selected one would die along with the rest in any case.

In another text from this period, the survival of the community norms within a wilderness of violence is what is at stake. Both these texts speak to the power of language and text to set the parameters of the most horrific human terrain. Both testify to the power of methodology and reason, of language that gives shape to the possibility of human order and relationality in the very middle of the anarchic world.

> Rabbi Meisals describes a "selection" conducted by the Nazis at Auschwitz in which some 1400 boys of less than an arbitrary height were singled out for death. Some camp inmates sought to ransom certain boys by bribing the guards. However, the guards would not release any boy without capturing another to take his place. This trading in lives went on throughout the day. The father of one of the boys, aware that his son could be ransomed only at the expense of another life, asked R. Meisals whether under the circumstances the Torah permitted a father to save his son's life. R. Meisals did not wish to render an explicit decision in a capital case, especially without access to books of law, the counsel of other rabbis, or the calm objectivity necessary to make such a ruling. . . . From the rabbi's refusal, the father concludes that the ransom of his son is *halakhically* forbidden.[44]

This terrifying text represents both the uses and the limits of words, or text. The rabbi stands before the man unable to give him the word that he seeks, "for I cannot say anything at all to you without studying a book." The rabbi cannot say, "Go, do anything, use the money, the corruption is in the system itself, all is permitted," because it is not permitted in the texts of the system to which they both are committed. Yet he cannot speak the words of restraint either. Perhaps he is overlooking a source; perhaps there could yet be found a way in the text. But both know that the saving of one is the death of another.

What adds particularity to the horror of this situation is that the rabbi's own son was also in the camp, spared this time only because of his height. It was the first day of Rosh Hashanah, the day on which in the Jewish liturgy "all pass before God to be written in the book of life or death for the coming year."

Both the rabbi and the father merely stood witness to, and the rabbi was mute in front of, the extraordinary maintenance of the system itself. The men understood the event in terms of the narrative of which they were a part. The larger relationship between God and the Jewish people and the mystery of the sacrifices of fathers and sons represented by the story of Abraham and Isaac were evoked. The responsum ends with this comment: "And you, my dear brother, look closely and consider the righteousness and perfect piety of this Jewish man. I have no doubt that his word caused a great commotion among the celestial host; and the Holy One, blessed be He, gathered together all the host of heaven and was, so to speak, very proud: 'Behold the creatures that I Created in my world.' Justifiably it is said of this man (Isaiah 49:3): 'thou art my servant Israel in whom I will be glorified.' "[45]

It is only in a theological context that such choices ultimately can be made, say such texts, understood in light of a systematic language and a story that is fundamentally one of justice, hope, and redemption. All of the siege texts, and the Holocaust texts as the most extreme example, are related to faith. The voice that they add to the discourse insists on the possibility of human ordering in the face of random and desperate chance.

•

The Rodef

The siege texts are linked to yet another halakhic argument. Raised as a linked text in several of the discussions noted above, the rabbinic discussion of the *rodef* offers other insights on the problem of distributive justice. Embedded in these debates are several key issues that address justice concerns.

Baruch Brody, a leading contemporary Jewish philosopher and bioethicist, offered a perspective on the traditional sources different from that which Dorff had suggested. Rather than basing proof texts in the siege texts, Brody argued for the use of the *rodef* texts in grounding a theory of distributive justice in health care resource allocation.[46] A *rodef* is defined as a case where one is in pursuit with the intention to kill. Hence we must kill the *rodef* or allow the death of the pursued innocent. The texts that discuss the *rodef* ask the following question: If a *rodef* is in pursuit of another person, what are the appropriate limits on the attempt at rescue? In his use of these texts Brody did not focus on the use of the "*rodef* defense," the question of the acceptability of homicide in these circumstances, the amount of force to be used, or the duties of the *rodef* and the rescuer toward property that might be destroyed in the general flurry involved in the chase, which is the focus of much legal commentary.[47] Rather, he considered the text as establishing the basis for the mobilization of community resources to rescue from injury, death, or dishonor the one who is pursued. Brody suggested that the condition of illness itself, being a patient, is equivalent to being pursued.

There are three relevant parts to the Gemara that discuss the economics of the laws of the *rodef*. Brody suggested that one is of particular importance in the discussion of allocation of public funds for health care. It is as follows:

Sanhedrin 73a:

MISHNAH: The following must be rescued [from transgression of the mitzvah not to murder or abuse another] even at the cost of their [the *rodefs'* own] lives: He who pursues after his neighbor to kill him, [or] after a male [for sexual abuse], [or] after a young woman [to dishonor her with sexual violence].

Gemarah: From where do we know that if a man sees his neighbor drowning, mauled by animals, or attacked by robbers, he is bound to save him? From the verse, "Do not stand idly by the blood of your neighbor." But is it derived from this verse? Is it not rather from elsewhere [in the Torah]? From where do we know [that one must rescue his neighbor from] the loss of himself? From the verse, "And thou shall restore him to himself." From that verse I might think that it is only a personal obligation, but that he is not bound to take the trouble of hiring men [if he cannot rescue the neighbor himself]: Therefore, this verse teaches that he must.[48]

Brody read the passage above as "placing significant economic burdens on third parties who are obliged to spend money to save the party who is being pursued."[49] Brody considered this central to a general philosophic debate about the limits of autonomy, noting that the greater one's moral obligation to spend resources of time and money on other-centered projects is, the less resources and freedom exist to pursue one's own projects. If the pursued one cannot escape, if his life, freedom, or dignity is at stake, then this text necessitates a rescue, a putting aside of the business of one's life to undertake an all-out rescue.

The urgency of the situation is suggested by the text. It allows for special dispensations: rescue yourself; if you cannot succeed alone, enlist the help of others; pay them if they will not consent to act freely; destroy property if you must, for you will not be liable; kill the pursuer without a trial; do what you will to save the hunted. Taken alone, this text might suggest that no expense ought to be spared, that even the laws of the land (normative justice) ought to be suspended if life, health, or freedom is at stake. Yet Brody suggested that this is too simplistic a view and that the intention of the texts was to be read in light of others in adjudicating any particular case. "Jewish casuistry is constantly engaged in assessing the significance for each case of many values, recognizing that not all of them can be satisfied in a given case."[50] Brody noted the impact that history itself has had on case law and suggested that in the sixteenth and seventeenth centuries, particularly in the Ottoman Empire, the custom was to disregard these laws and pay whatever was required. This link between oppression and lenient interpretation of the law is not absolute: witness the Holocaust text discussed above. As Brody says, "Quick answers are very dangerous in Judaism." Brody used the text of the siege to describe how community responsibility to rescue can be curtailed by the community's economic limits and by the problem of precedent—that we not sacrifice future lives to save current lives.

The text of the Gemara does not stop at this first passage. It includes two further stipulations that address the issues of the commodity relationship to rescue. The language they introduce into the debate is important for the issues that surround justice.

> 2. [If a man being pursued breaks some goods in his flight] he is not liable if they are the goods of the pursuer; he is liable if they are the goods of anyone else . . . because he saves himself through the property of another.

> 3. A pursuer who is pursuing a pursuer to save [the person the latter is attacking] and who breaks the goods of the pursuer or of the pursued, or of anyone else is not liable. That is not in accordance with strict law (*min hadin*), but unless you say so, it will turn out that nobody will rescue anybody from a pursuer.

The first text suggests that the rescued person, whether victim or innocent, is nonetheless also bound to both the community and the future. His or her use of community resources, in this case the resources ("utensils") used, must be compensated for. One cannot use up the resources to save oneself and then not repay, not acknowledge the existence of the other in whose world one has been. The notion that the rescued person has an obligation is parallel to the response of the imprisoned person of Rabbi Meiri. Here again, the victim is not viewed as passive, but as having the responsibility of the self toward the community that has rescued. It is not the victim's "right" to have unlimited use of this community's resources.

The second text raises yet another key point. Not only is the *rodef* defense accepted as having the equivalent stature as self-defense in Jewish law, but the law itself is altered in this situation to provide a version of what is currently called Good Samaritan language in modern law. Normally in Jewish law, if one destroys something belonging to an innocent third party, one is obligated to pay for it, as in the first quote above. Yet if in the pursuit of the pursuer the resources of another are lost, then the individual responsible is not liable. This dispensation, the text tells us, is allowed in order to encourage the very act of rescue. In a deeper sense, however, this clause lifts a portion of the gesture out of the normal relationships of the marketplace—transactions between two individuals whose obligations can be expressed in the halakhic terms of *what is owned*—and asks instead, *What is the community obligated as a whole to provide?* It is not specified in our text who will pay for the damaged property, the loss incurred in the rescue. It may be that the third party must also become involved. This may be the cost of living in a world of social order where all will be aided. Or it may be that the community as a whole will repay the damages. In any case, the loss is a collective responsibility, as it were.

The three excerpts from the *rodef* texts offer yet another vocabulary for the discourse about the commanded individual in a community that is obligated and commanded, a vocabulary without the framing language of rights, but of obligation and duty. Yet the sense of this text, as in all the texts heretofore discussed, is of the desperate moment, the forced choice situation, or the life-for-life justice appeal. The next text addresses the rationing issue but stems from a different textual location; it is rooted not in extremity, but in daily life issues.

•

A Community of Moral Order

If the text on the flask in the desert provides the extreme example of the individual and the fatal consequence, and the texts of siege explore the extreme limit of the permissiveness of a community on behalf of the individual, then perhaps another text could tell us something about less dramatic choices. Is there a text that moves the discourse into the world of the ordinary choice? Moshe Tendler, a contemporary Orthodox rabbi who is considered to have special expertise in bioethics, has cited the text of Sanhedrin 17b as useful in discussing an issue not tangential to health care allocation: how a Jewish physician determines his place in the health care crisis.[51] In particular, Moshe Tendler raises the question, "What is a just wage for a Jewish physician?"[52] Further, the text stands as another response about the collective responsibility to provide for health care as a basic decent minimum.

At issue here is the notion of a basic decent standard. The physician, like the butcher, is a necessary part of the standard. As such he can expect a decent wage but not more than is necessary to live. This is one of the few rationing texts that addresses the issue of limits of benefit for the provider, not simply the rescued. Further, cities and other social orders, to be just in the real sense of the term, have obligations in addition to those of the commanded individual. The collective makes it a fit place. Justice can occur only if the physical and spiritual needs are met and if the children are taught. Good medical care does not stand, moreover, at the top of a hierarchy of social goods. All the needs must be addressed, and resources drawn to the health care system must allow for the social reality of competition between many needs.

In exploring this, Tendler relied on a text that is located within a larger discussion of the nature and parameters of justice in the form of the adjudicating court (the Sanhedrin). The Mishnah considers the size and the function of the rabbinic court. It reviews the scope of responsibility and authority of adjudicating courts of various sizes. Courts of three judges can decide monetary disputes, courts of twenty-three can decide capital crimes "for men and for women and for beasts,"[53] and a Great Sanhedrin of seventy-one is required to decide justice in matters of the most gravity or that affect great numbers of people. In connection with this, the question of the size of a city that needs a formal court of twenty-three judges is raised. Since the Great Sanhedrin is a national body, then the next highest body is this "lesser" Sanhedrin. But the formulation is curious. It raises issues of how much of a society is needed to call forth a court and how much of a court is needed to create a city. Both are definitional. At issue seems to be the problem not of mere size, but of the relationship of rationality or sociability to justice. For justice to be public and for the social order to be just, what is required?

Sanhedrin 17b:

It has been taught:
A person of wisdom should not live in a city that is empty of the following ten things:
    1. a court of justice that imposes flagellation and decrees penalties
    2. a communal charity fund, collected by two and distributed by three
    3. a Synagogue
    4. a mikvah
    5. a toilet
    6. a mohel
    7. a surgeon
    8. a scribe
    9. a butcher
    10. a schoolteacher
Rabbi Akiba is quoted "Also several kinds of fruit, because these enlighten the vision."[54]

Tendler's suggestion of this text to address the issue of distributive justice allows an interpretation of the language that surrounds the setting of a standard of cityhood. A city that is acceptable, that is thus named as a just habitat, has a corresponding obligation to provide these ten specific things for the citizens. Tendler posited that the citizens and service providers are in a relationship of mutual obligation. Tendler further proposed that what is provided is a "living wage" for the scribe, the schoolteacher, the butcher, and the mohel, and there is no hierarchy of being in that list. Indeed, the theme of solid equity of status is reinforced by the listed aspect of the text itself, providing a comment on the relative status of physician (after toilet). Such a wage would be guaranteed, according to Tendler, but shaped by the norms of other needs of the community.

To parse the text more slowly, it is important to note that it is rooted in the problem of social justice, of the creation of the *moral community* of judgment itself. How large a body is needed to decree penalties? There is a dispute in the text. The majority opinion is that three judges can suffice, yet the minority position is upheld. Rabbi Ishmael called for twenty-three, as flogging may involve flogging to death. Thus, a heavier sentence requires more certainty. Justice in social disputes (unlike matters of kashrut) is not a singular act, as noted in the previous chapter. Three may not be enough to set decrees that involve even the chance of capital punishment, even if the death is consequent and unintended.

Hence, in respecting the order of the text the first need for the social order to exist is the formation of the court itself. This leads to another interesting detail of this text. For the court process to proceed properly, it needs a specific number of rows of witnesses, twenty-three rows of twenty-three people. In addition to the defendant and two accusers, this is a large number, quite possibly all of the town's males.[55] This suggests that the sitting of a court, the making of justice, actually requires the entire town to witness the acts of justice, in the same way that all who witness both the funeral procession and the wedding celebration ought to stop and participate. To "make justice" requires the judgment of the entire social order. Justice does not happen in some isolated and distinctive location, but in the center of a discursive community where all have a vital role.[56]

Next on the list is the communal charity. Second only to justice is charity, *tzedakah*, the obligation to repair the world that is unredeemed. Note that charity comes from *caritas*, which is not the root in Hebrew. The concept of *tzedakah*, as noted in Chapter 6, is based on the principle that the poor are, in fact, owed a portion of God's land that is temporarily held and used by a tenant commanded by God to dispense the proper amount to the poor person. Without such a fund, the community is not whole. Note that the text does not call for righteous individuals to give *tzedakah*, but that it is a requirement of community.

The next requirement is a synagogue, a house of meeting and study, that would contain a copy of the Torah. This necessity suggests that while justice and righteousness and allocation and public policy are the first choices that a community ought to make, they are not separate from a spiritual life.

A *mikvah* is a ritual bath that is used in the practice of traditional Jewish life as a marker between states of encounter with death and the resumption of sexual relationship in marriage. It is required for all married women to bathe in the *mikvah* after each menstruation and childbirth.[57] Thus, sexuality and procreation are the next priorities.

Next are the demands of health and the embodied experience.[58] For these one needs a public toilet, a circumciser, and a surgeon (the work done by the non-surgical doctor in Talmudic times was closer to the work of nursing, and hence was done by relatives). The placement of the surgeon suggests that his work was no more redemptive, or more or less necessary, than that of a *mohel*.

The *mohel*, the surgeon, the scribe, the butcher, and the schoolteacher are persons who function in part as technicians and in part as spiritual leaders.[59] Each has the responsibility to know the halakhah as it affects the others who are dependent on him or her. Each is to be paid a living wage, and each must be provided for by all if the whole community is to stand (that is, if it is to be fit). Each represents the elements that are a part of the establishment of a collective conversation about what is the basic decent minimum for daily life in a community of others. The placement of the whole discourse in the Gemara that discusses justice is a further recognition of the link between sustenance, justice, fair distribution, and daily social life that occurs often in the text. Nothing about the private is entirely private: the public arena is both a responsibility and an expectation. The life of the individual self cannot be lived without the presence of the other, and the other and his or her needs are what trace the map of the terrain that is habitable.

The variety of classic texts that I have suggested addresses the issue of distributive justice in the tradition in a way that is not comprehensive. Nonetheless, it responds to the current critical hermeneutics of modern commentators on bioethics. The next chapter advances a text that is not normatively described in the canon of mutually referential texts of justice. The narrative of the Book of Ruth involves a community applying and interpreting the biblical norms that the rabbinic leadership argued over in the texts just described.[60]

However, this narrative account of justice offers a different vocabulary for the discourse, and it re-creates the discourse itself, even as it assumes the method of collective address that both creates and is created by the halakhic system. What do I mean by this? I mean that to create the possibility for an ethics of encounter we have to do more than have the right words. We have to have, as founding narrative, a practical case that recalls for us the method of discourse itself. We are not looking for principles; we are looking for a new way to talk justice, a new alphabet whose shaping insists on new relationships. The hard work of policy gives us one example. The radical encounter with the other that is found in the Ruth story offers us our organizing narrative.

CHAPTER EIGHT

DEVELOPING
THE COMMON LANGUAGE
The Book of Ruth

The first years of modern feminist scholarship have offered an extraordinary wealth of literature reinterpreting the Jewish tradition. Feminist scholarship has uncovered voices lost to the canon, has validated alternative ways of hearing and speaking in the discourse, has uncovered and re-created women's prayer, and has both offered sharp critique of the issue of praxis and suggested renewed ways of spiritual return. This chapter seeks to accomplish something different: the beginning of a Jewish ethics rooted in feminist and social justice concerns. Such a development must begin with new language and new theory, ways to hear and speak of social justice different from the current claims of individual rights and individual entitlements. It is by the application of Jewish texts read through such a lens that a new language can be constructed. Such a task is, of course, very large, and this chapter describes only a beginning, an outline of the project that can make possible such an ethics of encounter. It is a setting of the philosophical and theological context for the implications of actual justice considerations.

Three things are assumed by this chapter. First, the insights of feminism are part of the scholarly tools of the discourse and need not be discovered or defended. That work has been accomplished by many other capable scholars. Second, and sometimes in tension with the first assumption, the Jewish textual and legal tradition, the halakhah, is a valid place to begin the search for ethical response. Finally, central to this chapter is the premise that what is at stake in all ethical discourse, including the discourse of feminist ethics, is the radical encounter with the other, the apprehension of his or her claims in the collective conversation about justice.[1] Justice is at its heart relational, and relationship implies social discourse.

One way to develop collective language is through the lens of the text itself. If the way to the truth of an action and the cut to the core in ethical decision making is via the shared narrative, then the text is the first place to begin when rethinking moral language (and certainly alternate moral language) in the discourse of justice and public policy. This is, of course, the traditional starting place in the halakhic method. By use of such a method, normative scholarship begins the reflection on justice: case by case, arguing by analog to the present problem. The discursive and argumentative halakhic method itself suggests that a richer, deeper account can be given of the problem of allocating scarce resources. If we are to develop new language beyond individual entitlements, it must be language rooted in story and community that draws from a method that is *itself* dialogical and communal. The Talmudic method itself, larger than any specific text, describes the relationship between the individual and the collective that creates the social and shared ground for justice. I remain committed to the halakhic methodology, the careful placing of the story of any particular contemporary choice beside the shared biblical story. This methodology is the place (to use Jeffrey Stout's metaphor) that is the vantage point within the tradition from which I evaluate and reason.[2] However, the suggestion—the insistence—that other texts are needed to explore an argument is well within the traditional method itself, namely, the search for other accounts on which to base law, morality, and public policy.

The texts examined in the last chapter lead toward an answer. Ultimately, however, they offer only a partial answer. It is partial, first, because simply stated, the language is taken from textual experiences that are not fully attentive to the reality of women's lives. A feminist stance claims that this consideration is neither petty nor foolish nor a relatively minor concern in the justice debates at the public policy level or the life-and-death decisions at the bedside. But why should we quarrel at so basic a level with the tradition? Many scholars have already noted that the Jewish textual tradition is replete with the notion of women as other, as dangerous, or as simply less valued than men. Although troubling, we have been assured that this notion is historically consistent. Traditional halakhic method would have us take the variety of these texts (and surely there are enough variants when speaking of social justice and the allocation of scarce resources) and quote them as the central and strongly argued sources of the collective and community-based moral language I am seeking. Surely, we are told, the textual casuistry can be meant to apply to all persons, not only to men. Yet despite this answer, the quarrel remains. Even if it is historically explainable, the value of women as diminished (as we saw in the texts of rescue) and the persistent address to the male is unacceptable in the modern application of halakhah for our ethical purposes.[3] This is especially true if we are seeking the sources of language, where exquisite attention to nuance is demanded. Hence the first reason to look for alternate narratives emerges.

Feminism insists that the political is at its heart personal, and that intimacy, the encounter with the other, is central in the world of social discourse and public policy.[4] Such a consideration leads directly to two sources for a feminist ethics that inform any text we examine. The first is the philosophy of Emmanuel Levinas, which demands as the first act of philosophy the regard of the "naked face" of the other.[5] The second is the lived experience of the women's movement itself, which begins with the small-group encounter with the story of the other. Both of these sources act as the theoretical ground for a distributive justice based in ordinary friendship, the dailiness of a life that is noticed as a series of choice-gestures among the competing needs of many.

This is cautionary work. Ethical analysis is not a sermon. The text is heterogeneous. The story is told in different voices, heard in different ways, and spoken from different points of view; the gaps in the text signal that the text is in this way interactive. The work of the analytic reader is to honor all of the readings, noting what in the tradition makes certain voices traditional and others variant. Ilana Pardes, writing in *Countertraditions in the Bible*, noted that attention to other voices or other stories (even within the textual account itself) suggested both the legitimacy of these voices and the relative arbitrariness of the version that was understood as singular. She called for a closer examination of the language and the story as a way to "call for a consideration of the heterogeneity of the Hebrew canon, for an appreciation of the variety of socio-ideological horizons evident in this composite text."[6]

Pardes and others cautioned against "reading into" in a way that obliterates the text itself. A text cannot mean whatever we need it to mean.

> [One must] try, in other words, to avoid an all too common tendency of feminist critics to turn the remote past into a fulfillment of current dreams. This does not mean that the present has no bearing on [the] endeavor. Quite the contrary. Like any hermeneutic pursuit, [our] own pursuit entails an attempt to make sense of the present in light of the past, to explore a distant mystery which includes our own . . . to strive to listen to the otherness of past voices, though I realize, with Stephen Greenblatt (1988), that in our most intense moments of striving to listen to the dead, it is often our own voices that we hear.[7]

Pardes was discussing biblical criticism, but I am asking the text for more. I suggest that her work could serve as a road map that delineates the terrain that is contested, places of tension and paradox within the text, and what is both said and unsaid in the text as the key geography of the use of the text in ethical reflection. I raise both the question of how aggadah or story can serve as source for new understandings of halakhah and the question of how sources newly understood as portraying a feminist voice can be used within the ethical tradition. Finally, I assert that without this critical voice, the use of halakhah as guidance in public policy is still incomplete. The tension between the ancient voice, heard with clarity and respect, and the demands of the society in desperate need of moral direction forms the crucible reforging the language called for in ethical debate.

But the specific search for the female voice in moral reflection is only the first reason to seek further texts. In looking carefully at other justice texts, I found that in some way each text was unsatisfactory. Each addressed only one part of the problem of allocation, and none offered direct explanations or direct solutions. Each left me with some disquiet: Can ownership really account for the right of survival, as in the text of two travelers and one flask in the desert? Can a community rank human value based on power, status, or gender, as in the texts that address the redemption of captives? Many of the classic texts on distributive justice are derived from extreme situations: war, hostage crisis, siege, or the Shoah itself. What is missing in the halakhic debate is not simply a non-hierarchical ranking system, but more about the fullness of what makes a society function as it addresses the daily struggles of justice. Hence another reason to seek alternate texts emerges.

The texts of the pursuit of the *rodef* also seem impartial, as do the siege texts. In critical ways illness is both like and unlike a brigand band, and the *rodef* that seeks out a victim is like and unlike death itself. The methodology of casuistry requires attention to what is morally relevant about the case situation. Illness and accident are not caused by human evil, and death cannot be bargained with or outwitted.[8] The *rodef* texts are fundamentally about the uses of power. Illness and death require an understanding of the essentially uncontrollable, uncertain nature of the world. Further, is the provision of health care services morally distinctive from the more general "giving of assistance"? Are cases and metaphors of war the most useful in the adjudication of healing? The texts about the Holocaust, remarkable in their power, raise the question of the difference between emergency and normative status. Gerald Winslow, in *Triage and Justice*, made the point that societies cannot function always in crisis; they must have rules that apply in extraordinary situations that would not necessarily apply in daily life. The text about the requirements of a just city are closest to this model, but in this text the actual roles and status of the categories of the persons needed and the contours of city life are quite altered by the modern world, and this understanding must temper the use of such texts.[9] Each text cited gives us a measure of an answer, but ultimately none is completely satisfying.

This leads to the third reason to seek other texts. The halakhic debate lacks a complete perspective on how a society functions as it addresses the problems that confront it in the health care and public policy setting. "Friendship also seems to hold states together."[10] In the *Nicomachean Ethics* Aristotle has a chapter on friendship, an oddity in a book about the ethical relations needed within the polis. A central topic in the discourse of civic structure, however, is civic friendship.

Walzer, Bellah, and West reference the importance of civic friendship and the centrality of relationships among the citizens as solidifying the state itself. What the Aristotelian formulation suggests is the understanding that the political is at its heart personal. All of this leads us to the necessity of reflecting on how intimacy, Levinas's face-to-face encounter with the other, is central in the world of social discourse and public policy.

Looking for another text that would act as a template for ethical reflection on the issue of justice, I sought a biblical text that would place women at the center of the story. I wanted to find language that was rooted not in the marketplace or in war; hence, what would be at issue in interpretation would be relationality and the problem of commitment. Further, I needed to find a text that came to terms with the issue of scarcity and sociability. I wanted a language in which what was at stake was the vision of the community life as a whole, a language that took seriously the reality of human finitude and human limitation in the context of the possibility of prophetic call.

Finally, I wanted to analyze the text closely, listening to the words and the sense of the story. It will not "solve" the problem of justice. Like the texts examined in the last chapter, it will push us toward a view that is newly possible if attention is paid to the particulars. Like the other texts, it will be subject to the argument of commentary.

Finding scarcity in the textual world of the ancient Near East was no problem. The history of the community of Hebrew people is marked by two major famines that shaped the Genesis story and acted as mirrors for each other in the Torah. These famines of the patriarchal story were recalled by all other accounts of famine in the biblical text. In a larger and more telling way, however, the entire biblical text is enclosed in a drama of scarcity, more specifically, in a tension between scarcity and blessing. The expulsion from the Garden is a banishment from the last moment of human abundance to a world of work.

The first famine, the famine of Abraham, sends the newly chosen Abram and Sarai to Egypt out of the land that is promised: "There was a famine in the land, and Abram went down to Egypt to sojourn there, for the famine was severe in the land" (Gen. 12:10).[11] The next is the great famine of Joseph and his brothers.

The famine, however, spread over the whole world. So all the world came to Joseph in Egypt to procure rations, for the famine had become severe throughout the world.

When Jacob saw that there were food rations to be had in Egypt, he said to his sons, "Why do you keep looking at one another?" "Now I hear," he went on, "that there are rations to be had in Egypt. Go and procure rations for us there that we may live and not die" (Gen. 42:1).[12]

I chose to examine the Book of Ruth because although the famine in the Book of Ruth is an echo of these earlier famines, it is *intertextual* because it evokes famine linked with covenant and generativity. All three famines have the same elements: all are desperate moments of scarcity, all mention leaving the land, and all pose the choice to stand with the community or to abandon it. I argue that justice needs to work in the face of that choice.

The Book of Ruth's mirrored famines and their associated behaviors are considered extensively in rabbinic commentary of the midrash. What marks this aggadah, like all rabbinic texts, is the assumption that normative daily rules of action ought to be required despite crisis. It is the commanded acts of justice, *tzedakah*, that ought to guide the behavior of the moral agents in the world of the text. Hence, this text addresses the tension between the extraordinary crisis and the normative problem of just allocation as a fact of daily life. It is the logical consequence of living in the human world of the finite, and I know that justice also required this discourse of ordinary life.

I began this research, frankly, with no definitive defense about my use of the Ruth text as another source for the language of justice. I had an intuition about the "fitness" of the narrative and an attachment to the story—hardly defensible hermeneutics.[13] I was looking for a text that addressed justice issues and a text that was widely familiar to both Jews and Christians, something with the cultural resonance of the Good Samaritan story. Research for the proof text of the Talmudic argumentation between Rabbi Akiba and Ben Petura in the pivotal text of the two travelers in the desert with one flask of water led me back to Ruth via Leviticus 25:35. This link to the Bava Metzia text occurs because the problem of how one lives with one's neighbor, the issue of distributive justice, and the tension between the marketplace economy, human desperation, and compassion are the organizing issues behind the call for the Jubilee in Leviticus. But the text asks, short of the Jubilee what can we do? How does one live on the road, in the interim generation, in the meantime? The text of Ruth is one answer to this question, and the Bava Metzia text is another. The relationship between the two is complex. Ruth predates the text of the Mishnah by perhaps 400 years.[14] Of course, Rabbi Akiba and Ben Petura knew the story of the women who traveled on the road alone in famine and scarcity greeted by kin who knew the laws of redemption. And, of course, the literate reader of the Talmudic debate ought to know the story too: the very words "two travelers on the road" evoke the Ruth text. It is my contention that the story around the story—the reference back to the Jubilee as the prophetic answer to the problem of distributive justice—and the details of the halakhah as the practical answer to the same problem link the two texts. I contend also that this story is meant by the author of the text to be held in tension with the other narratives, and that this tension is part of the methodology of temporal simultaneity of the system itself.

·

The Marginal as Central

In the Book of Ruth, the centerpiece event is a (rare) inside look at an intimate relationship between women. In contrast to some of the problematic female interior relationships in the Torah (e.g., Sarah and Hagar, Rachel and Leah) where women compete for the scarce prize of a relationship with a man, the decisive ethical gesture in Ruth actually has little to do with a male figure. It speaks instead of a responsibility to a larger community. In fact, as Pardes noted, the only men mentioned in the first chapter are dead.[15]

Judith Plaskow's critique of the Torah is telling: in most stories the women stand outside, in the peripheral vision of the teller. In the Book of Ruth, the story of women is central, and Elimelech, Mahlon, Chilion, and even Boaz are either dead or nearly silent to the central passion of the story about women's loyalty to each other outside the safety of a relationship to a man. The details, the verbal action of the story, is women's work of the time. It is this work—eating, gleaning, producing, homemaking, and nursing babies, and not war making, sacrificing, marching, or destroying—that is honored.

Two women travel alone in the desert, shawls in the wind, thirsty, mourning, and walking in silence to Bethlehem. The city of bread is "all astir" when they enter. The women are at the point of utter despair, having nothing; they are without men, without children, without land, and without community. Yet their coming is a public event, not simply some private tragedy, which will be taken into account by the public community and for which the community will bear responsibility.

Ruth's ethical gesture, which makes all that follows possible, is to embrace the angry old woman not out of love or compassion—it is certainly not that simple— but out of a sense of recognition that she and Naomi are fundamentally bound. In Levinas's language, Ruth recognizes the self in the other and, as such, recognizes her responsibility not to turn from the vulnerable face of her former mother-in-law. She is not compelled to stay; the death of her husband has unbound her as it has unbound Orpah. And yet Ruth sees herself *as* Naomi, as paired as surely as Adam and Eve were paired, a coupling of similar selves in the darkness of the world.

The halakhic details that follow the facts of harvest and widowhood, and the exchanges of commodity for commodity, are recognized by the larger community as Ruth's choice, the Rutharian alternative of relation over self-actualization, the recognition that self-becoming is not possible in isolation from obligation. My life, says this Rutharian gesture, cannot continue with you, other, lost in the darkness of the desert of Moab. The rain would not fall and the grain would not grow if it were so. It is proven by our text, by the bursting fecundity of the barley harvest and by the fecundity of the widow Ruth in the next year.

The language of the story is critical. It is about going from isolation—no family and no community—to a specific place, to a specific listening to the voice of the most vulnerable, in the context of an actual relationship. The ritual act of the release of obligation (the shoe ritual) is making the connections public (face-to-face).

After the birth of her son, who is linked to the future and to the largest vision of community, Ruth maintains the strongest possible relationship to Naomi: she gives her the child. Naomi thus becomes parent in relationship to the child via the female rather than through the male kinship bonds. These female bonds are spiritual rather than hereditary.

In other words, the Rutharian choice is to understand that one's personal story is part of the collective story of movement of a people in history. It is also a choice at every moment about gesture as intimate, as fragile, and as ordinary as a child passed between women. It is a prophetic act that suggests, "Look, the world can be like this." But it is a prophetic act wrapped in the context of the daily, difficult world—as if to say, "The prophetic act is obtainable, it can be yours."

That is the outline of the story. Embedded within it are seven moments/scenes on which I will focus. It is by a close examination of these moments, the lacunae in the text, the narrative, the commentary, and the language itself that an ethical challenge can be most clearly drawn.

1. *To leave the community at a time of scarcity/danger is wrong.*
There is no personal escape from collective scarcity.

> And it came to pass
> in the days of the judging of the judges,
> that there was a famine in the land.
> And a certain man of Bethlehem in Judah went
>   to sojourn
> in the field of Moab,
> he, and his wife, and his two sons.
> And the name of the man was Elimelech,
> and the name of his wife was Naomi,
> and the name of his two sons Mahlon and Kilyon,
> Ephratites of Bethlehem in Judah.
> And they came
> into the field of Moab
> and remained there. (Ruth 1:1–3)

The text begins oddly, in paradox. It will be a text about justice. Plain words tell the reader where to place the text historically, in a time prior to kingship rule of the Jewish people. What is the justice of the judges, however? The midrash and commentary say that it was chaotic, capricious, and the opposite of justice. "The judging of the judges" is taken to refer to the era of lawlessness, when the judges ought to have been judged themselves. The following rabbinic midrash makes this point: "*And it came to pass, in the days of the judging of the judges.* Woe unto that generation which judges its judges, and woe unto that generation whose judges are in need of being judged! As it is said, *And yet they harkened not to their judges* (Judges II, 17)."[16] This is wordplay in Hebrew as well as in English. The eighteenth-century Yiddish language commentary on the biblical text, the *Tz'enah Ur'enah,*[17] explains this midrash further:

> The verse lets us know two things. The episode of Ruth and Boaz took place at a time when there was not yet a king over Israel, only judges who led Israel. The verse says *shfot hashoftim* (lit., "the judgement of the judges"), which can be interpreted to mean that the judges themselves were judged. The judges were wicked, and they, too, needed to be judged and rebuked. Or, it may mean that the people were very wicked, and did not want to heed the judges. When a judge found them guilty they would mock him and say: "You punish us? Punish yourself." The word *vayehi* ("it was" [in the days] . . .) hints that Israel shouted *(Oi) Vay*! ("woe"). They had many troubles, because they did not want to heed the judges.[18]

The troubles were not only physical, linked to the scarcity, but spiritual as well. This was apparent because famines were understood to be linked to God's own judgment of the failings of a people,[19] and because of the historical moment described in the text. As Jack Sasson argues: "Time is at once specific and diffuse ('When the Judges used to judge'), conveying more than the actual words imply, since during that period—as any Hebrew would know—people were constantly losing God's grace before earning it again."[20] It is in this generalized chaos that the famine occurred, in a society so driven by individual greed,[21] say the rabbis, that it was unable even to regulate the systems of agriculture or to forestall ecological havoc.[22]

From this disaster the leadership flees, abandoning the community. In the *Midrash Rabbah*, the compilation of the midrashim that surround the scriptural texts, the rabbinic commentary is extensive on this spare verse. Why does such disaster fall upon this family? Who is this Elimelech? The rabbinic response is that he must have been a man of substance, who abandoned Bethlehem at the first sign of trouble. Note how the following selected midrashim (there are two chapters of midrashim in *Midrash Rabbah* on this first paragraph of the story) uses the verse in Psalms to locate the text morally and explains the meaning of the tragedy that is to come. Concerning Elimelech, the commentary reads,

> "*And the name of the man was Elimelech*" (1, 20). Because trouble has came to thee, thou hast forsaken them? "*And a certain man of Bethlehem in Judah went*" (1, 1). That is the meaning of the verse "*Whose leaders are borne with. There is no breach and no going forth*" *(Ps. CXLIV, 14).*

> R. Johanan said: It is not written "who bear," but "*who are borne.*" When the young bear with the old, *there is no breach*, i.e., there is no breaking out of the plague, as it is said, "*And no going forth . . .*"

> R. Lakish transposes the verse (as though it read "Our leaders bear"). When the great bear with the small "*there is no breach of exile*", as it is written, "*And ye shall go out at the breaches*" *(Amos IV, 3)* "and there is no going forth into exile," as it is written, "*Cast them out of My sight and let them go forth*" (Jer. XV) . . .

> R. Lulianus said: When the small hearken to the great, but the great do not bear the burden of the small upon them, then the verse applies, "*And the Lord shall enter into Judgment*" (Isa. III, 14).

> *And the name of the man was Elimelech.* When trouble came, thou hast departed and left them. [This is the meaning of the verse] "*And a certain man of Bethlehem in Judah went.*"[23]

What troubles the rabbis that comment in these midrashim is how a man of substance and position, a man capable of undertaking a significant journey in the midst of a cataclysmic famine, could have so thoroughly misunderstood the meaning of his obligation. Note how the psalm used as a proof text is a text about the mutuality of dependency between leaders and people. What causes the disruption of the social fabric of the exilic community, the disaster and the plague? ask the rabbis. Is it the refusal of the people to "bear with" the elders, the small to listen to the great? asked R. Johanan. No, the contrary is true, responds R. Lakish, it is when the great do not bear with the small. R. Lulianus concurs: It is when the most vulnerable depend on the leadership and the leadership flee from this obligation that the judgment of Isaiah 3:14 applies: "The Lord will bring this charge against the elders and officers of His people: 'It is you who ravaged the vineyard; That which was robbed from the poor is in your houses, How dare you crush my people, and grind the faces of the poor (in the dust)?' " The verse from Isaiah links the cause of desperation and poverty to the exploitation of the poor by the ruling class. Famine is a direct result of this sort of social plunder. The midrash connects the Ruth text, by means of the multiple layering of text, to this judgment. Another midrash continues the theme of the rabbinic condemnation of leadership that protects itself by denying essential obligation:

> And a certain man . . . went. Like a mere stump! See how the Holy One, blessed be he, favors the entry into Eretz Israel over the departure therefrom! In the former case it is written, Their horses . . . their mules . . . their camels, etc. (Ezra II, 66) but in this case it is written, and a certain man went like a mere stump. The reason is that in the latter case, since they were leaving the country for another land, Scripture makes no mention of their property, [but states simply] And a certain man went—as though empty handed.[24]

This midrash is sensitive to the judgment of the text. Since the verse does not speak of Elimelech taking anything with him, the plain meaning is that he left Israel and went to Moab empty handed, "like a mere stump." The midrash contrasts this to the return of the Hebrew people as they enter the land from their exile in Babylon. Here "the sum of the entire community was 42,360 . . . ," and they not only travel as a community, they travel heavily laden, with each horse, mule, camel, and household object elaborately inventoried (Ezra 1:9–11, 2:64–66).

Cynthia Ozick, commenting on this verse, was even harsher. She, too, filled in the text with an interpretation that is supported by the midrashic material.

> Elimelech turns his back on the destitute conditions of hungry Bethlehem, picks up his family, and because he is rich enough to afford the journey, sets out for where the food is. He looks to his own skin and means to grab his own grub. . . . This is the Rabbis' view. They are symbolists and metaphor seekers; it goes without saying that they are moralists. Punishment is truthful; punishment is the consequence of reality, it instructs in what happens. . . . The man who throws away the country of aspiration, especially in a lamentable hour when failure overruns it—the man who promotes egotism, elevates the material, and deprives his children of idealism—this fellow, this Elimelech, vexes the rabbis and afflicts them with shame. Of course there is not a grain of any of this in the text itself—not a word about Elimelech's character or motives or even his position in Bethlehem.[25]

The text may be silent on motive, but the names of Elimelech and Naomi's sons translate as "sickness" (Mahlon) and "vanishing" (Kilyon), hardly neutral signifiers. Further, the land they depart for is the land of Moab, which is associated with idol worship and licentiousness, and whose people are enemies of the Israelites and with whom marriages are prohibited. In fact, the midrash supposes that the text says the family lived in the fields because the cities of Moab were too sordid even for these exiles.

The text that will address the responsibility for the other begins with the negative example. Elimelech is the prudent libertarian. He uses what means he has to craft an individual solution. One does not need to position him as a leader or even as a man of extraordinary duty to suggest that the text sees his flight as problematic. A crisis emerges. The individual chooses his individual solution, leaves the land and the community, and disaster strikes. Rather than turn his face to the face of the other, he turns away and heads in the opposite direction. Like Jonah, off to Tarshish, his flight is to no avail.

> 2. To resume responsibility, even if one
> is powerless, is the just course for every citizen.

> Elimelech, Naomi's husband died,
> and she was left,
> and her sons.
> And they took to them wives
> of the women of Moab. (Ruth 1:3–4)

Where is Naomi in the moral moment of the first chapter of Ruth? She is without voice and without name, anonymous in Judah until the flight to Moab is begun.[26] Yet she does not protest; she goes without question to the disaster ahead.

> Until Elimelech's death, Naomi has been an exemplum of the normal. She has followed her husband and made no decisions or choices of her own. What we nowadays call feminism is, of course, as old as the oldest society imaginable; there have always been feminists: women (including the unsung) who will allow no element of themselves—gift, capacity, natural authority—to go unexpressed, whatever the weight of the mores. Naomi has not been one of these. Until the death of her husband, we know nothing of her but her compliance, and it would be foolish to suppose that in Naomi's world a wife's obedience is not a fundamental social virtue.[27]

Even after Elimelech dies, Naomi does not suggest a return to the land, nor does she speak a word in the story when first one, then another of her sons marries the prohibited Moabite strangers. She lives in the silence of the text for ten years, and it is only when her sons die that she finds language and, with it, both moral imperative and action in the center stage of the public arena.[28]

> Then she arose with her daughters-in-law,
> that she might return

> from the field of Moab;
> for she had heard
> in the field of Moab
> how that the Lord had remembered His people
> in giving them bread. (Ruth 1:6)

She arose because she remembered that God's remembering has a meaning for her. It is the first time in the narrative that God is mentioned. The text, despite the midrashic embellishments attributing great wealth to Elimelech, now portrays Naomi as the ultimate widow. Stripped of all social standing and surrounded by death, she is not only without land, but without support. There is no mention of any community that either surrounds her or takes account of her worth or responsibility for her plight. There is mention only of the daughters-in-law. There is also no social provision made for her destitution. A pagan land, a place of stark individualism, offers no social welfare for the needy. In the Moabite culture, the only option for widows is to return to the family of origin.[29] The act of return is not only the righting of an old wrong;[30] it is an echo of earlier biblical decisions: of Abraham, Jacob, and the Israelite people themselves back from depravation, enslavement, and the pagan world of exile. The return to the world of justice begins with the recognition that each person is responsible for the commitment to community. It does not matter how poor or how disempowered one's gender is; each person is a subject, not an object, of another's gaze. The textual language makes this point clearly: Naomi, the anonymous speechless one, the generic widow of the mitzvot, the other that one is to account for, moves to the center stage and sets the opening for all dialogue that is to occur in the text.

Note that Naomi's language is theological; it is a prayer.

> Go return each of you to her mother's house;[31]
> the Lord deal kindly with you,
> as you have dealt with the dead and with me.
> The Lord grant you that you may find rest,
> each of you
> in the house of her husband. (Ruth 1:8–9)

In Levinas's terms, the gaze between the self and the other is a mutual one requiring a recognition (a remembering) that the other is also a self. It is Naomi's radical claim of self that makes possible Ruth's response to her. Naomi's journey is taken in isolation. She assumes that she will be traveling alone. The midrash compares her to the "remnants of the remnants" (of a meal offering: waste, scraps, and ashes).[32] Yet, as empty as she is, she is complete, certain of where she is headed. She is not begging. She is with God, with the movement of history. "One of Levinas's most creative contributions is to call attention to the asymmetry of the interpersonal relations that marks the commencement of moral consciousness. The person I meet in a moral mode is both higher and lower than I am: higher in the sense that she summons me to conscience and judges the arbitrariness of my freedom; lower in the sense that she approaches me not with power to coerce, but in destitution and supplication, offering no resistance other than a moral one."[33]

3. To have a face-to-face encounter makes
generations and redemption possible. It is the encounter
with the face of the other that makes possible the ethical choice.

> Then she kissed them;
> and they lifted up their voice and wept.
> And they said to her:
> "No, but we will return with you to your people."
> And Naomi said: "Turn back, my daughters;
> why will you go with me?
> Have I yet sons in my womb, that they may be
> your husbands?
> Turn back, my daughters, go your way;
> for I am too old to have a husband.
> If I should say: I have hope,
> should I even have a husband tonight,
> and also bear sons; would you wait for them
> until they were grown?
> Would you shut yourselves off for them and
> have no husbands?
> No, my daughters;
> for it grieves me much more for your sakes,
> for the hand of the Lord is gone forth against me."
> And they lifted up their voice, and wept again;
> and Orpah kissed her mother-in-law;
> but Ruth cleaved unto her. (Ruth 1:9–14)

Naomi describes the reality of their situation. They are not actually kin; they are free to go home.[34] Naomi is clear about the limits of their responsibilities; they are to go home to their families. She cannot physically be connected to them because her use value, in a social sense, is now ended. What makes a woman valuable? It is her husband, her ability to bear children, and her ability to organize a household. All features that define personhood and role, all her rights, are gone. Even, as Naomi fantasizes briefly, were she able to start again, bearing sons, with her body restored, it would be of no use. For the work that her daughters-in-law must give their bodies to is immediate. If they are to have identity and value, they must marry quickly and bear children of their own. To wait for Naomi's new sons would be to wait beyond the uses of their bodies, both sexual and procreative.

Orpah sees the tragedy in this. Her response is to weep, to grieve, and to add not a word to the discourse. Interestingly, most translations add the words "and she left" to Orpah's reaction. But it is not in the text.

Cynthia Ozick described this moment clearly.[35] Orpah is a loving and faithful daughter-in-law. She has already done much. She married outside convention, lived for ten years in childlessness, and held fast against death and death and death. She does not abandon her chosen family, but she "goes nowhere." In staying home in Moab, she falls out of our text and, thus, out of the ethical moment itself. She performs the normal and generous act, and it is not enough. Naomi is offering a repeat of Elimelech's original choice: Here there is nothing; abandon loyalty and go your way into the singularity of your own life.

Orpah is like most of us most of the time. Radical monotheism and all that it implies is an enormous concept. What Naomi is really asking is easy to turn from and deny in the dailiness of existence. Orpah is faithful within the rules we live by—family, birth, and death. Orpah is sympathetic, alive to the pain of homeless-ness, poverty, and desperation, and she has cared for Naomi within the limits of the law and the boundaries of her rights.[36]

More is being asked. The text is subtle here, issuing a call covertly and without comment. It is a cloaked call; but Ruth hears clearly, and the call evokes the extraordinary language of Ruth's reply. The narrator calls the women daughters-in-law (*khaloteha*). But Naomi repeatedly calls them her daughters (*b'notai*) in her actual speech. In the Hebrew text, she is both pushing them away and binding them at the same time. Orpah is "gone" because she is not present to Naomi's real, embodied situation or to her actual ethical call. Ruth hears differently. It is this tension in the language, to the opening of the discourse, to which Ruth responds. Ruth hears the prayer behind the speaking and understands the magni-tude of the spiritual choice embedded in the social decision. To hear in this way is to hear ethically. It is to understand the language behind the language.

But Ruth cleaved to her.

> And she said:
> "Behold, your sister-in-law is gone
> back to her people and unto her god;
> return after your sister-in-law." (Ruth 1:15)

Ruth cleaves (*dbq*) to Naomi. This is the same word used to describe the coming together, both the physical and the spiritual clinging, in Genesis (2:24) of Adam and Eve.

The Book of Ruth is the only Biblical text in which the word "love" is used to define a relationship between two women. And once such love is represented, an intriguing rewriting of Genesis takes place. From the very beginning of the Book of Ruth, "clinging" between women determines the movement of the plot. Rejecting the option of returning to Moab to seek a new husband, Ruth chooses to "cling" to her mother-in-law. The verb *dbq* first appears in Genesis in the etiological comment which follows the depiction of a woman's creation out of Adam's body. "Therefore shall a man leave his father and mother, and shall cleave (*dbq*) unto his wife: and they shall be as one flesh." "To cling" in this case means to recapture a primal unity, to return to a time when men and women were literally "one flesh." . . . "To leave one's mother and father" is the recurrent phrase that links the two texts. Yet while in Genesis such leaving and cleaving defines the institution of marriage, in the Book of Ruth it depicts female bonding, a hitherto unrecognized tie.[37]

Cleaving represents the radical encounter with the face of the other. Far beyond civic friendship, it is the "going with" that Naomi is actually demanding by the mere presence of her tangible human face.

In Levinas's terms, it is the very vulnerability and actuality of the face of the other that commands us. It is the skin of the face that stays the most naked, the most upright, and without defense.

There is first the very uprightness of the face, its upright exposure, without defense. The skin of the face is that which stays the most naked, most destitute. It is the most naked, though with a decent nudity. It is the most destitute also: there is an essential poverty in the face; the proof of this is that one tries to mask the poverty by putting on poses, by taking on a countenance. The face is exposed, menaced, as if inviting us to an act of violence. At the same time, the face is what forbids us to kill. The face is signification and signification without context. I mean the Other, in the rectitude of his face, is not a character within a context. . . . Here, to the contrary, the face is meaning all by itself.[38]

Ruth comes to understand that she is whoever she may be, but she is also the "first person," the one who must find the resources to respond to the utter need of the face of Naomi. This ethical premise is the precursor to what Pardes described as the theme of female bonding in the text. What makes the bond possible and, hence, moral and meaningful is that Ruth has recognized Naomi as a self, has taken on the responsibility of the entire capacity of her being, and in that moment truly has been able to be a Self in the text. It is only after this recognition, or by way of this recognition, that Ruth finds her voice in the text. Levinas posited that full confirmation of self emerges only in radical transcendence of all of our concern for self, including rights. The moral encounter involves a decentering of being, an opening up to plurality and, indeed, to the infinity of possibility in the presence of the other.[39]

This encounter is the responsibility of the subject; the mutuality of response is not the concern of the self. Naomi, in fact, does not respond. The text has Ruth and Naomi continue afterward in silence, calling attention to this silence between them. Naomi will not respond for several more verses. When she acknowledges her responsibility toward Ruth, she takes an extraordinarily active role in the plot, advising Ruth what to wear, how to anoint herself, and what to say to seduce her protector. But this moment will come later, and it is the healing embedded in the text that allows that doubling of the moral encounter to occur. At this juncture, it is a moment of pure remembering on the part of Ruth.

> The readiness to learn from the other, to be a disciple, is thus a crucial moment in the ethical relation to the other. It is the moment by means of which the moral imperative gains its material content. Levinas sums up his analysis by saying that justice is prior to truth, or better, justice is the essential precondition for gaining the truth. In the commencement of moral experience the other is not only higher than I. He is also in important respects lower, the destitute one who entreats me to have regard for his condition. In this dimension the prototype for the other is the widow, the orphan, the poor, the stranger at the gate. . . . In this modality the other is manifest as the one who is in no position to bargain or negotiate fair exchange, as one who has no power to coerce me to give him his due.[40]

What is critical about this text is that both Ruth and Naomi are destitute. Ruth has nothing to give but the infinity of self—infinite responsibility. She recognizes the inalienable responsibility of subject: No one can substitute for self in this responsibility toward the other. Even while the reader is at all times aware of Ruth's destitution, her widowhood, her orphanhood, her poverty, and her estrangement, we can see her acting as subject. While the hearer of the text is aware that none can be more the stranger than this Ruth, at the moment that Naomi is telling Ruth to go home to her own, the Ruth in the text is at that moment beginning the moral recognition that makes her human, voiced, a free moral agent, and a commanded Jew. The rabbis, in clear recognition of this nuanced interplay in the text, explain midrashically that Ruth's conversion occurs at that instant, on the spot, and on the road.[41]

> And Ruth said:
> "Entreat me not to leave you

and to return from following after you;
for where you go, I will go
And where you lodge, I will lodge;
your people will be my people,
and your God my God;
where you die, will I die,
and there will I be buried;
the Lord do so to me, and more also,
    if anything but death
part you and me."
And when she saw that she was steadfastly
    minded
to go with her,
she left off speaking unto her.
So they two went until they came
    to Bethlehem. (Ruth 1:16–19)

The two walk out of exile, wilderness, and hunger, out of the starkness and silence of the road, through the desert and into the City of Bread, to the Promised Land, into the yellow, ripening, and abundant harvest. In the year of the story in the text, it is just after Pesach.

As Levinas asserted, at issue is the death of the other. The nakedness of the face and the totality of the command always underlie the simple presentation of the mortality of the other. The embodied other confronts the embodied self with the reality of their shared mortality and vulnerability. It is the human fragile body that demands the not-killing, demands that the actions of the self not involve the death of the other. Ruth cannot be indifferent to this demand once she has gone beyond Orpah's choice, the legal gesture, and into the ethical moment of her own choice.

Ruth asserts in this language that the face of the other is her responsibility and, moreover, that the body of the other is in some way *her* body. It is this theme of doubling of self that Pardes recognized and that Levinas would claim *is* the ethical itself. In this verse, Ruth claims that it will be so. In the truth of the later text ("ethics is prior to truth") Naomi will share the fate, first, of Ruth's body via the pre-telling and elaborate planning of the seduction scene on the threshing-room floor. Second, she will share Ruth's fecundity ("to Naomi a child is born" is the cry of the village chorus of women). And, last, she will suckle Ruth's child, utterly merging the most intimate tasks of the body itself with Ruth.[42]

Pardes noted another way that the text itself is a comment on the theme of shared fertility in the intertextuality between this story and the story of Rachel and Leah.[43] Pardes's point was that the parallels between the two stories are intentional. The Ruth story, with its themes of barrenness and uprootedness (they are the same word in Hebrew, *aqara*), bitterness, harvest and sexual seduction, exile and return to the land, acts as both a mirror and a reconciled version of female competition for the matriarchal position in the history of Judaism. As Rachel and Leah, the younger and the older women, come to "share" Jacob, Ruth and Naomi come to "share" Boaz, albeit with a noncompetitive and loving relationality.

All of this intimacy, all of the language of the intense embodiment (the double embodiment) of pregnancy, is heightened by the extraordinary extremity of Ruth's position as the quintessential stranger. Ruth is more than estranged by Naomi's statement delivering her back into Moab. She is textually unbound from the moment of her entrance into the text. She is a Moabite. In the intertextual world of the tradition, she signifies the enemy, the pagan, and the forbidden sexual liaison. In Numbers, Balak, the king of Moab, recruits Bil'am, his own wizard and prophet, to curse the Israelites and so diminish them. The text assumes the power of the word to create social policy. But Bil'am the Moabite cannot curse. His speech is taken from him, and the animal he rides becomes empowered with speech and, by extension, with rational will. Bil'am is filled only with the word of God. He cannot hurl curses; he must hurl only blessings at the Hebrews. The intent of Moab is to destroy, to attack the hungry, homeless Israelites on the road back to the land. The way of arms, the way of speech, and finally the way of seduction are used to defeat the Israelites on their journey. It is the seduction of the Hebrew men by the Moabite women that, finally, nearly undermines the entire enterprise of return.[44]

Ruth offers a retelling of the encounter with the Moabites. In a private way, the Jew and the Moabite (the Moabite again speaking in the prophet's voice) meet again on the road back to the land. However, this time the exiled one will be helped; this time the pagan will come to see the holy in the other. This private act must take place before the public acts to follow. Once it is completed, they can be on their way to Bethlehem, where they will encounter the public chorus.

Since the text echoes with the depth, both in history and culture, of the stranger, it prompts us to hear the call of the stranger with greater attention. If this moral encounter can be had with a stranger, an enemy, then it must be available to all.

4. To count on social order for a decent basic minimum is a given.

The return to Bethlehem of the textual couple begins the emergence of the problem of scarcity and the allocation of resources not only as a private moral question, but also as a public act. Here the text asks, Can the private commitment of the face-to-face encounter have meaning in the wider world of social policy amidst a city of faces?

Bethlehem, the city of bread, is now the literal symbol of abundance (far removed from the empty Bethlehem of chapter 1). It is the moral order of this commanded community that will provide the concrete, redemptive scaffolding for the poor. The problem of allocation now shifts: How can the resource at hand be justly allocated?

A city will provide moral order. A chorus greets Naomi, who publicly proclaims her need. It is notable that Ruth speaks not a word here, and no one comments specifically on her presence. Despite the eloquence of her gesture of recognition, neither Naomi nor the text acknowledges it.

As soon as they establish need, however, Naomi, seemingly newly energized by her role in the community and by her public naming, sets about the task of justice. She knows she is owed a basic, decent minimum; she understands and remembers the rules of agriculture that provide for *tzedakah*. In essence, the mitzvah of *tzedakah* is to allow to the poor all that is lost through error, all that is left behind, all that is lost by the human design of the harvest itself, and all that is grown in the corners of the field. It is a direct gift from God, from whom all is being given on this land, to the poor, who do not own the means of production. It is, as it were, God's righting of the inequality that exists in human and, hence, limited societies that is enabled through the hand of the reapers. It is not charity; it is the part of the harvest that actually belongs to the poor by right and obligation. If properly given and not expropriated by the landowners, it is enough to feed all widows and orphans, not lavishly but sufficiently.

The basic, decent minimum is reparations. It acknowledges that not all are equal, that some are weaker, others stronger. What is given is given out of responsibility for this difference.

The texts assure that all know of the laws. All citizens are part of the system of justice in the way that the Talmudic text (Sanhedrin 17B) assumes all inhabitants are part of the judging court. Ruth and Naomi will not starve. Further, the private choices made by each participant will be part of the public acts of recovery of the vulnerable. Ruth's gesture toward Naomi will become part of the public discourse, the language that defines the narrative of this problem. Boaz sees Ruth; like the village women, who respond to Naomi's call to name her Mara, he names her too, calling her *bitti* (my daughter) and acknowledging her history. She is known by her deeds in the community. Her name, her daughterliness, is acknowledgment of this chosen role.

> Then said Boaz to his servant that was set over
>   the reapers,
> "Whose young woman is this?"
> And the servant that was set over the reapers
> answered and said
> "It is a Moabite woman

that came back with Naomi
out of the field of Moab;"
and she said:
"Let me glean, I pray you. . . ."
Then said Boaz to Ruth:
"Hearest you not, my daughter?" (Ruth 2:5–8)

5. *Intimacy/family is seen as an obligation beyond justice and the law.*

The measure of this redemption is far beyond the dictates of the law. Boaz demonstrates his supererogatory actions by allowing Ruth not only to glean in his field as
a stranger with entitlement, but to eat at his table as a member of his household.

And Boaz said unto her at mealtime:
"Come here, and eat
of the bread, and dip your piece in
    the vinegar."
And she sat beside the reapers;
and they passed her the parched corn,
and she did eat
and was satisfied
and left. (Ruth 2:14)

It is this act of sitting at the table, the acknowledgment of kinship, that allows
all that is to follow. The language that responds to Ruth's call in the wilderness to
be kin to Naomi is linked to this, the first meal in the text after the accounts of
famine, hunger, and loss.

Ruth actually wants permission to gather the grain from among the
sheaves, a privilege (we learn from 2:15) reserved for members of the clan,
which only a landowner can grant. Boaz notices the woman as she stands
waiting for his reply. . . . Boaz asks no question from this underprivileged
soul but readily offers advice: stay in my field, stick to my girls; even drink
a little water if you care to. However, he does not respond to her original
request. Ruth is not ready to give up. With a gesture of exaggerated
servility—usually only kings and gods receive such prostrations—Ruth
gently cloaks her expectations: "Why is it that I pleased you enough to
notice me? I am but a foreigner (*nokhriyah*)" (2:10). Boaz responds with
another speech but is now more personal: you are wonderfully loyal and
brave; God will surely reward you for seeking his protection. . . . Finally
grasping Ruth's intent, Boaz waits until lunchtime to make up his mind.
Then, in full view of his workers (an act which may have a legal

implication), he seats her among them, personally fills her bowl with grain and mash, and gives her the permission he has not granted previously.[45]

Boaz will give Ruth not only what is her basic decent minimum, the gleaning from his harvest, but he will reach into his own portion and give from this as well.

> Let her glean even among the sheaves
> and put her not to shame.
> And also pull out for her some of purpose
> from the bundles, and leave it,
> and let her glean,
> and rebuke her not. (Ruth 2:15–16)

This is beyond the basic requirement of the halakhic system. His acceptance of Ruth, the stranger, as family offers a model of justice language similar to what the text makes plain in Ruth's speech. In fact, Boaz's action is a playing out of Ruth's pledge: "I will give fairly to you, not because I am contracted to but out of bonds of the community, out of familial love."

Further, the female relationships continue to deepen at this moment in the story. Here is the rare example in the biblical story where seduction is not a competitive struggle, but a cooperative venture. Here again, it will be the recognition of family that makes generation of the Jewish people possible. "The antithetical completion of female bonding and initiative turns out to be unexpectedly essential to the prosperity of the House of Israel."[46]

6. Trust that friendship/family will make generation/redemption possible (again) and that this action is mutually a duty and a right.

Finally, Ruth is acknowledged, and the text describes a burst of activity on Naomi's part. No further laments about her status or loss will appear in the text. From now on, she purposefully directs Ruth toward what she understands is her entitlement. The text now depicts Naomi as face-to-face with Ruth. It is a moment of reprise.

> And Naomi her mother-in-law
> said to her: My daughter
> shall I not seek rest for you,
> that it be well with you? (Ruth 3:1)

Whereas before Naomi had implored God to find rest for Ruth, here Naomi takes responsibility and moral agency for this work. It is surely not a turning away from God. Naomi does not speak in this text without reference to God lacing her syntax. Rather, it is acknowledgment or recognition of responsibility for responsibility.

At this moment, when Ruth has returned to feed Naomi, her skirt full with ripened barley (the literal image of fertility restored), Naomi pledges herself to concrete action. A new turn is taken in the text, and the story moves to conclusion in a rush of swiftly told scenes. It is when Naomi can actually return the gaze of the stranger—when she can "see" her, name her daughter, and know her as kin—that a curious thing occurs in the text. At this moment the reader first hears of a field in the possession of Naomi, an inheritance that, when sold, could certainly relieve the destitution of the women. It is as though this inheritance is somehow evoked by the recognition of the kinship, as though metaphorically the "inheritance" is, in fact, the commitment of kin to kin made tangible. Nowhere in the text up to this point is there language to suggest that Naomi has inherited anything. She is portrayed as unrelentingly bereft. Clearly, this field could have been claimed and sold much earlier, and Naomi and Ruth need not have been reduced to gleaning.

What seems to bring the physical inheritance into the language of the story is the understanding that it has real meaning, that Ruth the stranger is *bitti*. It is an odd moment when scarcity simply drops away. There is enough; the poorest have their own resources. It occurs only when all seem to trust that it is possible to redeem again land, self, and vision after tragedy (tragic error and bitterness).

The intimate, solitary encounter between Ruth and Boaz in the darkness of the threshing room at the end of a long harvest season is an encounter involving a woman who can claim her full personhood. In the language of this speech, she is no longer the stranger. She offers (quite literally) her entire self and asks for the entire self from Boaz.[47] In terms of the moral encounter, Levinas would argue, this is what is being asked at all times. These are the stakes of all recognition and relationship, and the encounter in the text is merely this enormity made tangible.

> And it came to pass at mid-night,
> that the man was shaken
> and turned
> and, behold!
> a woman lay beneath his legs.
> And he said:
> "Who are you?"
> And she answered:
> "I am Ruth, your *amah*[48]
> spread therefore your cloak
> over your *amah*
> for you are a near kinsman."[49]
>   (Ruth 3:8–10)

Ruth is asking for more than the obvious straightforward sexual encounter here. She is asking for Boaz to "spread his cloak over her." Spreading the cloak is a metaphor for the act of marriage itself, comparable to spreading the *chuppah* over the bride in the traditional Jewish wedding ceremony.[50]

7. Trust in community and the language of community to name and define the future.

Finally, the text ends with a recommitment to the health and well-being of each person as intrinsically tied to the health of the community and citizenship. After the intense, powerful, and startling intimacy of the private encounter, every-thing—every act, every gesture—in the conclusion of the story happens in the public realm. All of the acts occur in the broad daylight of the city, within the gates of the city, with the community as witness, and with community taking responsibility for the framing and naming of the final acts of justice.

> And Boaz said to the elders and to
> all the people
> You are witnesses this day,
> that I have acquired all that was Elimelech's
> and all that was Kilyon's and Mahlon's
> of the hand of Naomi. . . .
> You are witnesses this day. (Ruth 4:9–11)

> And all the people that were in the gate,
> and the elders
> said: "We are witnesses
> The Lord make the woman that is come
> into your house
> like Rachel and Leah,
> which two did build
> the house of Israel." (Ruth 4:11)

Justice is done by public acts in full view of all at the gate, but these acts are echoes of promises made in private human encounters. In both the (repeating) scenes of Ruth-Naomi and Boaz-Ruth, the private face-to-face encounter is made whole and actual by moving the text, language, and, hence, commitment to the public discourse.

Finally, the text ends with the swift conception and arrival of the child Oved, named in public by a chorus of women neighbors of the village and nursed in public. Once again, men fall out of the story. In fact, one midrash has Boaz conceiving the child on the wedding night and dying shortly thereafter to explain his curious lack of presence in the text.

Naming and nursing are the ultimate signifiers of parentage, yet the language is clear. These are public acts. The doing of justice, the restoration of Naomi, is a matter of public discourse. It is also crucial to history and foundational for the founding of the Davidic kingship.

> And Naomi took the child
> and laid him on her bosom
> and became nurse to him.
> And the women her neighbors
> gave it a name,
> saying:
> "There is a son born to Naomi";
> and they called his name Oved,
> he is the father of Jesse,
> the father of David. (Ruth 4:16–17)

•

Justice Is Prior to Freedom

The convention of the midrash is that Ruth and Naomi enter the community from their exile prior to Pesach. The barley harvest is begun; the winter is past. Ruth stays in the fields with Boaz for the full harvest, into the wheat harvest, about three months.[51] The convention continues that Ruth marries Boaz at Shavuot and immediately conceives her son, Oved (*ovd*, meaning "one who serves"), who is born about nine months later, again near Pesach.[52] The name he is given cannot help but reinvoke the image of Passover, the theme of service/freedom being a central motif of the Exodus story.

The name Oved alone might be a slender thread on which to hang this intertextual allusion if the connection and conundrum expressed by the word were not so strong, and if the Ruth narrative of return from the land of exile, a land fled to in famine, were not so parallel to the Exodus narrative. We were slaves, *avadim*, in Egypt, but now we are free. Free to do what? Free to be servants, *avadim*, to God. The word is the same, one of the interior puns of the Passover liturgy that trembles with meaning. To be free, in the words of Michael Walzer, *is* to be able to be commanded, to accept and accede to a life of justice and command, to acknowledge an order of responsibility, and to understand the responsibility of Exodus itself—that each of us is a stranger in a strange land and that the challenge is to remember to act as though each were himself or herself a recently freed slave (*ovd*), each one of us, Oved.[53]

The rabbinic structure is subtle and unfolds after the close, as it were, of the story. The Ruth story is read aloud yearly in the liturgy cycle at Shavuot, both for the agricultural relationship to the story and for the theme of marriage, and for the taking on of the Torah, given to the Jewish people at the time of Shavuot. The hearer is meant to remember not only the faithfulness of Ruth and the generosity of spirit of Boaz, but the self/servant/slave, who is to come as a result of this story. It links the Messianic with the personal and makes the covert but radical claim that it is the face-to-face encounter of the poorest and the most outcast, the female stranger, that makes possible the continuance of the Jewish people and each self.

Hence, the story ends with a reflection on the text after the telling. Justice and reparations are about the move not only from famine to feast, but also from enslavement to service and from exile and displacement to community and place.

•

Clinical Applications

Of what use is this? If the language of the text offers a radical shift in worldview, then we must be able to look to the insights and the call embedded within it to be of use in the actual, difficult world. The contentious debate that surrounds the allocation of resources in the real famines that engulf our modern sensibilities—the scarcity of resources in health care, education, and social welfare—must be the terrain of the discourse, the place of real use of this language. The language must be of use in the world to real strangers, widows, orphans, the vulnerable, and the homeless on the road.

The point of the detailed search in the text just described is to recount with care the texture of the actual gesture in Ruth, to claim the prophetic in the act, and to claim the possible. What Ruth teaches is that citizenship is solidarity, that meaningful discourse starts with the recognition of the other, and that justice is prior to any human freedom. The text insists on the radical recognition of primary responsibility as calling into being a community that is both prior to and responsible for the just flourishing of any human self.

Ruth comes to conscience by the moment described in the text as her "cleaving" (*dbq*). It is a moment of understanding that the "flesh of my flesh and bone of my bone" is the other who stands to face me. It is this moment that makes conscience possible. The conscience can be said, then, not to be the speaking of the voice within, but rather the hearing of the quiet voice of the other.

This is the first gesture of human community. Ruth's story is central because it is her language, at the instant of her human recognition, that frames relationality as primary to ethical choice. The second gesture is, of course, the response of the commanded community that surrounds this gesture. For while recognition and cleaving are essential, they are not enough. It is a foolish and solitary gesture in the arena of public policy if it is not embedded in the community that sequences and interprets ethical gestures. It is the community that gives public voice, that names, and that itself recognizes and insists on the human connection that is the context for language of an allocation based in relationality.

This is the language that I claim is the best for the application of justice. It argues for the association of justice with encounter, with response: in short, with friendship, the deep and enmeshed friendship, *dbq*, that characterizes both this text and the actuality of the human experience. Using this language as a starting pattern for a public response to scarcity allows a reframing of the basic pattern of isolation and self regarding action that now is the dominant tone of contemporary policy discourse.

The lessons of the relationship embedded in the Ruth story are not unique to this one text in the Jewish tradition. The texts that I examined in the classic rabbinic tradition of scarcity, siege, rescue, and pursuit also teach critical lessons about community and the mutual nature of responsibility. The legal texts of the halakhic tradition are a source of justice and basic civil order. The Ruth text is certainly not the only text that will give us framing language for the discourse on health care justice. The texts suggested by the Talmudic and responsa sources each have contributed to this new language. The texts offer suggestions about basic decency and the obligation to minimal standards of sustenance for the poor, for essential links between the justice promises of a city and the provision required by its citizens, and the response of a believing community when confronted with the starkness of tragedy and crisis.

The Ruth text adds to Jewish thought, however, in significant ways. It does better than the other texts in providing a basis for talk about health care as a social, daily experience that will define the nature of community in major ways. While it acknowledges scarcity, it transforms its power: scarcity, the famine that lurks beneath every abundance, does not threaten the fabric of human community if the demand of relationship is consistently heard. It is not a text about violence; it is a text about the experience of aging, vulnerability, and solidarity in the face of death. The Ruth text deals with the most difficult issue of agency, that of the limits set between the self and the *ger*, the other, the stranger in the land.

The Book of Ruth adds another voice to the rich and complex tradition of Jewish ethical response to the rationing of the scarce resource. It is a text that is firmly rooted in the story of women as central actors and insists on the primacy and power of women's choices to remake the world. The halakhah is not the only way the tradition admits new framing language into the ethical discourse; as we have seen, other ways include midrash and *minhag* or praxis. The method of the telling of the Ruth story is midrashic, lyrical, and narrative. It suggests rather than directs; rich in detail and context, it thus opens us in a dramatically new way to the ability to see what seemed to be given, fixed, and immutable about legal and political relationships.

But the work of philosophy is to make sense of ordinary trouble, of real policy debates, of real fields of grain. The issue we now face is how to return to the specifics of the clinical context. Having found the vocabulary of relationality that I offer in response to Churchill's call for such language, I argue that we could begin immediately to recast the discourse in its terms.

COMMUNITY AND CONSCIENCE
Public Choices and Private Acts

This book began with the actual stories of the clinical world, with the voices of specific families and the dilemmas of particular patients and providers as they struggled to make meaning of the tragedies that confronted them and to make sense of the complex health care system intended to serve them. These narratives raised the question of justice and the relationship of justice to public policy. These narratives made plain that the question of what is just is at once both deeply political and intensely personal, that the sense of justice, of rightness of our actions, is shaped by a variety of encounters and discourses.

I spent the last several years both writing about the theoretical tasks encountered in the discipline of ethics and justice theory and struggling with the clinical reality of justice, as I have helped families and providers choose and reflect on the best possible course of action in a health care system that is increasingly competitive, costly, and chaotic. The real struggle for health care reform is going on daily, even hourly, in the American clinical encounter. There is not a gesture, not an order, not a touch, that is not painfully rationed. When one by one American families face their deaths and their losses, they come to know this.

In many ways, the situation has worsened since I began this project. The debate about health care justice, once marked by creativity and promise, has faltered. In response to the crisis, in the face of intellectual and political paralysis, marketplace forces have only consolidated their definitional grip on the rhetoric of medicine. Every month 100,000 families lose their health insurance. When I began this research, there were 37 million uninsured Americans; now 43.2 million are uninsured. In two years, the entire health care climate in California has been revolutionized far more radically than we would have expected. Radical changes have occurred in patient choices, the closure of hospitals, the advance of home care, the role of the family, and the income of physicians and their ability to make unilateral decisions. Some changes have happened in perverse ways: for example, a physician may share interests not with the patient but with the patient's benefits manager. These shifts have taken place with speed and effectiveness. Health care costs are no longer increasing at a rate of 17 to 20 percent a year, but even this change is now stalled. In the fiscal year that ended in October 1996, federal Medicaid spending grew at just 3 percent, probably because of the greater use of managed care and because of the use of these systems to deny health care services, to restrict coverage, or to eliminate coverage for dependents or retirees.[1] Newspapers are full of stories about the rapidly diminished quality of health care for even those with insurance. Medicare recipients are being gathered into competing, free-market-inspired HMOs. These HMOs are actually being marketed, and for the first time, advertisements (all featuring persons of color) for plans have appeared on inner-city buses and soul and rap stations. In inner-city Emeryville an ad for the Blue Cross HMO for Medical recipients is displayed next to a cigarette ad with a smiling couple, calling out "healthy living."

We have decided that managed care is very good for the very poor at least, and the much-advertised necessity for choice is not so critical. Even for the employed who are covered by robust health plans, the marketplace reorganization has affected all health care delivery. The for-profit HMOs have complex problems of their own, hundreds of details that create ethical dilemmas for caregivers. For example, the formulary for pain medication for Medical patients, in many cases a dying child at the pediatric medical center where I used to consult, is different from the formulary for private payers. In states such as Georgia, epidurals are not covered—they are not considered medical necessities. Much of what we focused on in the field of bioethics, for example, the primacy of the physician-patient relationship, has become nearly comical in the face of the advent of the seven-minute office visit. And finally, as the much-touted "Secure Horizons"-type plans for seniors proved too costly to turn large profits for some HMOs, millions of senior citizens with Medicare HMO coverage were simply dropped from the plan. We have much to worry about. But I contend that we cannot realistically begin to comment on our needs unless we first reflect on our essential responsibilities.

Something fundamental must be challenged if we are to change seriously significant aspects of health care delivery. There must be a change in the ideological paradigm of health care itself, and there must be a concurrent change in the process and language of the discourse of public policy. There must be a change in how Americans perceive health and illness, cure and death. Finally, there must be a serious collective and public reflection on the question of justice.

It is to this last task that this book is directed, for it is only by shaping the language of the discourse that a moral community, a nation with the habit of moral gesture, will develop. The development of an attributable conscience—a reflective knowledge, feeling, sense, moral sense, a knowledge or feeling of right and wrong, with a compulsion to do right[2]—about the problem of sharing what we have, within the social world that we inhabit, must first be addressed. The problem of reforming the chaotic world of the national health care system is so large, so mesmerizing in its detail, and so vulnerable to technological and mechanical jury-rigging, that the moral questions must be addressed first or they will not be addressed at all. The necessary fundamental and transformational justification for radical moral choices and paradigmatic changes must be addressed prior to the mechanics of access, delivery, or payment. It is with the problem of conscience that justice must begin, and in the insistence on justice that health care reform must be rooted.

The text of Ruth provides a metaphor for how these necessary changes might happen. It is a Jewish metaphor, but not exclusively. In placing a language that is Jewish and feminist at the center of the framing discourse, I risk the perception that I propose a marginalized, particularized response to the problems held in common. Precisely the opposite is the case. I am proposing an ethics of encounter that has a clear expression in the Ruth text but the application of which, when insisted upon, can be the moral notation that undergirds public policy. The Rutharian encounter on the road, the portrayal of the self and the stranger, provides a pattern of interpretation that allows one to locate the gesture within a cosmic framework.[3] It allows us to create a template for justice that is at once intimate, possible, and personal, a first location for our actions of conscience.

In an important article published in 1990 in the *Hastings Center Report*, Lisa Sowle Cahill made this point explicitly. Theologians could introduce into the civil discourse insights "borne by their own tradition" on the assumption that a common moral language could be fashioned on the "common meeting ground" of the diverse moral traditions that made up our society. There was no privileged secular realm, asserted Cahill, no reasonable neutral vantage point that was not indebted to a particular tradition. The organization of autonomy and the association with individual rights, the theories of the virtue of independence, and the language of justice itself, as I have shown, were not neutral; they were a specific language from a specific historical tradition. Moreover, it was a tradition that excluded many voices and much of the experience of those whom it hoped to describe and for whom it hoped to create normative standards.

The necessity of mutual discourse was created when members of a society settled on a common life together in the actual and pragmatic world. This fixed point, the situation of common practical interest, "a dilemma about the nature of a practical moral obligation," is what gives a "common starting point."[4]

Bringing the pattern and language offered by the Ruth text into the debate challenges the discourse of health care reform and the allocation of scarce resources in several ways. It was, to create a visual metaphor, stepping into the auditorium late, after the actors had begun to testify. But insisting on making new testimony deepened Cahill's critique further. The common discourse of ethics was not only assumed to be secular and objective, but Christian. When one speaks of religious inclusion, the unspoken assumption of the bioethics literature is that the inclusion is Christian, that the faith principles of Christianity are shared and mutual among all religious people. In fact most of what are accepted as the fixed and core principles of bioethics and justice are in reality core assumptions about the human capability, spirit, and horizon described by Christian tradition in particular. The text of Ruth, not interpreted as a general religious inclusion, but viewed through the particular lens of the methodology of Jewish textual tradition, asserts that important new insights can be brought into the discussion from language and faith principles that are significantly distinct.

The Jewish textual world, the historical tradition, and the method of halakhic debate teach us this lesson of inclusion. If we are to develop a new language beyond that of rights and entitlements, this language must be rooted in story and community that draw from a method that is dialogical and communal. The method *itself* ultimately suggests the relationship between the individual and the collective that creates the social and shared ground for conscience. Because of the near-hegemony of the assumption and power of autonomy in clinical ethics, it is important to offer some reflection on the tenuousness of that central claim. Jewish thought struggles not only with the nature of the self relative to the other and the self relative to the community, but with whether the embodied self has at all what post-Enlightenment thinkers described as rights. The notion of the good in this formulation rests not on the promise of voluntariness, but on the promise of obligation. A Jewish theological approach explores the robust debate on the problem of informed consent with a reflection on the difficulty of the model of the unencumbered disconnected patient engaged in neutral rational discourse as a template for either clinical ethics decision making or attendant social policy. Such an approach would insist on the community of others that are dependent on and responsible for one another. As part of the process we will need to question if voluntariness itself is either possible or the ground for human freedom. Elsewhere I have argued that the Talmudic method itself is one such template of such a discursive community.[5] I posit here the Talmudic notion that coming to truth is a process of debate, a conversation, and that this method can be extrapolated to bioethics.

Further, reflection on both the content of the story and the Jewish hermeneutics of Ruth means focusing on texts that can be said to be from "the female gaze." This gaze is not only rare in any canonical or authoritative texts, but rare in the debate on health care reform, where the stories of women are admitted primarily as objects of pity, illustrations of injustice, or barometers of need. The Ruth narrative teaches not from the position of victim but, rather, from the position of woman as subject, as central player, and as enmeshed in a successful community event of encounter, obligation, and response that changes the facticity of what would appear to be historical inevitability. To allow this is to allow the entirely radical notion that the centrality of the view of the other is possible. This method both uses and demonstrates the possibility of discourse where the ability to reverse is the gesture at the heart of the encounter with justice itself.

This reversal is not unique to Ruth but is a methodological reality of the form itself. The quality of an alternative reading is present in all midrashic interpretation. Midrash is exegesis that by its very nature fills in the lacunae in the textual account. It assumes that the reality of human conversation—that glance, that nuance, and that interiority of reflection—are also relevant to an account of full moral action. Rabbinic midrash brings attention to the voice of the excluded, finds glimpses or overt references to rabbinic discontent with standard halakhic text, or places troubling questions in the mouths of midrashic characters.

The application of textual narrative is a technique of applied theology that is at the heart of the halakhic method. Embellishment of the aggadic source to achieve a template for action is central to Jewish method. What is distinctive about my use of the text is a persistent insistence that the theological pattern has a pertinence to the actual contemporary public policy debate. This example of an alternative feminist gaze is interesting in its own right in Jewish studies and academic reflection. But it is imperative that the possibility of the pattern, in all of its quirky and idiosyncratic Jewish particularity, is seen as requisite to the reordering of the philosophic stance. Without this view of the other, the ground of justice will be impoverished. There is not only poverty in the assumption that the public discourse is Christian; there is the certainty of error in describing the very terms of encounter for public debate.[6]

Looking at the established debate through another lens creates the possibility for many alternate readings and many contributions to the common language. This is of particular importance when the multicultural, multiclass, and multiethnic setting of clinical medicine and public distribution is addressed. Hearing the language of a particular discourse from such a distinctive tradition allows the radical apprehension of the discourse itself. The entrance into the public debate requires that the actors must turn from the ongoing nature of the conversation to notice, to admit the incoming of the other. Before the content of the story, the presence of alternate narrative changes the terms of the discussion. Further, the Ruth narrative is rooted in the assumption not only of faith, but of a particular faith, and a faith that asserts itself not as ethnic color or vague blessing, but of practical and tangible use in the setting of policy.

•

Health Care Reform and an Ethics of Encounter

The policy of reform must emerge from what I have come to call an ethics of encounter. What I mean by this term is described in part by the insights of Levinas, in part by the communicative ethics of Benhabib, in part by the acknowledgment of a specific other asserted in Gilligan's feminist philosophy, and in part by calls for community and responsibility from communitarians such as Churchill, Hauerwas, and Bellah. The ethics of encounter implies a process that is most elegantly illustrated in the Ruth story of encounter. In this story, the Hebrew term *dbq*, meaning "to cling" or "to cleave," most fully expresses the first principle of the ethics of encounter. Concretely, the seven moments that I identified as central in the texts can be used in the health care justice debate.

1. To leave the community at a time of scarcity/danger is wrong.
There is no personal escape from collective scarcity.

The text of Ruth reminds us that there is no personal escape from collective scarcity. The health care debate is quickened by this reality. Unless one is prepared to build a fully equipped hospital with a separate blood product supply on one's own premises, there is no escape from the collective fate that crisis and scarcity imposes on all of American society. To live in New York City in the 1970s was to draw from the very blood of the poorest and most desperate. To travel on the freeway across Los Angeles in the 1990s is to share in the risk that an accident could bring you to an emergency room that serves as an outpatient clinic to the poorest and the uninsured. It might be closed, full beyond capacity, no matter how exquisite your car or provident your health care coverage. To walk in the subway or shop at the supermarket means that your child will share the very air with the homeless woman and her child beside you. There is no escape to Moab.

2. To resume responsibility, even if one is powerless,
is the just course for every citizen.

Hence, it falls to each person to resume responsibility, even if one is powerless. It is the just course for every citizen. Even the one who has been silenced, like Naomi, who had never been trained to speak, must become a part of the discourse. Each citizen must be asked the question that Martin Benjamin suggests: "What is the most just plan?" And each answer must be taken into account.

3. To have a face-to-face encounter makes generations and redemption possible.
It is the encounter with the face of the other that makes possible the ethical choice.

Any plan must begin with face-to-face encounter. The selective survey will not do; the advice of many experts will not be enough. One needs the radical recognition that what one chooses for the body of another will happen also to one's own body; it is the physicality and the *dbq* character of the encounter. The encounter itself must be insisted upon.

4. To count on social order for a decent basic minimum is a given.

The initial recognition will be of little meaning unless there is a concurrent commitment that allows each person to count on the resultant social order for a decent basic minimum. It must be a given that certain basic protections, analogous to the minimum standards for the poor in the Ruth story, are respected. A world in which health care access is defined by a market metaphor is inevitably unstable, to say nothing of immoral. First, access that is universal must be assured.

The question of the justification of such a basic decent minimum and the content of such a basic minimum can be answered, in part, by the response of the community to the vulnerable in the Ruth text. In the story, the provision for the poor can be assumed—by Ruth, by Naomi, and by the community. Unlike the society of Moab, where there is nothing and no one in the field, the fields in the Ruth story have a mandated portion, a corner in each that is reserved for the poor in the text of Leviticus. It is not out of pity that Ruth is allowed to glean; it is out of the halakhic requirement that a fixed percentage of the crop belongs to the poor, given from God's hand via the work of Boaz. The access is universally available and guaranteed to all, the citizen and the resident alien alike. In part, the response pattern between the women in the story, the language itself, and the tradition of discourse support a principle of respect for community that must be adhered to if we are to be faithful to the centrality of the encounter that is prior to all justice. Once there is a commitment both to universal access and to a process of decision making that involves each citizen, there must be a conversation that centers around the ends and goals of medicine. What is it that works? What is the outcome? What do we think is fair? The questions must be geared to the establishment of the standards to which each person will be entitled. In the case of Oregon, the standards were hardheaded yet rich—more generous than what was currently provided.[7]

5. Intimacy/family is seen as an obligation beyond justice and the law.

Structuring health care reform in this way allows for the setting of limits on a coherent package of benefits to be intimate, to involve the personal reflection of conscience in a collective setting. It allows small moral communities to recognize the stranger as sister or daughter, to see inescapably the stranger who sits across from you as the fellow traveler on the road. The impulse for a system of justice and the language of justice itself must recognize justice as intimate and familial, as an obligation beyond the law and a formal equality, to include relational ties to the specific other.

6. Trust that friendship/family will make generation/redemption possible (again) and that this action is mutually a duty and a right.

In fact, as was patterned for the reader in Ruth, only the mutuality of friendship and relationality make even simple continuance possible.

7. Trust in community and the language of community to name and define the future.

Finally, the language of Ruth teaches that the child of the most vulnerable and excluded really is the salvation of each of us. The child will be called "one who serves," and thus he or she will be born into an obligation of his or her own. His or her name will define the work of a free person, which is to respond with faithful action and to pick up the task that is unfinished and that is sacred, the task that is mundane and thus deeply human. It is our mutual responsibility, as citizens of this moral community that is our own America, to name that child, to call him or her ours. To trust in community and the language of community, to name and define the future, means that we must begin with the name of a single child.

Cleaving to another, recognizing that the other is the bone of the bone and the flesh of the flesh that is given in common, locating the mutual body as the site of the moral gesture, is fundamental to ethical reflection. First, it pulls the discourse to the specific, the limited and the mortal self, insisting on mortality as the inescapable frame for all moral gesture. Next, it requires a radical rethinking of all that occurs to the other; all of the yearning, all of the loss, is in fact my loss. This responsibility for the narratives great and small, for the dreams of the other, for the temptations of the other, and for the responsibility of the other creates a mutual commandedness in the language of Levinas. The encounter is intensely personal. The death of the other, the illness of the other, and the vulnerability of the other are your own ("and where you will die I will die"). *Dbq* is a requirement of intensity that precedes and deepens the language of citizenship. It insists that citizenship, even with the stranger most foreign, could be and ought to be experienced with the intensity of family. Unlike citizenship, the term *dbq* suggests to us that human beings are, by absolute definition and design, relational. Justice is then personal: it calls for no less than the totality of re-membering, of re-call, of the person who walks at your side.

The ethics of encounter has a second defining vocabulary. It is the language of community. I began this research in 1991 with a certainty that the principle of autonomy, so dominant in the field of bioethics yet so painfully limited in the clinical encounter, was also of limited use in addressing the allocation of resources and that talk of individual rights was of limited use in addressing the problem of health care reform. The case stories of the Gallos, the Lincolns, and other families were reminders that despite the theoretical constructs of the field, humans were not simply or even primarily autonomous. Rather than living in a world described and defined by the necessity of autonomous choice, freely made, most people live in the relational, obligatory, and interconnected world, a world far messier and heavily freighted, far more passionately loving and passionately hating, than that described in philosophic texts. I began by postulating a principle that would counterbalance autonomy: the encounter. This term expresses the next step in the process of justice. It is the response and recognition of the community that contextualizes the choice for *dbq*, the encounter, that would otherwise simply be an act of personal conscience, a good act, but a limited one.

In the clinical world one sees this principle in action at all times. Persons speak in the collective voice of tragedies that seem to be individually embodied. Although often their work is invisible to clinicians, families are counted on to mediate and rename the indignities of medicine. It is a powerful clinical truth that, despite the forbidding and sterile world constructed around illness, despite the clinical efforts to make the hospital look as much like a laboratory as possible, families make efforts to personalize and deconstruct the "text of scientific management." Even the tiniest neonate in the most modern ICUs, where arguably the machines far outweigh and outnumber the actual patients, is bedecked with little ribbons, cards, and stuffed animals. Even when the parents of such infants are not present at the bedside, these decorations stand as mute testimony to the power of relationality, of naming, and of the signifiers of inclusion in human community. Prior even to the conceptualization of the self, of the autonomous being with rights and bodily integrity, there is a self-in-relation, a self-in-connection, a child born from the body of a woman, into the waiting hands of another. Community is prior to autonomy. We know this is true from the commonest details of an ordinary life, and it is from these details that the language of justice must also be created.

•

Community and Conscience

Thinking of community as prior to autonomy raises the issue of how one comes to know the good act. How does one come to conscience? Martin Benjamin suggested that conscience is socially derived. The benefits and burdens of conscience, wrote Benjamin, are a "reflection of the inescapable tensions between the individual and the social dimensions of human existence."[8] Conscience in this sense is the response to the interior voice of the self as a whole, understood temporally—as having a beginning, a middle, and an end—as well as at a particular moment.[9] The chorus of Bethlehem women who greet the travelers Ruth and Naomi on the road, and who name the child they create, is such a moral community. The existence of the pattern made available to us in this way reveals that such work is also possible in actual communities of moral encounter, deliberately created and maintained. The reflective sense of integrity spoken of by Benjamin does not only occur because one reflects on the effect of action on the self, and on the notion of the good self that is interiorly constructed. It occurs because, as Levinas would argue, there is always the presence of the other. Conscience is shaped by the human experience of relationality. There is no atomized self that hears only its own voice and its cause. The possibility of internal, reflective dialogue of a self that is capable of response assumes a relational being. Such a self then struggles with the problem of the effect his or her choice has on tangible, identified others. The sense of temporality present in the reflective sense of integrity depends on such dialogue and such narrative, and on the human propensity to experience life as a story told to a circle of others. Narrative assumes community and the listening presence and reciprocity of the other.[10]

Bioethics has a prophetic responsibility that is inescapable.[11] Describing "what is" cannot be the entire task of ethics. It is the role of the ethicist to point out what ought to be, how a world ought to look (rather than how to achieve only the pragmatic). This is never meant to depreciate the first step toward the future (that is in part why the Oregon project can be supported), but it is also why it is imperative never to lose sight of the vision in light of the possible achievement. Ruth's is the story of the necessity for prophetic voice in bioethics. The seven moments I have identified in the text can be specifically lifted up and reflected upon as the critical gestures of choice and justice. It is remarkable that the terrain we are drawn to again and again is the terrain of collective moral reflection, of the inescapability of the other, and of the relationship between self and stranger. Linked to this alterity is the necessity for advocacy rather than neutrality on behalf of the most vulnerable. As the theological stance of the Jewish text is that of the outsider, the theological claim is for the stranger and the powerless that dwell within our gates. Extrapolated into the world of the clinic, this becomes, again, nearly dangerous, for it assumes an advocacy that in this era becomes political. But to take seriously either the text or the history or even the vaguely expressed "value" of Jewish thought means to take a partisan stand in the name of *tzedakah*, righteousness; this will of necessity have ramifications in the clinical world. In California, in the children's hospital where I consult, this will mean civil disobedience to a law that forbids the offering of care to the children of the stranger. But the regard for the stranger as central to the social world offers a much needed corrective to the problem of sharing the resources of the common. The texts of Ruth or Leviticus and of the Talmudic interpretation of the same call for the encounter between the self and the stranger to be the place for ethics, and for the geography of encounter to be more fundamental than the entitlement of property. Focusing on conscience allows a language to develop that is accountable to the reflective sense of integrity. It is a language that takes account of the yearning toward the good. It is in light of this language, of a differently apprehended understanding of justice, that all health care reform policies must be apprehended.

•

Applying the Language

There is no simple solution to the problem of American health care reform. The application of the language of justice and the delineation of the philosophic ground that must undergird such efforts will be extraordinarily difficult. The focus of this book is not to craft public policy in detail but to reflect on the aspects of the language of the discourse both as it emerges and as I believe it ought to emerge in this debate. Nonetheless, this work has always been rooted in applied philosophy and theology. It is important to address the actual changes as they emerge contextually.[12] But what has become of the carefully crafted reforms debated in this book? In Oregon, the plan is moving ahead with vigor. But in the rest of the country, especially in financially devastated California, the real revolution in health care is made manifest by a for-profit HMO-driven system that made $1.8 billion for its shareholders in 1994 alone. In light of the public discourse for which I have argued, the approach currently popular—managed care as marketplace competition—is troubling. First, it is troubling on purely linguistic grounds. Rather than using the reclaimed language of community, it uses the language of the marketplace. Clinicians are reminded to "watch the bottom line." Patients are bought and sold from one chain to another, spoken of as covered lives or as capitated "heads." Such a system reifies the competition of capitalism with an odd mix of metaphors. We are to imagine the hearty entrepreneurialism of the nineteenth-century businessman, seeking through earnest enterprise and industry to win in a free-trade market. This vision of competitive practice is overlain with the powerful metaphor of a mutual fund, the quintessential financial instrument of the 1980s. This ought to come as no surprise. Health care became a hugely successful for-profit enterprise in the 1990s. To make this happen, the for-profit HMOs and insurance companies used and built on what is successful in the world of economics to address the problems of health care delivery.[13] In a mutual fund, many individual investors with no particular relationship among them are artificially pooled into groups that share the risks and benefits of larger group buying power. Diversified investments are selected by experts in money management who seek the best deals, based on long-term financial success for each investment. What matters to the expert manager is the financial outcome, not the individual story of the investor or the actual quality of the products or properties in which he or she is invested.

Similarly, in managed competition, individuals are pooled into risk groups in the same fashion. There are experts—usually far removed from either the clinical context or any democratic restraint—who negotiate the package of benefits. The outcome is what is at stake, and outcomes are judged successful or not by the cost-benefit formula. Plans are rewarded with "investment," as it were, by offering the most health care commodity or product for the lowest price per unit. Physicians and hospitals are encouraged to consolidate into cooperative ventures because that is the best way to manage them as a commodity.

An examination of some aspects of this emerging system is instructive. First, there are problems with the assessment and use of outcomes. There is an assumption that real science can accurately measure outcomes of medical intervention, that "real" is scientific and quantitative and can be only assessed and adjudicated by what is measurable as altered. This further assumes that the choice of such measures and subsequent observation are free from the values of the observer. Second, outcomes research assumes that justice means impartiality and consistency, which, as demonstrated in Chapter 4, is a most challenged assumption of liberal theory. Much of the current outcome study upon which the success or failure, and thus worth of treatment, is judged is based on QALYs. These supposedly set a standard by which all treatments can be rated.[14] As discussed by some commentators, however, these QALYs are to be used by the expert negotiator, much as a market analyst would use dividend size to assess the value of an intervention to each investor. At issue here is the not inconsiderable problem of difference of values, which is to establish a purely tautological argument. Quality is so thoroughly in the eye of the particular beholder that it is hardly more than a restating of individual desire.[15] The dilemma exists because most people would agree that they would not want to experience a particular fate, but a minority does not agree. Giving a qualitative number to this conflict will ultimately do little to resolve it.[16]

Must private insurance companies be part of the permanent landscape of the American health care delivery system? The emerging system is often put forward as one that "makes all the players in the health care system happy," assuming that insurance companies are a necessary part of providing health care to people, and that the profitability of this particular industry must be maintained. That assumption can be critically examined. As I pointed out in Chapter 3, there is not an intrinsic, organic link between insurance funding and the delivery of medical or nursing care: this assumption is a historical veracity, not a structural one.

Further, the justice of the current health care system rests on the assumption that the few large entities competing for "business" will compete honestly. There is no readily observable benefit to this assumption. It makes economic sense to expect such a competition along the margins in products whose differences are primarily a matter of taste—to see the sort of minor cost and content variances one notes in the American car or soft drink markets, for example. But it is more than likely, given the market metaphor, that these companies will develop community standards that are virtually identical and similarly reimbursable. The alternative is for one system to outbid all the others, resulting in a single provider system with multiple payers. This would maintain the forest of insurance coverers while reducing the choice in health plans and providers that competition is designed to preserve—exactly the opposite of what most Americans say that they want.

The issue of who will serve as the experts is similarly problematic. Will these persons be economists? Will they be medically trained? What will be the standards they follow, and who will oversee their work? Who will pay them, and how much? Most importantly, how will they decide what is contained in the package for which they will negotiate? If there is no role for a public voice, then the package negotiated will be subject to the same competing interests to which public funding is subject now. Without a careful building of consensus about the public priorities of social provision, any package will be more influenced by market forces than social forces. While managed competition would certainly address the problem of access mentioned in the cases in the first chapter, the conflict of values that emerges in the difficult cases will have to be addressed by the community as a whole.

At issue always will be the problem of limits. As long as rationing focuses on the limitation of care and not the limitation of profits, it will continue to burden the most vulnerable disproportionately, shifting the cost of the solution onto those individuals least able to bear it. Justly to address the problem of limits will mean subjecting to scrutiny each aspect of the medical system, not simply the appropriate limits of a basic decent minimum health care package. It will mean that there must be a serious discourse about how much physicians should charge and how much income it is fair for them to make. It will mean asking if private health insurance is an appropriate part of the system at all.[17]

The discourse on cost effectiveness is itself driven by assumptions that regard cost as a fixed entity. In the common discourse about neonatal care, it is often cited that "for every $1.00 spent on prenatal care, you save $3.00 on intensive care." While this may be conceptually true (the claim itself has now been nearly completely discredited), the problem deconstructed reveals that little is known about the origins of either figure. What is the real cost of prenatal care? How is this number arrived at? What is the cost of a day of prenatal intensive care? Upon what is this based? How is the profit margin of the company that manufactures ampicillin and gentamicin (two antibiotics given at some point to nearly every neonate in the critical care unit in which I worked) determined? Who decides the cost of arterial blood gases collection supplies or of phototherapy technology? Who decides how much advertising revenue is justified in marketing the product and hence needs to be built into its price structure? Further, what if the time of the nurse practitioner who might see the prenatal patient were more highly valued than the time of the specialist in neonatal cardiology? If prenatal care were determined to be *more* costly than intensive care, would this be a reason not to offer prenatal care? The market value that sets cost is based on what it is possible to charge. Since there has been no external limit on this amount and no records of health care expenditures have been kept at the national or state level, there is no mechanism for knowing if a charge is just. We cannot judge if the cost is even relative to the labor involved in the actual construction and development of technology. Even the construct that says that ill persons ought to be cared for in large hospitals emerges not out of a reflection on what is best for their healing, but on what made profitable sense at a certain historical period.[18]

Reinventing health care delivery represents an enormous subject for critical social discourse. It is far beyond that attempted even by the Oregon plan. Yet it must be addressed justly to decide how much and what type of treatment can be part of our expectation of health care. Unless the discussion is begun in the most straightforward terms and language possible—in the language that assumes a common good that must extend to each person—the real reforms cannot begin to be addressed.

There is yet a larger subject that will need to be a part of this discourse of citizenship as well. I have argued elsewhere in this book for its inclusion, but I will mention this point again here. In part, the ethical dilemmas faced in the narrations described in the first chapter grew out of a yearning that is central to the American collective understanding of medicine. We have been encouraged to accept, and have come to believe, that an entitlement to health care is equivalent to eluding death. In the clinical context in which I practice, this is expressed repeatedly: Families are faced with what looks like a scene from a television series on catastrophe, but this time the drama is their own lives, and this time there is no recovery. What we yearn for is the miraculous, the redemption once promised by religion and now promised by medical science. The last fifty years in medicine have been remarkable. But the issues that face us now as a society are the plain inescapability of death and our persistent efforts to deny its force and power.

The discourse of health care reform needs to start with honesty on the part of physicians and other providers as they confront their own limits. They need to learn how to fail in public, admitting that they are at the limits of understanding, ability, or courage. They need to do this in full view of their particular patient and in full view of a society that pays them very well to keep us from death.

The discourse needs to be continued in a central way by the religious community. The blessings of friendship in the human endeavor and the responsibility for bearing the collective burden of the ill and the vulnerable must be borne by the theology and purpose of the faith communities. That the Reverend James Lincoln and Paulie Gallo and Mary O'Connell will soon die is inevitable; what must be understood as miraculous is our ability to love them and bear their weight in fellowship.

The discourse needs to be deeply social as well. The Oregon project's founders understood this, and their earliest work reflected this. This model must be made imperative. The serious attention to the ends and the goals of medicine must begin with a direct address of our culture's denial of death, devaluation of the elderly, and dishonoring of the bodies of the discarded and despised disabled. Only by encountering the most vulnerable on the road, and only by remembering that the vulnerable stranger is you and that you must travel exactly his or her road—"whither you go, there will I go"—is this address possible. Only when the other is understood as myself is it licit to speak about limits on his or her life. The dialogue is moral only if it is understood that all speech is about one's own death as well the other's. To allow the limits to be set by some corporate, neutral entity is to absent ourselves from what is at the core of our human existence.

•

Daily Practice

Ultimately, this book would be simply promising philosophy if I could not demonstrate that, in actual practice, small-group discourse can be a starting point for significant historical and cultural shifts in the consideration of values and ethics. I can reflect on three specific examples where this model has worked to make remarkable changes in history written small and large and in the American health care system.

First is the Oregon model that I have described as the focus of this book. Here, the small conversations over a ten-year period have resulted in a conscious and aware citizenry making specific changes in the law and in health care delivery.

Second is the model of the feminist small group. Women's consciousness raising groups began in the late 1960s within the culture of the antiwar and civil rights movements of that era and quickly spread into a broader constituency. The groups typically met weekly over several years. Women came together simply to share their personal narratives. By so doing, they recognized that what had been previously understood as a series of individual and personal events of one woman's life could be seen and identified as a socially constructed and systematic public narrative. The personal, went the slogan that accompanied this insight, was political. This meant that the individual story of any woman's life was really a collective story, and that she was "named" by the collective experiences of her community as surely as Naomi had been named. This realization enabled millions of women to change significant aspects of what until that time had been accepted about the "place" of women, about gender, and about personality. Changes in the nature of the family, the movement toward reproductive control, and concurrent structural legal changes all began in this intimate, rather modest way, in living room after living room. An ideology that has come to shape our American history began with these small conversations, the encounter that was face-to-face. This movement in its own way changed the face of American medicine as well, spurring a women's health movement that paralleled the consciousness raising movement, encouraging thousands of women to enter professional medicine for the first time.[19]

The final model of small-group discourse is emerging now. It is the extraordinary development of hospital ethics committees. Not all ethics committees are models of moral community—far from it. In many, however, the moral community that is established by such an encounter is remarkable.[20] In such communities, the moral communities deliberately created by the staff members and ethicists of the Kaiser Permanente HMO, I encountered the Lincolns, the Gallos, and Mary O'Connell. In each case, the committee was able to create a human discourse that allowed each to see the full humanity of the other. The committees were not only able to reflect on the ways that each of us shared the story of the family thus encountered, but they were able to draw on this reflection in the continuing life of the committee. Thus was created a moral casuistry that in turn created the actual perimeters of policy set by this particular moral community. The narratives represented the concrete others to whom we were responsible in every deliberation that followed this work. It allowed the development of both the courage to say no to some demands and the compassion to know how to see community and relationships where only autonomous rights had stood before. Each committee, a small group meeting over time, committed to one another and to a discursive process of encounter and response, thought through cases that were noted, reflected on, and honored. It is the accumulated experiences of each such moral community that will also begin to change what it means to be taken care of by the American health care system.

Thus it can be shown that even in large, pluralistic, anonymous societies such as the United States, long prior to a utopian conclusion, these small models can not only thrive but can affect social reality. Even in a society of strangers, amidst other indices of despair and anomie, this has occurred. This has happened in ordinary life despite little or no encouragement from the state or popular ideology, an ideology that, in fact, argues for the primacy of the individual and the unrelenting fear of the stranger.

This phenomenon of the possible is what encourages the discourse of the prophetic. The confidence that discourse itself has a power cannot be overstated; it is a different way to view the limited world. The confidence that Gilligan described ethnographically in her female subjects reflects the textual optimism of the Ruth narrative in the Jewish theological and textual tradition. The women's chorus of naming in the Ruth narrative provides a textual parallel to the face-to-face development of each of these moral communities I have described.

•

Reflection on the Oregon Health Care Reform Process

This book began in part as a prolonged attempt to analyze the case study of policy in the State of Oregon and to reflect on the rightness of this plan. Ultimately, one must decide: Can this plan be considered a just model, a just pattern, in setting the standard for national health care policy reform? Finally, after all the arguments are considered, is this plan helpful in moving the United States toward justice in the actual distribution of this resource?

I contend that it is, for a specific reason. At this time, the Oregon plan represents one of the best examples of a public reflection on what is just and what is needed in health care reform. It is an attempt to encounter and take responsibility for the other in building moral community. What is best about the Oregon health care plan is ultimately the community process that has been developed over a ten-year period that involves large numbers of citizens at the most intimate and intense level. Over time, this process has shown itself to be a force of tremendous energy and passion for collective conscience in that state. The details of the plan, the levels of care, the amount of monies, and the inclusion or exclusion of specific procedures are the result of political compromise and can be read as the historical account of victories and defeats along the road. But the direction of the journey is principally just. It is one that is being taken with the end goal, the prophetic "ought" clearly in mind, as the participants stumble along the inevitably broken way from now until then. The debate in Oregon has been far reaching. The organizers have been sensitive to issues of race and class and gender. The effort has consistently been to focus on grassroots efforts, both in style and in content.

The process reflected two critical things. First, it reflected a deep faith in democracy. While the answers that emerged in the first years of the process were not always complete, they were always answers that had been struggled with and debated. They reflected the passion and moral reflection that surrounded the moral community that was made. It was, finally, the creation of moral community itself that made meaning of the discourse.

Second, the process reflected a willingness to ask a question that is uncommon in our American moral life, where the habit of the moral gesture is too often rare and where we often lack moral vocabulary altogether.[21] It asked not "What can I get?" but rather "What is just? How are we to construct the most just society together?" The Oregon process allowed the encounter between actual lives and stories and languages, vividly described as theoretically possible by Benhabib and the theorists of the communicative ethics school. It allowed citizens to come to terms with the encounter theologically described in the Ruth text, in the ordinary meeting halls of their towns. It was the moment of significant encounter, coupled with ongoing and committed location in a specific community, that was the best aspect of the Oregon project. As I noted in my assessment of the resultant health plan, there was much that was problematic about the effort. However, I do not believe that the issues that cloud the implementation of the plan are as salient as its considerable achievements.

The plan was also notable in its essential commitment to universal access, to community-based decision making that led to a basic package of benefits. That the benefit package reflects other social needs expresses both in content and, most importantly, in process what will be necessary for any morally successful health care reform. Finally, a fundamental contribution of the Oregon plan is that it is a reform plan and an allocation scheme that is not based around the premise of autonomy and individual rights, but around the organizing principle of community. The plan is constructed around the premise that to do justice means to pay careful and prolonged attention to the fact that people live in, are responsible for, and are obligated to communities. It recognizes that it is the provision of the entire community that makes for good health, and that health is never an individual willed effort.

Further, the Oregon plan recognizes that there will be burdens on a community. The vulnerable, the elderly, and the helpless will burden a society, and it is in large part to bear precisely these burdens that societies are constructed. Human persons depend on one another. The template for this is the dependability of the family, but the social extrapolation is the necessity for dependability and dependence of the stranger. Humans live socially to depend upon and to be dependable to one another, and it is this recognition, and not the recognition that persons are primarily independent and entitled, that is the moral location upon which to begin to build a just health care reform plan. We know this in part from the daily truths of our own experience, and we can be guided by specific insight and language available to our discourse from the particular tradition that is my vantage, the Jewish tradition, which is largely organized around the principle of community itself.

This book was not only clinically situated; it was also temporally situated. For Americans, 1992 was an election year, and the election was in part a referendum on the national health care debate. I first wrote the conclusion to this text as a new administration pledged to change utterly how Americans get health care. There was talk of the significant restructuring of insurance, of payment, and even of the principle that links employment to health care services.

Yet all of this changed in the next two years. A protracted acrimonious debate about funding and choice left the Clinton proposal in shambles. The elections of 1994 were everywhere interpreted as a final resounding defeat for health care reform. Why such a failure? And what role and responsibility ought to be taken by ethicists and policy theorists? Why the relative silence of ethics in the public square?

It was my hope in constructing research for the ethics of health care reform that the debate on such reform would have been at its peak just prior to the elections in the fall of 1994, and that such debate would stimulate the widest discourse about the topic of ethics and public policy. But that summer, when I thought that Americans would be following the making of the reform package, the news was preempted by reports of the trial of O. J. Simpson.[22] By the time we collectively turned, a little dazed but sated, from this drama, the health care debate had reached a sudden denouement: every day brought the news that less could be brokered. It was suddenly common wisdom that nothing would change—not one goal would be met prior to the end of the year, not one more American would be granted access to care, and not one less infant would die from treatable causes. Each day the national press bought us news of the compromises.[23] Last to be denied were extended benefits for home health and hospice care, then health care for pregnant women and children, then finally only care for children. The loss of the democratic majority in 1994 threatens to close the books on health care reform, a reform that less than a year earlier seemed certain. Now polls tell us that the enthusiasm for reform has been diverted to other concerns: what is taken by the state in taxes rather than what must be distributed by the state.[24]

The fault for this diversion lies beyond the obvious villains. That the crisis in social welfare remains unaddressed is a challenge not only to the makers of policy, but to the intellectual leadership—theological and philosophical as well as political—in this country as well. If we are to take seriously the call to participate in the public square,[25] to claim the notion of a religious citizenship, it will mean taking a rigorous look at our own role in the production of ideology and social capital. There has been a frenzy to seize the arena for a particular genre of religiosity, that of fundamentalist evangelical Christianity usually associated with the far right. I want to describe this carefully, in part because it has been so randomly vilified. I believe that such religiosity has its claim on the public arena. I disagree with their arguments in nearly all respects, but not with their voice; what I am arguing for is a substantive answer to this challenge. Is it surprising that persons of faith have passionate, political fervency of a conservative, reactionary nature? That the calls for a return to earlier values include a certainty about the threat from the vulnerable and the poor? That the poor are despised, then targeted? These calls should not be startling; they are part of the familiar and, for Jews, the lethal history of Europe. In large part they are the central drama of the prophetic texts, wherein are located the earliest struggles about the meaning of scarcity in a fecund world, about responsibility for the widow and the orphan, and about the ethical treatment of the stranger. What is surprising is not these new voices, but that the texts of traditional religiosity have been so unspoken for, leaving the contention between the right and the left roughly comparable to the contention between the religious and the secular. A rigorous defense of the meaning of the common good in this context requires a hard shaking down of the theories of social justice suggested by differing interpretations of religion. This will mean a reclamation of the difficult, demanding calls of the text, and in large part this will mean a reappraisal of our fondness for such central concepts of the liberal vision that emerge more or less in a direct line from the Enlightenment as privacy, safety, and autonomy. A reassessment of the theories of social justice will entail a robust reclamation of the necessity of the stranger for the workings of justice in a society held in common. This insistence on social justice for the most vulnerable is the traditional, unpopular role of the theologian; it is a battle that must be waged over and over again.

We cannot simply accede to the commonplace pronouncement that health care reform and health care justice are politically dead. At the minimum, we need to reopen the debate about why we must have universal access to health care. In our states, in our publications, and in our teaching, we need to turn our scholarship toward this ordinary drama and to insist on its possibility. There is precedent for such an attention. In part, thoughtful reflection on the nature and meaning of slavery in the 1850s undergirded the abolitionist movement, and in part, the scholarship of theologians undergirded the Progressive era. In bioethics itself, the intellectual calls for informed consent, for advanced directives, and for confidentiality precede the clinical practice of the acts that we argue are theoretically necessary. In much of the debate around the issue of transplants, for example, Arthur Caplan and others remind us that the system cannot be made fair without a recognition that the existing differences in access to medical care itself are deeply unjust. Susan Wolf, Alexander Capron, and others remind us that the calls for physicians to assist in suicides take place in the context of a system that is structurally skewed. We must frame our ethical reflection with this dark border; we must insist that there will be no justice in health care and no ethical course in individual decisions unless the central and abiding issue of basic access is solved. Unless we trouble the discourse, our focus will be indefensibly narrow. But theory will not be enough. We must build a praxis of bioethics as well. Bioethicists must act ethically in such a way that extends the access we call for.

Embodiment and the nature of befallenness and fragility are human realities. Theorists are paid to teach, write about, and research the clinical act; to comment on it; and in many cases, to recommend and evaluate its virtue. Yet how many bioethicists have the privilege of touching and caring for the body of the stranger?

Can we envision such a thing as bioethicists volunteering to sit in a pediatric ward or a nursing home and read to a real patient? If we theorists are trustworthy, we might be allowed to braid the hair of the old woman or feed the man who cannot feed himself. We might, by our work, teach medical students and administrators to act in this way as well.

We are at the beginning of a new period in bioethics. As I write this, a new national bioethics commission is in place, and a second-term Democratic president is in office. Much of our collective history will be shaped in the next few years. The construction of the basis for the discourse will depend in large part on what we have the courage, the clarity, and the integrity to speak about.

·

Privacy and Private Choice: Morality in Full View of the Other

Choices held personally and made privately have their costs. When we flee from public discourse, the public space physically and spiritually becomes a place of shadow, disrepair, and even danger; the indistinct figures of the other appear, but their faces are turned from your own. Privacy in such a place rests on an odd notion that what one does can actually be covert, as though one's actions have no bearing on the ground that we know to be shared. Privacy is linked with individuality, as though dozens of little private decisions, made like so many purchases, add up to freedom. Nothing could be further from the truth, and nowhere is this more apparent than in the arena of health care reform. Each decision made in private does matter and becomes public. The privacy we attest to is a delusion. Each separate act becomes an act in conversation with its precedents. Each person is a neighbor to another; the challenge is how we will live together.

Of all the issues that now haunt the American common ground, the most motivating seems to be fear. The world is no longer safe or sane, goes the cry; the defense of the self is ever more desperate. Guns are only the most visible symbol of this retreat into a kind of Hobbesian darkness. The return to fundamental religious values is one more turn away from the chaos and danger of the social world into the imagined privacy of the family. But even the family offers no safety.[26] For ethicists and theologians the need for safety will have to be carefully considered even as we celebrate, rightly I believe, the restoration of the life of faith. While we all yearn for peace, the promise of this world as without risk is distinctly un-Jewish. The world is troubled, unredeemed, and demands a lot of work, and its Messiah is only due to arrive, the Talmud reminds us, on the day after the world is perfected. The Jew is obliged to seek peace in the family and the larger circles of city and nation. But peace is risky; this is true in the world of health care reform as well as in the political world of border treaties. Inviting the wretched poor into one's home will be a challenge to privacy; this is why autonomy, privacy, and safety are linked and must be so seriously challenged. Being personally and socially defended, safe from the assaults of others, cannot be the normative end of a human life. It is a denial of the fragility of the embodied self, of the sorrow, surprise, burdensomeness, and ecstasy that we must encounter as humans. To keep faith is to bear witness to what is possible, a gesture as chancey and as ordinary as the recognition that the stranger beside you is on the same road.

Meanwhile, every time I rework this manuscript, the enthusiasm for health care reform is less vital and central. In 1999, as we became mesmerized by cloning and postmortem sperm donation, and as ethicists were interviewed eagerly on television, the issue of universal health care seemed in peril of slipping completely out of our public gaze. And it was not only the academic literature or the trade discussion that had shifted. In the *New York Times* database of the fall of 1996 and the spring of 1997, there were 298 articles about health care; most were from the business page, and most concerned the new (big) business of health care. There was not one article on universal access for the uninsured. The *Los Angeles Times* ran one significant story in 1997 about the issue. Reporting the closing of the County-USC hospital, the story raised critical issues about the continuing needs of the uninsured. But here, too, the bulk of the coverage was on the shifts of quality for the insured population, changes in conditions for physicians and the business success of the merger marketplace in the health care industry. In one memorable piece in 1995, salaries for CEOs of HMOs, all in the several millions of dollars, were compared, and one CEO, Malek Hassan, was quoted as saying that his remuneration of $8.8 million was too low, since he and others like him had "saved health care."

Finally, and perhaps most telling, was the observation, now a media commonplace, that the presidential debate of 1996 barely mentioned the crisis in the U.S. health care system, a topic that had dominated the contest in 1992. An observer of the U.S. political election campaign would not have known, for example, that 9.8 million children, or 13.8 percent of all American children, have no health care coverage, an increase of 1.6 million (.9 percent) in the last decade, and a rise even from the time of the 1990 elections. One might think, in doing a scholarly review of the campaign coverage or the literature in years hence, that a critical health care issue concerned the number of hours that health insurers allowed a new mother to stay in the hospital.

Not long ago, the terms for the public discourse were set quite differently. The loss of the public discourse has meant quick and deep shifts in the very gestures of medicine. It is with some bitterness and much grief that I recount the dramas of the clinical world. In California, because even the Clinton plan has failed, the managed competition model reigns unfettered by any social policy. In the years since managed competition was implemented, we have seen just what this turn from the stranger has meant: the closing of the county systems, as they are driven into insolvency by a competitive marketplace, and the deepening of some epi-demics that affect the poor, including tuberculosis and measles. But other signs are more subtle. For example, last year there were a few signal cases of meningo-coele meningitis in the local county children's hospital. The families were poor, uninsured, Hispanic, and largely undocumented. Although the catastrophic out-comes in the ICU were treated and, after the amputation of several limbs, the surviving children were saved, the prophylaxis, rifampin, for the rest of the family was not covered by public funds. As the winter wore on, more and more children, all with Spanish surnames and all with the same form of meningitis, came from all over the Bay Area and entered the hospital. The senior physician who told the story recalled, "Finally, the residents had enough; they went to the pharmacy and bought the preventative drugs themselves, which cost $187 for a family of six, and handed them out." But by then it was too late. Now cases come in from everywhere—insured, uninsured, Hispanic, black, and white.

In the emerging clinical world, as providers consolidate and compete, patients are at risk of simply being given less care. Fewer staff members are in attendance, fewer days are allowed in the hospital bed, fewer procedures are approved, and fewer hospitals are as well equipped as they need to be. Patients are discharged earlier, but as the family structure has changed, there is no one at home to care for the ill. Often there is no mother at home, no daughter, no nurturing community of women or men, and no extended family. Mutuality and intergenerational interdependence vanished in the social and economic choices made a generation ago, buttressed by the generalized flight from difficult obligation. We need to turn truthfully to Naomi, angry and gesturing on the road. How much of her journey will each of us share? Or will we claim that her death has no hold on us?

•

Speaking Truth to Power: The Necessity of Prophecy

The period that we now face offers us another chance at the health care reform that has eluded us in the past. It is important to remember that this new organiza-tion of prepaid capitated HMOs is not the only way reform could happen. In other work, I have reviewed the remarkable history of HMOs, a history that began with staunch commitment to the poor.[27] If we could take seriously such a responsibil-ity, our collective voice might have an impact. New bills in Congress seek to build on the Kennedy-Kassebaum effort. The White House has released plans for pro-posals for small-business support whereby companies can purchase health care for their workers through voluntary purchasing coalitions. The Labor Depart-ment has released plans to protect retiree benefits. HMO executives discuss their expectations for federal regulation and reconsideration of the way that Know Keene waivers have allowed full-risk contracting. Gag rules are under rhetorical attack, and the rise in surgical outpatient procedures—such as mastectomies—are finally being noticed. Representative Bill Thoms of California, the Republican chairman of the Ways and Means health subcommittee, is expecting a "detailed proposal" from the White House addressing the need to expand coverage to more children.

These are all good efforts, and they should be supported, as the efforts in Texas to expand pediatric coverage, for example, need our support and analysis. But I contend that we can and ought to do more. We need not merely to follow and analyze this legislation, learning what is "politically expedient" from the commentators. We must restate what we know: that there is in fact a basic ethical principle and a fundamental ethical value, and that everyone must have secure health care coverage.

Calling the ethical question in the political world of health care reform is of necessity very difficult. Both the political process and the clinical setting are steeped in the tradition of the hierarchical relationship and the foregone conclusion. The role of the ethicist is nearly always that of a curious outsider, and the political claim of pragmatism is seductive. Yet the prophetic tradition can tell us much about the imperative of the outsider who can see an alternate vision and stubbornly cling to it despite the imperiousness of the task. Challenging the "is" with the "ought" leads to fruitful understandings about the role of the alternate claim, leads to questioning the givenness of the relationships as presented, and leads to an ironic view of political certainty. Such language is neither safe nor endearing. That the historical place of the philosopher as well as the theologian was to remain the outsider can easily be forgotten.

The notion of the commonweal suggests a venue for citizenship, or moral location that is the place of such a society. But this terrain is contested, and it is imperative that a voice for ethics be clear about our responsibility toward and our necessity for the stranger. At stake here is the problem of the citizen and the stranger. What do I mean when I say that the stranger is necessary for a just place? In part this is reflected in the idea that the citizen of a moral community is a person of temporary potency. Each of us is born necessarily into the waiting arms of the other, and each of us, with luck and blessing, will die from the waiting arms of the other. The estrangement and the wondering that may fill the center of our lives are a tragedy, and in large part the point of living in community is to cobble together a human social life that allows protection from vulnerability. In the texts of the Torah it is clear that the intentional design of the very seasons of crop, harvest, and production belong to God, that the structure of the harvest allows for abundance that creates a bounty that must be shared, and hence that the gleaners are fed not from charity, but from the righteousness that is inherent and inescapable. They are entitled to the corner and the tithe by virtue of their vulnerability itself. The flight from this is hastened by a collective panic about one's own frailty,

I believe, and not from inherent meanness of spirit. But the stranger stands beside you as you are given the law and the land, and the word of faith is clear on this point: The poor one is to be valued far above the king.

> This is the fast I desire:
> To unlock the fetters of wickedness,
> And untie the cords of the yoke
> To let the oppressed go free
> To break off every yoke.
> It is to share your bread with the hungry,
> And to take the wretched poor into your home;
> When you see the naked, to clothe him
> and not to ignore your own kin. (Isa. 68:2)

The meaning of the last line should be apparent: The stranger who is beside you can be seen as your kin, the startling recognition of the breath that you share, the ultimate reversibility that you must count on. Ethicist Larry Churchill's call for a new language is answered by the process of developing the language of the encounter on a road other than that which was traveled by the Good Samaritan. It is the encounter on the road to Bethlehem, City of Bread, and in the Jewish textual tradition that surrounds and defines this encounter. The model of the Ruth narrative, and the very method of its telling, honors the discursive relationship, the ethic of encounter and principled community response. It is on these methodological grounds that policy can be resolved: through the actual case story, the actual face of the other, and the return to the collective that will surround every gesture. The moral discourse modeled in the language, content, and method of telling that I have described here allows for a renewed certainty that the truest public policy, the most just plan, and the best vision for American health care reform will be created by the development of collective conscience. This conscience can only be made actual in the moral communities of citizenship, of obligation discourse. It will only come into being in the full and public encounter between our most private and vulnerable human selves and the extraordinary and actual human face of the other.

NOTES

•

Chapter 1

1. The names in the real case stories that follow are fictionalized, including that of Ray Cates, a California assemblyman who represents Alameda and Contra Costa Counties. The characters in the James McElveen and Millagan case, which was reported in the *New York Times*, January 1993, as summarized are an exception. The other cases come from my clinical experience as a consulting ethicist for the national Kaiser Permanente Health Maintenance Organization. While difficult, they are by no means exceptional; they are representative of many more that I have encountered in the twelve years I consulted there.

2. Lewin, "Health Care System."

3. Hilps, "Public Hospital Wait"; Spiegel and Wielawaski, "Care Rationed."

4. This point is extensively made in Stout, *Ethics after Babel*, p. 13. This is not to ignore the new works in ethics, especially feminist ethics, that take a radically different view. By this comment, I, like Stout, intend the classic tradition, which advocates a language of moral disengagement as critical to evenhanded viewing of both sides of a dispute.

5. "The men, whatever their condition, lie there, and patiently wait till their turn comes to be taken," Winslow quotes Walt Whitman, poet and nurse, as recording. He adds that no rationale is offered for this system of treating a casualty on the basis of his place in the queue. See Winslow, *Triage and Justice*, p. 3.

6. Gerbert, "Why Fear Persists."

7. Molly Cooke, as reported in a speech at the conference "AIDS and Ethical Issues," a satellite conference of the 5th International AIDS Conference, San Francisco, June 1990.

8. Attributed to Phil Gramm by the *New York Times*, 29 December 1995, but heard all over Washington, D.C., in the fall of 1995 by this author.

Chapter 2

1. Ironically, when I began this work in 1991, I had a professional, white collar job with insurance that covered complete health care for myself and my dependents. As I wrote the final draft of the work, in the California depression of the winter of 1992–93, my employer decided, first, that he could no longer afford to cover my dependents on my health benefit plan and then that he could not provide health care benefits at all. I am fortunate to be married to someone who did have health coverage. My coworkers, however, were not so lucky. In fact, co-payments and deductibles increased for my spouse's coverage, since the

amount that the insurance company charges his employer rose steadily over the past years. What was an abstract problem has assumed very real proportions for millions.

2. Lumberg, "National Health Care Reform."

3. Late in the process of writing the dissertation that evolved into this book, another dissertation completed just ahead of mine came to my attention. Written by Mary Enid Pinkerson, it focused on the Oregon project, and, like my work, it identified the citizen-based initiative that generated the governance model as the key feature of the ethical importance of the work. (We both have lived for long stretches in Los Angeles. It is an interesting further parallel that when visiting Oregon in the process of doing research, we both were struck immediately by the intensity of the natural beauty of the place and the civic spirit of the participants in the project.) Pinkerson's work and friendship have been indispensable to my parallel project of searching for the philosophic grounding for the historical process she so eloquently described. I draw heavily on her interviews for the "thick narrative" she described in tracing the history of the health decisions movement. See Pinkerson, "Oregon Health Plan."

4. The timbering industry was affected by a combination of factors, including some federal regulation of cutting in response to a growing environmentalist movement horrified by the finality of the cutting of the old-growth forest, the destruction by clear-cutting of the most available and most accessible forests, and significant changes in the milling industry. The milling industry, created to do on-site conversion of the timber into lumber, faltered. There was a huge Japanese demand for Oregon timber, but milling costs in Japan were lower, in part, for the same reason that Japanese cars are cheaper: health care costs that need to be "built into" each job are lower because the Japanese worker's health care is covered by the Japanese government. A market developed for raw lumber that was shipped to Japan, milled, and then either used in Japan or shipped backed to the United States (even with shipping costs, the Japanese mills were competitive) for use in the housing industry. Meanwhile, the entire American milling industry was adversely affected by a decline in housing starts and construction in the late 1970s. Riding through the Oregon backcountry today, one sees small mills abandoned everywhere.

5. Some unemployed or underemployed workers managed to get jobs in the service sector, but the service sector, traditionally nonunion, has never offered health benefits to its workers. In California, for example, 93 percent of all workers are employed at sites with fewer than fifty workers. Hence, most employees work for small companies that can neither afford nor be forced under law to offer benefits. Fast food chains, franchises, and industries at the margin rely on a transient workforce outside the usual union profile. When large numbers of laid-off workers compete for these jobs and stand in long lines in the freezing cold to apply for them (as the news media documented again and again in the deepening recession of the 1990s), employers feel no pressure to offer increased benefits to lure workers.

6. Pinkerson, "Oregon Health Plan," p. viii.

7. In 1965, prior to laws prohibiting mandatory retirement age, the bulk of all workers actually retired by age sixty-five.

8. This percentage keeps climbing, as noted elsewhere.

9. And many do. In whole counties in the western United States, it is not possible to

obtain prenatal care by using Medicaid vouchers. In many cities the only option for care is in local hospital emergency rooms, an increasing number of which also do not accept Medicare patients after immediate stabilization.

10. Pinkerson, "Oregon Health Plan," p. 7.

11. Jane Brody, "Doctors Admit Ignoring Dying Patients Wishes."

12. Golenski, "Oregon Prioritization Experience."

13. Government Accounting Office, *Medicaid Expands*, pp. 2–6.

14. To some extent the legislators were not prepared for the volatility of the debate. When I met John Kitzhaber in the summer of 1988, he seemed confident that the logic of his plan would prevail. Armed with clear and beautiful slides neatly graphing the economics of the plan, he was enthusiastic about getting the necessary waivers and eager to hear what others thought of the ideas. Kitzhaber was direct and thoroughly engaged, proud of his work as a physician and a creative legislator, and ready to be taken on his own terms. He was a member of a variety of social and political organizations and wore lapel pins signifying his support of projects to end nuclear war and to defend endangered species. We met after a speech he gave detailing the Oregon initial proposal to a health care ethics conference sponsored by the group with which I then worked as a consultant, the Bioethics Consultation Group, in Berkeley, Calif.

15. I can speak with firsthand and ironic familiarity about experiences with the HSA. In 1977 I was a citizen representative on the local board in Berkeley, Calif. Like Crawshaw, I was a miserable participant in endless meetings to convince providers how little each hospital really needed their own individual CAT scanners and how services that *were* needed were not being provided.

16. Pinkerson, "Oregon Health Plan," p. 51.

17. Ibid., pp. 43–50.

18. Ibid., p. 50.

19. Garland and Hasnain, "Community Responsibility and the Development of Oregon's Health Care Priorities," p. 195. Quoted in Pinkerson, "Oregon Health Plan," p. 54.

20. Hines, "Health Policy on the Town Meeting Agenda."

21. Crawshaw, Garland, and Hines, "Oregon Health Decisions."

22. Pinkerson, "Oregon Health Plan," 26. Pinkerson cited Elazar, *American Federalism*, pp. 115–22, as quoted in Fox and Leichter, "Rationing Care in Oregon," p. 16.

23. This has been a major source of criticism of the formation of these "moral communities," as we shall discuss later. Charles Dougherty, among other critics, asked the question about difference: Would the process have been so sanguine if the citizen groups were not so neighborly or so homogenous?

24. Lynn is an ethicist and physician expert in issues of geriatrics and the end of life. She recalled this initial training session for me in 1991, in private conversation.

25. Crawshaw, Garland, and Hines, "Oregon Health Decisions."

26. Hines, "Health Policy on the Town Meeting Agenda." Hines's article was widely read and discussed by many persons interested in bioethics at that time. In it Hines noted and considered many of the issues that would later be pointed out as "new" critiques of the OHD—the problem of structural lack of concern for the poor, for example.

27. Pinkerson, "Oregon Health Plan," p. 62.

28. Jean Thorne, quoted in Pinkerson, "Oregon Health Plan," p. 65. Pinkerson also revealed how the pressure from the prospect of the university becoming a transplant center, the fact that only nine of the last nineteen patients had survived, and the expected need for thirty-four transplants at a cost of $2.2 million over a two-year period influenced the decision. It was, in effect, the first allocation decision.

29. Kitzhaber, "Oregon Experience."

30. O'Neill, "State Denies Funds for Two Transplants" and "Profiles: Oregonians Awaiting Transplants."

31. Egan, "Oregon Cut in Transplants Aid."

32. Golenski and Thompson, "Impossible Solution."

33. Rather than discontinue the transplant funding alone, he noted, the committee should review all the procedures that Medicaid was currently funding in light of outcomes data, professional medical judgment, and social values.

34. Ibid. The story has been recounted in great detail in a series of speeches made as reports to the Kaiser institutional ethics committees, at which the author was present.

35. Pinkerson, "Oregon Health Plan," p. 82.

36. Hines, "Health Policy on the Town Meeting Agenda." In a sidebar to Hines's report, Bruce Jennings of the Hastings Center staff detailed the several states where Health Decisions groups had been regularly meeting to discuss ethics and public policy.

37. Pinkerson, "Oregon Health Plan," pp. 76–77.

38. Crawshaw, Garland, and Hines, "Developing Principles for Prudent Health Care Allocation." Also as quoted in Pinkerson, "Oregon Health Plan," pp. 77–79.

39. Jonsen, "Bentham in a Box."

40. The highly nuanced and highly charged relationship between Golenski and the Oregonians, among them Kitzhaber and the leadership of OHD, and the relationship of all to the national ethics community and press corps are long and complex. These relationships are not the subject of this book, which is focused on the values emergent in the community-based process that shaped the Oregon project and how the notion of the common good in health care can be addressed. The story of how Oregon faced its health care crisis is as fascinating as it is detailed, however. Pinkerson's extraordinary doctoral dissertation retains both the cinematic quality of the entire narrative (she believes in thick description) and careful, thoughtful documentation of all the personalities and stories involved.

41. I was a consultant with the Bioethics Consultation Group from 1986 to 1993. I was not a direct part of the Oregon project, which occurred contemporaneously with the birth of my third son. The project was staffed principally by Golenski with support from Stephen Blum and Daniel Shostack.

42. In September, Golenski and some of his staff met with Kitzhaber to outline a plan for allocation.

43. In November, Golenski had met with Kitzhaber and with RAND corporation theorist David Hadorn (like Kitzhaber, an emergency room physician) in the Colorado offices of then-governor Richard Lamm. (Lamm had just received media attention for a controversial remark that the press interpreted to mean that the elderly had an obligation to "make room" for the young by voluntarily forgoing their access to health care.) Also present was

Gail Wilenski, then director of Project Hope and later head of the HCFA. Kitzhaber listened to all of their suggestions for additional details for his legislative proposal.

44. They would be working on a small pilot project with Golenski, Steven Blum, and the Medical Research Foundation of Oregon.

45. This effort was staffed by Golenski and Steven Blum, from the Bioethics Consultation Group, and the Medical Research Foundation of Oregon.

46. The plan was to rank all existing services and health care interventions that could be provided, whether covered or not, and to assess how to use tax dollars to render the greatest good to the greatest number. This purely utilitarian ranking was based on two different teleological goals. First, health care was ranked in order of its outcomes as reckoned by the providers, senior physicians, nurses, and social service administrators. Hence, a "good" health care service was one that accomplished a *provider* goal of an efficacious outcome. Its relative necessity was based on a largely intuitive sense of "what really worked in the field" (Golenski, "Grand Rounds"). Second, a health care service was ranked by a utilitarian criterion in which "good" was judged by the satisfaction or dissatisfaction the service was thought to have provided the consumer.

47. Service providers were grouped according to the patient population they served. These groups, roughly approximating stages in the life cycle, covered obstetrics and gynecology, pediatrics, adult medical/surgical (including trauma and mental health), and geriatrics (including chronic and long-term care). First, providers collectively gathered data and created an exhaustive listing of all services furnished to all patients in their service group. Services included those actually provided and those the providers themselves thought to be necessary to offer optimal care (e.g., nutrition supplements for all pregnant women and transportation vouchers for making clinic visits). At issue were the following questions: What do we do? What really works? What do we really need? The ranking was done first by provider intuition alone and then with input from the community via the values statements developed from the extensive work done by the OHD, and added to the health decision movement values clarification project. The Golenski project took three months to work through the extended lists generated by the providers. Most services, 82 percent in all categories, were assigned ranks of ten (90 percent were assigned ranks greater than seven, and 98 percent were ranked greater than four). Once again, transplants were ranked low at level three, which generally meant that they probably would not be funded. Golenski has said in later accounts that he came to disagree with this, adding that transplants were often efficacious, especially in pediatric cases. But at no time did he attempt to critique this problem, claiming later that he "felt he could not interfere with what he felt must be the fairly and democratically agreed upon process that he had created" (Golenski, "Grand Rounds"). There were other problems that became immediately apparent. In particular, his list included the ranking of all services to the disabled, the mentally ill, and the aged, along with the rest of the population. These most vulnerable populations were taken out of the Oregon Health Services Commission listing in response to citizens' groups concerned with the impact of these populations on the rankings. The ranking of services to these vulnerable groups was planned to be phased in more slowly, argued Kitzhaber after Golenski and Blum's report was submitted.

48. The plan was, first, to send the list of ranked services for actuarial accounting to

quantify the exact cost of each intervention based on the standard diagnostic codes already used by the Medicaid system. Then the costed and ranked list would be submitted to competitive, managed-care bidding. Half of all Oregon Medicaid recipients, under a previous waiver, were covered by HMO contracts.

49. This was one of the very few features of this plan that was actually retained.

50. Pinkerson, "Oregon Health Plan," p. 119: "The distrust of the grassroots for Golenski's project helped ensure that the plan which eventually emerged would involve an open and democratic process."

51. Ibid.

52. Hines, *Quality of Life in Allocating Health Care Resources.*

53. Ibid.

54. Ibid., p. 4.

55. Ibid., p. 5.

56. In Bellah et al., *The Good Society*, the authors make the point that it is a peculiarly American choice to tolerate such poor public space and services. In other societies, they note, "quality of life" hinges more on what is held in common rather than what is possessed by the individual. Hence, while they diminish individual income, high taxes provide superb parks and day care, for example—things that are shared—while in America public parks are places of at least some squalor and danger.

57. Hines, *Quality of Life in Allocating Health Care Resources*, p. 7.

58. Jennings, "Grassroots Movement in Bioethics," pp. 22–23.

59. Hines, *Quality of Life in Allocating Health Care Resources*, p. 6.

60. Ibid. The problem here is glaring. What if your ability to care for yourself has nothing to do with your assessment of life quality? What if you *like* to be bathed and shopped for? Why, further, is "shopping" not a category that interests or delights? Linking a good quality of life with the extent of successful, individuated self-sufficiency is a cultural decision, not a truth of the human spirit. It is temporally based and rooted in particular Western traditions about rugged individualism.

61. Ibid., p. 14.

62. Ibid., p. 9.

63. Here is a problem that the plan does not address and that will be discussed at length in Chapters 3, 4, and 8. If the majority is defined differently, the utilitarian principle changes. Hence, the majority could be, for example, people on Medicaid, the poor in the state, all taxpayers, all sick people, or all people potentially helped by health care services.

64. Jennings, "Grassroots Movement in Bioethics," p. 13.

65. This was Rawlsian choice without the veil of ignorance that Rawls thought necessary for rational actors to make completely equitable choices. This is an acontextual note: Rawls's work is the subject of the chapter on liberalism, but the reader may wish to refer back to this point to reflect on one possible application in practice. See Rawls, *Theory of Justice*, p. 136.

66. Hines, *Quality of Life in Allocating Health Care Resources*, p. 12.

67. Much of this coverage did not actually discuss the reality of the process or the ideas of the plan but reacted to the specifics of the list or the mere mention of rationing health care.

68. Again, for a complete account of the relationships and personalities involved, see

Pinkerson, "Oregon Health Plan." Pinney was disturbed by the Golenski project's reluctance to conduct its meeting in full public view and wanted both increased citizen and
media scrutiny of the details of the ranking decisions. Pinkerson wrote that it was the "elite"
nature of the Golenski project that led to a far broader view of citizen involvement in all
subsequent legislation. The decision to change significant aspects of the Golenski list was
clearly related to this increased involvement. First, the exclusion of the elderly and the
disabled for the first period (until 1993) and, next, the use of quality-adjusted life years with
costing as consideration differed from the Golenski idea.

69. Pinkerson, "Oregon Health Plan," p. 141.

70. Ibid., p. 142.

71. Ibid., p. 67.

72. Ibid., p. 147.

73. Hadorn, "Setting Health Care Priorities in Oregon."

74. Senate Bill 27, section 4a, codified under ORS 414.036. Pinkerson, "Oregon Health
Plan," also quoted these sections of text, clearly the central ones for defining the content of
the bill.

75. Eddy, "Oregon's Plan."

76. Golenski and Thompson, "Impossible Solution," p. 43.

77. Critically, however, an amendment linking the benefit package of state employees,
including the legislature, to the same level as the package available to persons on public
assistance was defeated.

78. Garland, "Justice, Politics, and Community," pp. 67–68. Garland was a pioneer as
well as a leading theoretician of the Oregon project, involved from the first with the
founding of the OHD and active as a representative throughout each step of the process.
Throughout the work, his clear-sighted view of the ethical conception of the process
enabled a high degree of consistency and history to illuminate the work. His article in the
Journal of Law, Medicine, and Health Care, cited above, is the clearest single summary of
both the history and the values of the project and demonstrates how his commitment to
communitarian philosophy continues to shape the work.

79. Ibid., p. 68.

80. Democratic governor Neil Goldschmidt selected the first panel.

81. Oregon Health Services Commission, *Prioritization of Health Services*, p. 4; also
quoted in Pinkerson, "Oregon Health Plan," p. 166.

82. Pinkerson, "Oregon Health Plan," p. 161.

83. Garland, "Justice, Politics, and Community," p. 71.

84. Pinkerson, "Oregon Health Plan," p. 170.

85. Garland and Hasnain, "Community Responsibility and the Development of Oregon's Health Care Priorities," p. 190, as quoted in Pinkerson, "Oregon Health Plan," p. 174.

86. Private conversation with the author and a speech to the annual meeting of the
Oregon Pediatric Nurse Practitioners Association, Portland, 1990.

87. Pinkerson, "Oregon Health Plan," p. 188.

88. Some of the initial criticism came from a helpful source, Hadorn, "Oregon Priority-
Setting Exercise," p. 13. Hadorn had been involved and supportive from the first meeting in
Denver, prior to the legislative session. Hadorn had long advocated a process that would

balance quality-of-life considerations, some understanding of the implication of cost, and a "hand adjusted" common sense intuition that included judgments from provider and consumer value discussions. The final listing relied more heavily on Hadorn's methodological suggestions.

89. Garland, "Justice, Politics, and Community," p. 69.

90. Ibid., p. 72.

91. This last point is of considerable interest. It is a key part of the Oregon method that there is an acknowledgment that untreated as well as treated conditions have a social and personal cost.

92. Pinkerson, "Oregon Health Plan," details this in full. The political debate has involved policymakers at the highest levels of the federal government, most notably the (unlikely) coalition of forces that spoke strongly against the waivers, then-senator Al Gore and the Children's Defense Fund on the left and the chair of the National Right to Life Committee on the right.

Chapter 3

1. What ought to follow from a determination of appropriate justice? Finally and critically, we persistently confront Churchill's question: In the face of competing needs and rights, what is the just choice?

2. Not all diseases are, of course, contagious. But I argue that most are irrationally perceived that way. See Sontag, *AIDS as Metaphor*, and others. AIDS, a disease with a relatively low risk of actual contagion, was at first widely perceived as casually contracted.

3. If it was not, all work would grind to a halt.

4. As I have noted in the detailed discussion of the Jewish tradition, this insight is at the core of the daily ethical practice.

5. As eternity receded in the popular consciousness, longevity moved to the fore. Among medieval Christians, eternity was a socially recognized need, and every effort was made to see that it was widely and equally distributed, that every Christian had an equal chance at salvation and eternal life. Hence there was a church in every parish, regular services, catechism for the young, compulsory communion, and so on. Among modern citizens, longevity is a socially recognized need, and increasingly every effort is made to see that it is widely and equally distributed, that every citizen has an equal chance at a long and healthy life. Hence there are doctors and hospitals in every district, regular check-ups, health education for the young, compulsory vaccination, and so on. See Walzer, *Spheres of Justice*, p. 87.

6. Hauerwas has noted this in *Naming the Silences*. Sontag has noted the power of illness as metaphor. But perhaps the most significant shift in this consciousness is the current trend to medicalize many conditions that in an earlier age might have been traced to spiritual depletion rather than to physical causes. For the problem of fatigue or generalized despair, we have seen a series of such namings: first low blood sugar, then PMS, then chronic fatigue syndrome, then environmental illness, allergies, and yeast in the body, for

example. All have been given as causes for very similar symptoms, but perhaps we should ask, "Why is it so tiring and at times so saddening to live in the modern world? And what can be done to change this?" My point is not that people "make up" fake symptoms, but that the naming of these experiences as "medical," and hence caused by something or someone and able to be fixed by something or someone, is a modern idea based in specific *language* about the body, about knowledge, and about what is real in the world.

7. This is Walzer's term.

8. On this basis Walzer makes his argument for an expanded welfare state where the standing and health of each person is not at stake in every medical encounter.

9. This issue is key. If it is largely unconscious discourse that produces such language, and hence such corresponding changes in the meaning of "needs," then what are the terms of the discourse itself? How ought this discourse to be conducted?

10. As a former clinician, I write this with painful certainty.

11. This last question is Churchill's Samaritan problem and the initial dilemma for any legislative body that addresses the issue. The Oregon legislature addressed the second issue in the most detail.

12. One could argue that one must be healthy to be a participant in a conversation, and the level of health required to meet this criterion would be the minimum level at which rights were set.

13. How this extends to public policy is also at issue. A multitiered system based on employment and income now exists. Ought this to be maintained, or ought a system of national health insurance to be instituted?

14. This is the principle of beneficence. Further, should this be decided by a direct health care provider or by someone further removed, such as a health plan manager?

15. This is the principle of autonomy or substituted judgment.

16. The issue emerges when organ transplants are performed. If the first organ transplant fails, then the patient is immediately placed on a priority list for a new (second) transplant because he or she is very critically ill, and the list is weighted by severity of illness and proximity to death. Some individuals get as many as three organs in this way. Each additional organ is less likely to work, tragically enough, because the body becomes progressively resistant to medication and deteriorated, and the organs themselves are from a differentially impaired pool. But the question remains: Is it the obligation to give each person a transplant, or is it the obligation to give each person a functioning liver?

17. Carol Robb raised a central point about rights when she read the first draft of this work. She advised me to be careful in my assessment of rights theory, noting correctly that Beverly Harrison and others have developed a rights-in-community conception that is distinct from the rights language of the (male) tradition and is central to some feminist theory, particularly the discourse of abortion rights and the right to be free of abusive familial relationships. In the field of bioethics, the rights language that has entered the discourse has been primarily from the classic liberal tradition. Harrison's use of rights is similar to Benhabib's. Here, the rights are the minimal requirements for entrance into a discursive community, rights to be equally heard and rights to be in a position of equal power in the discourse relationship. It is my contention that these rules for discourse are a

partial answer (they fall short of the conception of *dbq* in the Jewish tradition) to this problem. In the dialogue of the bioethics community, the term "rights" still means rights in relationship to the formal contract of citizenship and the authority of the legal standard.

18. As was noted by Hume in the discussion of distributive justice, there is no need for justice schemes in the Garden of Eden. The problem of distributive justice in health care emerges out of the recognition that there is not enough, ultimately, to allow for each person an unlimited and endless garden.

19. Churchill's most recent data reported that a full 60 percent of ICU survivors and families would want full-bore ICU care again, "even if the outcome were futile or the patient would be in a persistent vegetative state [PVS]." See Churchill and Danis, "Autonomy and the Common Weal."

20. As a consequence of this response, Carol Robb pointed out in comment on the first draft of this work, the freely functioning marketplace plus charity is the means of access to health care.

21. There are many sources that illustrate this. The most widely used is Beauchamp and Childress, *Principles of Biomedical Ethics*, chaps. 3, 5.

22. The doctor would be a torturer or an animal researcher. I do not mean to imply that these are the same! I simply mean that those are the only two options for unconsented care: either the intention of beneficence or the consent can be not a part of the relationship.

23. See Ramsey, *Patient as Person*. See also Spicker and Englehardt, *Philosophical Medical Ethics*.

24. This is referred to as gatekeeping in the extensive literature on the subject. See, for example, Veatch, *Theory of Medical Ethics*, esp. chaps. 1, 6.

25. See Chapter 2.

26. Not all Americans lived within the medical insurance safety net. For some, largely in the rural South, medical conditions have always been marginal, even in the 1960s and 1970s and times of relative abundance for most of the rest of the country.

27. Compare the Hippocratic origins of the principle of beneficence.

28. This includes the patient's responsibility to the community. Hence, as in Emmanuel Levinas's view of "responsibility to his responsibility," the provider must consider the citizenship of the other.

29. It was the power of the lobby of the American Association of Retired Persons that led to the creation of the federal Medicare program, the age-based entitlement programs to serve all Americans over age sixty-five, regardless of class status or accumulated wealth.

30. Callahan, *Setting Limits*, introduction and conclusion.

31. Hauerwas also used this language. His work is addressed extensively elsewhere, but I want to credit his similar critique of the Enlightenment as being largely responsible for basic errors in our way of perceiving medicine. See also Callahan. Callahan's position was made clear in a number of books and articles, but the most comprehensive account of this position is in *What Kind of Life*.

John Hardwig suggested that a further challenge to autonomy might be required. He indicated that the patient did not stand alone at the moment of medical encounter, but was linked to a family (variously defined) and a network of others whose needs ought to be considered. Hardwig called for a reexamination of the trumping notion of autonomy. See Hardwig, "What about the Family?," pp. 5–10.

Hardwig's argument was another compelling recognition that the philosophic premise of autonomy rests on a particular anthropological choice. In the system Hardwig suggested, the family's interest ought not necessarily to be trumped by patients' rights. No one member of the family could automatically prevail, even if he or she was ill. Hardwig's commonweal challenge was more limited: it was the smaller circle of the family that created a larger circle of responsibility. While not arguing for a principle of community, it is a related call for an examination of the problem of autonomy. Like Callahan's work, Hardwig's also suggested that the special relationship of the physician to the patient was more nuanced and permeable in the clinical setting than an autonomy-versus-beneficence relationship would explain.

Norman Daniels described the problem of justice as a function of lifetime commitments made between societies and individuals. He asked whether the "moral moment of medicine" could be seen as the extended choice over a lifetime rather than a series of choices made only at times of crisis. Daniels proposed that rational choices or "prudent judgments" could be made by agents concerned with fair shares over a lifetime. Daniels drew on Rawls's imagery of rational agents to suggest that persons could be asked to place themselves in a situation where they chose shares in lifetime provision. One could choose shares at the beginning of one's life or at the end, but not both. Underlying his language, however, is the assumption that resources are limited and could be adjudicated by a process held in common, that no one individual was "entitled" to every desire being met at every moment of desire, and that a fairly chosen process would enable a society to direct rationing choices. See Daniels, *Just Health Care*, pp. 56–59.

32. Churchill, *Rationing Health Care in America*, p. 57.

33. Locke, Rawls, and Nozick are contrasted with this: all shared the assumption that at the core of the human being is the necessity of rights, "holdings," and entitlement.

34. Ibid., p. 59.

35. Ibid.

36. He notes the use of the term "sympathy" in the work of Adam Smith and points to the tradition of sympathy in the works not only of Smith but of David Hume, Bishop Butler, George Herbert Mead, Harry Stack Sullivan, and theologian H. Richard Niebuhr.

37. Ibid., p. 64.

38. Ibid., p. 66.

39. Ibid., p. 101.

40. Ibid., p. 138.

41. Churchill and Danis, "Autonomy and the Common Weal."

42. All the respondents were over age fifty-five, and all had received extensive medical intensive care. The majority of the 160 patients and family members who were interviewed reported that they were "extremely willing" to undergo intensive care again for very brief periods of life prolongation: "Three-quarters of survivors who were interviewed were willing to undergo intensive care for one month of prolonged life." (Intensive care at this level costs nearly $10,000.00 a day.) Further, very few (4 percent) were unwilling to proceed with

intensive care at the outset. This is remarkable. Much of the assumption of the movement to codify autonomy in bioethics has been to insist on full informed consent of patients. In fact, there is a series of films and a cottage industry of publications to detail the complexity of the ICU for the uninitiated. Just beneath this effort is an unspoken assumption that an informed patient will likely refuse such dramatic and invasive technology. The research that Danis and Churchill cite tells us that the opposite may well be more accurate. Of course this means that ever more people will expect and desire ever more expensive technologies and that the pressure on the resources will be greater, not reduced, as some would argue.

43. It is the same critique that closes Churchill's earlier book.

44. Churchill and Danis, "Autonomy and the Common Weal," p. 27.

45. Ibid., pp. 25–31.

46. The plan's progress has at every juncture been given front page coverage in the *New York Times*.

47. One can only wonder what critiques would emerge if the actual in-place Medicaid system were to be proposed today.

48. For many years, it was my favorite argument.

49. Relman and Levinsky, "Is Rationing Inevitable?"

50. "Wasted Health Care Dollars."

51. Rothman, "Rationing Life."

52. Dougherty, "Setting Health Care Priorities," p. 5.

53. Dougherty, "Proposal Will Deny Services to the Poor," p. 30. This point was also noted in Pinkerson, "Oregon Health Plan," p. 312.

54. Caplan, "How Can We Deny Health Care to Poor?"

55. Many critics have pointed out this problem, potentiated because Oregon is named as an experiment in health care reform, and thus eligible for HCFA waivers. If it is an experiment, then are there controls and protection for the subjects? See Steinbrook and Lo, "Oregon Medicaid Demonstration Project," p. 342.

56. Menzel, "Some Ethical Costs of Rationing," p. 58.

57. Dougherty, "Ethical Values at Stake."

58. Steinbrook and Lo, "Oregon Medicaid Demonstration Project," p. 342.

59. Rothman, "Rationing Life," p. 36.

60. Friedman, "Rationing Healthcare," p. 13.

61. Meyer and McCormick, "Disability Law Fear," p. 8.

62. Bleich, "Jewish Entitlements of Valuing Life."

63. Hadorn, "Problem of Discrimination in Health Care Priority Setting."

64. This was the central reason for the ultimate denial of the HCFA waiver by the Bush administration: "Our principal concern is that Oregon's plan in substantial part values the life of a person with a disability less that the life of a person without a disability. The premise is discriminatory and inconsistent with the Americans with Disabilities Act." See Sullivan, "Oregon Health Plan Is Unfair to the Disabled." It is this aspect of the plan that appears to have been changed to win Clinton administration support.

65. Dougherty, "Ethical Values at Stake," p. 2410.

66. Winslow, "Watching Coby Howard Die," p. 24.

67. Menzel, "Some Ethical Costs of Rationing," p. 64.

68. Caplan, "How Can We Deny Health Care to Poor?"

69. Matthiessen, "Code Blue."

70. Capron, "Oregon's Disability," p. 19.

71. Dougherty, "Ethical Values at Stake," p. 2409.

72. Swartz and Aaron, "Achilles Heel of Health Care Rationing."

73. Relman, "Trouble with Rationing."

74. Menzel, "Some Ethical Costs of Rationing," p. 64.

75. Menzel, "Oregon's Denial."

76. Winslow, "Watching Coby Howard Die," p. 24.

77. Cleveland, "Redoing the Health Care Quilt."

78. Matthiessen, "Code Blue," p. 62.

79. Gillon, "Basic Ethics"; remarks as noted by the author from a panel presentation.

80. Jeane Friedman, former administrator for the Disability Rights and Education Fund, a national disability rights and defense fund, in a personal communication with the author summarized the reaction in the disabled community in the period 1989–92.

81. Steinbrook and Lo, "Oregon Medicaid Demonstration Project," p. 343.

82. Barber, "Role of the Responsible Citizen."

83. Garland, "Justice, Politics, and Community."

84. Callahan, "Oregon Initiative."

85. Roberts, "Bush Blows It on Health Care"; emphasis in original.

86. Paige R. Sipes-Metzler, quoted in a sidebar (unsigned), *Hastings Center Report* 21 (May/June 1991): 5.

87. Hadorn, "Setting Health Care Priorities in Oregon," p. 2224.

88. Carlson, "Doesn't Single Out the Poor."

89. Hadorn, "Setting Health Care Priorities in Oregon," p. 2224.

90. Crawshaw, letter to the editor.

91. Eddy, "Oregon's Plan," p. 2445.

92. Hadorn, "Setting Health Care Priorities in Oregon."

93. Eddy, "Cost-Effective Analysis." Eddy's main problem with the plan is that he believes that cost effectiveness ought to play a larger role in the ranking of services. But he stresses that effectiveness must have some sort of clinical measure.

94. Callahan, "Oregon Initiative," p. 16.

95. The problem of justice is not purely one of rational thought and will but is also a matter of sentiment and sympathy, as pointed out in Hume and Smith. This issue is given fuller treatment in the chapter on liberal theory.

Chapter 4

1. My claims are, I understand, perhaps larger than the claims of the organizers of the project.

2. Churchill, *Rationing Health Care in America*.

3. I wish to note that this account is deeply anti-Semitic, which was brought to my

attention by Daniel Boyarin. The Cohen and the Levy, honored among the Jews, ignore the ill person, and the non-Jew Samaritan, long the personification of the person to be feared and despised, is the one who in contrast helps. It is part of a long historical polemic against the "legalism" of the Talmud. Here, however, I believe that Churchill uses it in another spirit, that of crediting its potency as a folk tale of medicine, and it is in this sense that I respond.

4. In a critique of an earlier version of this book, Churchill pointed out that for many readers the following account will be a rehashing of ideas that have been presented over and over again. For some readers, it may be necessary to situate my next argument. For both reasons, my account will be a condensed review of the ideas presented.

5. Edwards, *Encyclopedia of Philosophy*, 3–4: 298.

6. Ibid.

7. Ibid., p. 301.

8. Ibid., p. 299. Stanley Benn adds, "and this is what distinguishes this from prudential judgment, in which the agent has a particular vantage point."

9. Lebacqz, *Six Theories of Justice*. In addition, I am grateful to Susan Rubin for her formulation of the issues in this chapter. Her suggestions on an earlier draft have been quite helpful. Rubin and I have used this formulation to explain justice theory to the professional staff of the Kaiser Permanente system since 1989. Her clarity and organization were invaluable in helping me to understand and construct this chapter.

10. Reading Aristotle, one is struck by the straightforwardness of the concept of justice: the unjust man takes more than his share. This notion of rationality, of knowing one's share, of limits on desire, seems particularly innocent to the modern sensibility.

11. We see this, of course, in the view of nonwhite peoples and women as "other" in systems of justice, such as in the foundational documents of the United States. Also see Lebacqz's work on justice and injustice. In *Six Theories of Justice*, Lebacqz reviews several theories of justice. Three are rooted in secular philosophy and three in theology. They illustrate what is central to the discourse.

12. What language is most useful to us in discussing this problem? There are limits to the currently available language. The recapture of older language, in which different cultural and social understandings of the person prevail, might offer a different answer to Churchill's call.

13. Churchill's question itself is not without a specific linguistic construct. Ought we to be asking more, or different, questions: the details of the journey, the condition of the road, the extent of social responsibility for that condition, the nature of violence in that society, and the moral meaning of wealth?

14. The purpose of the following section is not to effect a complete defense of each theory but, rather, to present the language of a representative figure from selected theories of justice in order to facilitate a more complete understanding of the context for the crisis in language that Churchill describes.

15. Veatch, *Foundations of Justice*, p. 143. Also see Sokel, "Allocation of Scarce Medical Resources," pp. 74–76.

16. Note that Locke lived prior to the historical veracity of absolute scarcity, since he was able to imagine a terrain of unlimited agricultural frontier: "31. . . . And thus considering

the plenty of natural provisions there was for a long time in the world, and the few spenders, and how small a part of that provision the industry of one man could extend itself and engross it to the prejudice of others, especially keeping within the bounds set by reason of what might serve for his own use, there could be then little room for quarrels or contentions about property so established" (Locke, *Second Treatise*, p. 17).

17. This theory is developed by the device of a male actor and springs from a specifically engendered self that is male as well as freely choosing.

18. Of course, the class was wildly larger than at any previous time in human history. I am grateful to Professor Samuel Haber on this point. For the first time in history, large numbers of men could actually hold property, a right not given to them by family heritage or theocracy, and participate in citizenship. That this right excludes most women and virtually all blacks does not diminish the power of the initial liberatory vision.

19. See Locke, *Second Treatise*, p. 54:

95. Men being, as has been said, by nature all free, equal, and independent, no one can be put out of this estate and subjected to the political power of another without his own consent. The only way where any one divests himself of his natural liberty and puts on the bond of civil society is by agreeing with other men to join and unite into a community for their comfortable, safe, and peaceable living one amongst another in a secure enjoyment of their properties and a greater security against any that are not of it. This any number of men may do, because it injures not the freedom of the rest; they are left as they were in the liberty of the state of nature. . . .

98. And this is done by barely agreeing to unite into one political society, which is all the compact that it, or needs be, between the individuals that enter into or make up a commonwealth.

20. It is critical to reflect at this juncture on the persistent problem of the gender identity of the self in philosophy. In Hobbes, Locke, and Rousseau, the self that is followed, whose life the reader is directed to be interested in, is the male gendered self. Jane Flax has been central in pointing out that the modern view of the natural law rested unequivocally on a view of the female that is passive and relegated to the role of sexual object and mother. Rousseau's state of nature is a description of a male free person who fathers children, then leaves women to raise them, presumably to be the next generation of leavers and leavees. Hobbes postulated a war of all against all, without consideration of the impossibility of the vision for women and children. And Locke described a human rational nature that had as its basis a disembodied rational being with no essential dependency demand, with only personal needs to fulfill. Women and children existed in this world as a part of the property relationship, as objects to be defended, hardly as independent moral agents. One cannot simply ignore this issue, reading "man" to signify "human," considering the moral agent to be a neutral, disengendered self. It is, of course, central to the flaw, the worm within the wood, as it were, to encounter this problem not simply as a historical necessity, but as a critical lacuna in philosophy itself.

21. Nozick, *Anarchy, State, and Utopia*, p. ix.

22. Nozick uses the example of crossing borders into other states. Since the state has no

simple right to compel this adherence to rules, even if they are required to maintain order, all such moments of the state's use of power ought be compensated for, using the market to address the problem of rights (note here the linkage of compensation and property with rights themselves).

23. Englehardt, "Rights to Health Care."

24. See Nozick, *Anarchy, State, and Utopia*, p. 8:

> The term "distributive justice" is not a neutral one. Hearing the term "distribution," most people assume that some thing or mechanism uses some principle or criterion to give out a supply of things. Into this process of distributing shares some error may have crept. So it is an open question, at least, whether re-distribution should take place; whether we should do again what has already been done once, though poorly. However, we are not in the position of children who have been given portions of pie by someone who now makes last minute adjustments to rectify careless cutting. There is no central distribution, no person or group entitled to control all the resources, jointly deciding how they are to be doled out.

25. In fact, the notion that there is a need for a system of distributive justice is called into question by this construct.

26. Nozick suggests that the natural order of things will result in the slow and inevitable creation of more and more "Protective Associations"; but still there would be many such, and there would always be other individuals whose particular choice would result in their being in some other minimal state.

27. Although one might offer the critique of the Oregon project as a problem with this theory, the citizens of Oregon are among the least taxed per capita in the country. This is one of the reasons that they are among the first to experience a budget shortfall in public goods and services. Several analysts have noted this and queried whether raising taxes could not more justly solve Oregon's problem. But all government is truly a balance of the consent of the governed and the public need. Witness the Boston Tea Party for the peculiarly American roots of such a struggle.

28. Of course, I believe in preventative health. I eat bran flakes, and I either exercise or feel guilty about not exercising. Yet it is philosophic principles, linked with Benjamin Franklin's homilies and the growing ideology of the mercantile class, that framed liberal theory that are at issue. For if one has the "ill luck" to become sick, there exists a faint sense of blame and a corresponding lack of collective responsibility for the outcome. Hence, if someone has cancer, it is not the responsibility of the EPA to change air quality, or pesticide manufacturing companies to explore nontoxic pesticide control; it is simply a just result of a series of fair exchanges that one person has made.

29. Lest one feel too incredulous at this point, one could reflect on the aftermath of Hurricane Andrew in the summer of 1992. Florida is a classic free-market, minimalist state. There are few regulations on housing, and safety codes, for example, are weak. The state had no power to compel people to evacuate for their own protection, and the state, despite being in the path of hurricanes, does not provide a comprehensive hurricane system. For days afterward, this laissez faire system played itself out: Floridians were reduced to hunting amid the rubble, with guns to protect their property. It was the war of all against all. The

much-resisted federal government finally sent troops days later. Yet, in the meantime, thousands of Floridians, as individuals, poured down the turnpike to donate baby formula and clothes—so many that there were traffic jams on the roads because "it could have been me" (in other words, because it was so unfortunate that this had happened).

30. There were several theorists associated with this particular language of justice. The focus of this review is not intended to address all of their work.

31. Mill, *Utilitarianism*.

32. Solomon and Murphy, *What Is Justice?*, p. 193.

33. Mill, *Utilitarianism*, p. 42.

34. "The feeling of justice might be a peculiar instinct, and might yet require, like our other instincts, to be controlled and enlightened by a higher reason" (ibid.).

35. Ibid., p. 407.

36. "The equal claim of everybody to happiness, in the estimation of the moralist and of the legislator, involves an equal claim to all the means of happiness except in so far as the inevitable conditions of human life and the general interest in which that of every individual is included set limits to the maxim; and these limits ought to be strictly construed" (ibid., p. 56).

37. Ibid., p. 553.

38. Ibid., p. 49.

39. Ibid., p. 50.

40. Ibid.

41. Each claim, appeal, or principle, from its own point of view, is unanswerable, and any choice between them, on grounds of justice, must be perfectly arbitrary. Social utility alone can decide the preference. See ibid., p. 53.

42. Ibid., p. 54.

43. Ibid.

44. "If everyone took one, there would not be any for all to use or to enjoy," one says to one's children. Of course, the tension in American society with the appeal of libertarianism is everywhere evident. Witness Yosemite National Park, so stripped of wildflowers (everyone has taken one) that some species have ceased to exist.

45. Mill honored not only happiness as a principle, but the notion of the common sense of humans.

46. Lebacqz, *Six Theories of Justice*, p. 29.

47. Baruch Brody, "Care of the PVS Patient."

48. Frankena stressed that deontologists can be "act-deontologists" or "rule-deontologists." Act deontologists stress internal intuition in each situation, trusting that intuition, a kind of universal internal conscience, will guide correct choice. Rules in this system are limited to "rules of thumb" or summary rules. Rule deontologists are the classic philosophical standard.

49. However, deontology has strong roots in the Jewish and Christian religious traditions.

50. "But what kind of law can this be the thought of which, even without regard to the results expected from it, has to determine the will if this is to be called good absolutely and without qualification? Since I have robbed the will of every inducement that might arise for it as a consequence of obeying any particular law, nothing is left but the conformity of

actions to universal law as such and this alone must serve the will as its principle. That is to say, I ought never to act except in such a way *that I can also will that my maxim should become a universal law*" (Kant, *Groundwork of the Metaphysics of Morals*, p. 73; emphasis in original).

51. Deontological theory is linked to the issue of rights. Brandt identified four kinds of rights: (1) prima facie rights, which are absolute if there is no competing duty or higher right; (2) moral rights, where somebody else is morally obligated (in the Kantian "ought" sense) to give you something; (3) legal rights, which create a sphere of autonomy; and (4) absolute rights, which, despite anything that anyone does, has, or says, are ideally yours. Rights assume obligation of others but power of the agent—they are a social promise.

52. While Nozick, as noted before, had strong elements of Kantian language in his work and drew clearly on the writings of Locke, it was egalitarianism, and social contract theory even more than libertarianism, that was associated with deontological approaches to justice.

53. Rawls, *Theory of Justice*, p. 3.

54. Ibid., p. 4.

55. Ibid., pp. 4–5.

56. Ibid., p. 5.

57. Ibid.

58. Rawls notes that this premise corresponds to the traditional theory of the state of nature in social contract theory but is hypothetical, rather than historical.

59. "One can say, in brief, that the circumstances of justice obtain whenever mutually disadvantaged persons put forward conflicting claims to the division of social advantages under the conditions of moderate scarcity" (ibid.).

60. Ibid., p. 12.

61. Rawls developed subsidiary principles: each generation would need to save for the next (just savings). Inequality would be attached to positions that would be changeable and available to everyone under condition of equal opportunity (affirmative action = equal opportunity).

62. "First Principle: Each person is to have an equal right to the most extensive total system of equal basic liberties compatible with a similar system of liberty for all" (ibid., p. 302). Rawls's first principle was based on the theory of equal standing of persons.

63. Note that in Rawls's language, it is the infringement of liberty that is key, not the economic or social well-being of the others, as in utilitarian systems.

64. This is the case because anyone could easily end up in the position of the least advantaged. Benefits accruing to a position are not enough; the mutability of position must also be assured.

65. "Second Principle: social and economic inequalities are to be arranged so that they are both:

a. to the greatest benefit of the least advantaged, consistent with the just savings principle, and

b. attached to offices and positions open to all under conditions of fair equality of opportunity" (ibid., p. 303).

66. This social contract allows for choices that will create a society that is fair in process, thus ensuring the greatest amount of both individual freedom and social cooperation.

Because liberty of the individual is prior to efficiency and welfare, Rawls argues that his principles of justice would be chosen lexically. Any compromise in equality, understood as access to liberty, must enhance the lot opportunities of those with the lesser opportunity. See ibid.

67. "The two principles mentioned seem to be a fair agreement on the basis of which those better endowed or more fortunate in their social position, neither of which we can be said to deserve, could expect the willing cooperation of others when some workable scheme is a necessary condition of the welfare of all. Once we decide to look for a conception of justice that nullifies the accidents of natural endowments and the contingencies of social circumstances as counters in quest for political and economic advantage, we are led to these principles" (ibid., p. 15).

68. Thus, this theory, in contrast to libertarian theories, identifies two lotteries when it addresses the problem of the distribution of health care resources. The first lottery is physical: the chance of the gene pool, of organ function, of good balance, and of t-cell resistance. Next is the lottery of the social and economic conditions into which each person, innocent and unchoosing, is born: the chance of parents, of neighborhood, and of the proximity to toxic waste dumps. The results of both lotteries are undeserved and, from the point of view of the infant, never selected.

69. For the health effects of being born black, see Stevens, "Racial Difference Found in the Kind of Medical Care Americans Get." For the differential effects of race on newborn birth size and corresponding mortality, see Wise, "Infant Mortality as a Social Mirror." In all health care parameters, from birth size, infant mortality, AIDS survival, cancer rates, and cardiovascular disease rates, being black is the single biggest risk factor. See also "Black-White Differences in Cervical Cancer Mortality"; "Life Expectancy Differences Widen"; Collins and David, "Differential Effect of Traditional Risk Factors."

70. "The principle of utility is incompatible with the conception of social cooperation among equals for mutual advantage. It appears to be inconsistent with the ideas of reciprocity implicit in the notion of a well-ordered society" (Rawls, *Theory of Justice*, p. 14).

71. There is no right to the details of human flourishing, or health care specifically.

72. Ibid., p. 21.

73. Veatch uses egalitarian theory for a specific application in health care, but his language provides a clear example of the application of this theory in general.

74. Veatch, *Foundations of Justice*, pp. 66–75. Veatch uses this term uncritically in his work, but I find it unacceptable. While Jews and Christians share some texts and some areas of theological agreement, the history, philosophy, and theology are distinct. The use of this term ignores syntactically the history of repressive persecution by some Christians of Jews on theological grounds and hence renders the term meaningless in any scholarly sense.

75. Ibid., p. 75.

76. The focus on process and motive marked both Rawls and Veatch as deontological, however, and distinct from either libertarians or utilitarians.

77. Lebacqz, *Six Theories of Justice*, p. 50.

78. How will secondary rules (derived from categorical imperatives) be ranked and competing prima facie duties categorized?

79. Hirshmann, "Freedom, Recognition, and Obligation," p. 1232.

80. Veatch approached this problem in his defense of egalitarianism, as noted above, but egalitarianism does not fully address the structure of a theory of justice he defended.

81. Hume, "Justice as Utility," p. 123.

82. Ibid.

83. The persistence of the philosophic necessity of scarcity is only one general parameter of the discussion. All theories are constructed to examine critically any single problem of distributive justice in light of the entire scope of all distributed benefits and burdens in any society. Any one problem of scarcity cannot be solved by manipulation of the distribution of other social goods.

84. Beauchamp and Childress, *Principles of Biomedical Ethics*. The authors certainly do not claim that the principles described in their work are exclusive, but it is to their work that an entire generation of ethicists has turned in seeking language of the discourse.

85. Often the discourse about justice proceeds as though justice is an abstract conception, a thing outside the text of the human story everyone (even philosophers) shares and lives out. Yet justice as device in the text of this story cannot stand alone as symbol and sign. As Lebacqz and others point out, the moral location of the actors in the social world determines the method of justice and its use. In fact, a critique of the Oregon process was precisely this: that the process employed by the policymakers in that state was to utilize a group of outsiders applying their values to problems of the actual embodied poor. The group of decision makers then remained external to the story and thus untouched by the results.

Hence, the first question must focus on this problem: *Who owes what to whom?* This is a restatement of whether there is a philosophic basis for entitlement and rights for social goods. Phrasing the question in this way creates a different paradigm because at issue is obligation that is prior to and, in fact, the ontological basis for rights.

Chapter 5

1. Taylor, "Atomism."

2. Hirshmann, "Freedom, Recognition, and Obligation," p. 1227.

3. Ibid.

4. The starting point for an understanding of liberalism is the notion that there is a distinctive liberal way of life, characterized by the aspiration to increase and enhance the prerogatives of the individual; by maximal mobility in all directions, throughout every dimension of social life (in and out of particular communities, in and out of particular social classes, and so on); and by a tendency to turn all areas of human activities into matters of consumer preference—a way of life based on progress, growth, and technological dynamism. See Beiner, *What's the Matter with Liberalism?*, p. 23.

5. Baruch Brody, *Life and Death Decisionmaking*, p. 78.

6. Benhabib, "Communicative Ethics," p. 333. Benhabib here is analyzing the school she is about to critique. She associates the three strains of this position with the neoconser-

vative (loss of moral bounds), the communitarian (loss of community), and Hans-Georg Gadamer (phronesis) and identifies this position as neo-Aristotelian.

7. According to Sandel, "Justice and the Good," p. 166,

> And insofar as our constitutive self understandings comprehend a wider subject than the individual alone, whether a family or tribe or city or class or nation or people, to this extent they define a community in the constitutive sense. And what marks such a community is not merely a spirit of benevolence, or the prevalence of communitarian values, or even certain "shared final ends" alone, but a common vocabulary of discourse and a background of implicit practices and understandings within which the opacity of the participants is reduced if never finally dissolved. . . . Insofar as justice depends for its pre-eminence on the separateness or boundedness of persons in the cognitive sense, its priority would diminish as that opacity faded and this community deepened.

8. Ibid., p. 167.

9. Ibid., p. 168.

10. Ibid., p. 170.

11. Bellah, *Habits of the Heart*. The following is a summary of the main arguments from the book. Note the introduction, pt. 1, and the conclusion.

12. It was Alexis de Tocqueville's question in his nineteenth-century analysis of American society as well, and Bellah used de Tocqueville's journey as an organizing principle and title for his work. Yet this focus raises its own problems. Bellah's method focuses on white, middle-class Americans. He notes this as a limitation but proceeds to discuss American culture as though there can be *an* American cultural norm apart from the deep divisions of race, gender, and class that so fundamentally construct the American character.

13. These themes appear consistently in American culture.

14. This model requires citizen participation and small governing units.

15. Whitman's radical departure exemplifies this latter model, as opposed to Franklin, the exemplar of utilitarianism.

16. The independent citizen represents a character based on mores, a fusion of biblical republicanism and utilitarian values whose moral life made the growth of small towns possible. The entrepreneur is a different character, capable of separation of self, of public and private, and of home and work. This character made possible the growth of capitalism and created the need for managers, a third type of critically competent American character able to manage effectively both things and people. The final model for Bellah's schema is the therapist, who manages the fit (or lack of fit) between organization of self and organization of work, relationships, and meaning.

17. Citizenship is both the place of success, which is individual and based in individual effort, and joy, which is the realization of human unity and fellowship.

18. Bellah then elaborates on this history. The 1880s solutions envisioned some change within an industrial society where public order, moral worth, welfare, and authority would be upheld. Two visions of this order were debated. An establishment resolution was suggested by the language of noblesse oblige of the ruling class, which had recently retreated

from stark competition and social violence to a settled consolidation of power. This language was rooted in large institutions, private donations, and personal negotiations by charismatic leaders.

Populism was another social vision. Its language stressed such constructs as "the people," face-to-face struggle, community of equals, biblical language, and mystical and sectarian religious groups as opposed to established religions.

The early twentieth century offered two other visions of the public good: neoconservatism and welfare liberalism. Neoconservatives had a "virtue theory" that postulated greed as the virtue. They organized a theory around this virtue, using the free market as the means of regulating the natural society.

Welfare liberalism trusted the government to balance the marketplace and create fairness. Compassion in this system was to be expected, but so was loss. All could be accommodated by economic expansion. Here the ideal was fairness (expressed in different ways by Rawls, Franklin Roosevelt, and John Kennedy) and justice. The notion was that a fair community could provide the social space to achieve private goals. Community meant personal security and free choice in the service of progress as a solution to scarcity.

As this economic reality diminished, two alternate visions were proposed: the administered society and economic democracy. Both these visions of the public good were basic to efforts to set up something new. Expertise and balancing of interest groups in the service of a great good were stressed by these competing world visions.

19. "Social ecology" is Bellah's term for this coherence.

20. Bellah and his colleagues followed *Habits of the Heart* with *The Good Society*. In this book the authors described the specific language of the discourse of citizenship more fully. They cautioned against possible misunderstandings of their use of the term "community" in their first book to refer to a narrow construct of "only face-to-face groups." The authors meant to include the larger social institutions "in which Americans live, like the state, and the economy," to be important in considerations of community as well. To address this issue they called for a politics of "attention" in public life. Democracy challenged our ability to call fully on the resources of intelligence, feelings, and moral sensitivity. See Bellah et al., *Good Society*, conclusion, pp. 254–87.

21. This is in the Niebuhrian sense.

22. To my mind the only communitarianism that allows us to escape the pluralist quandary that I have described is a community of discourse, where the very possibility of public talk about a world we share confers an experience of substantive citizenship. According to this conception, the public world itself as a locus of shared concern rescues us from the fragmentation and moral anarchy of a liberal-pluralistic universe. See Beiner, *What's the Matter with Liberalism?*, p. 35.

23. Carol Robb, in helpful comments on an earlier draft of this book, noted that this was a managerial viewpoint, certainly that of the dominant ideology and not a workers' viewpoint, which tends to have more appreciation for social solidarity. My intent is to note the power of the dominant ideological language.

24. The paradigm has particular meaning in the American context. It is helpful to look at literature for the elaboration of the U.S. moral agent. American literature and ideology are

paradoxical on the question of exactly who the agent ought to be. As Bellah et al. noted in *Habits of the Heart*, the language of individualism and the language of biblical republicanism exist as themes in contradiction and coexistence in the American character. In similar ways the outstanding moral agents of American fiction both coexist and compete as voices of the moral and of the just.

There is a tradition of the hero as individual, with Melville the first American writer to define it. He placed his Ishmael at the center of the sea, utterly alone, as isolated narrator. The hero, Ahab, is a complex, isolated, driven man. Ahab is the lone actor on a quest of rightness in the universe. The odds are impossible; the task, unstoppable. This tradition cuts a clear and unbroken path across the genre. The quintessential American hero is a cowboy, coming from beyond the horizon to confront injustice, single-handedly fixing the problem by an act of individual courage (the Aristotelian virtue of gentlemanliness in nineteenth-century garb), and retreating afterward beyond the (seemingly) limitless horizon. Where he comes from and where he goes is outside human community (indigenous peoples do not figure very highly in this schema). The members of the saved world—the farms, the children, and the rooted lives—continue living as before. They are not the moral agents; they are the subjects of agency. Justice is made for them, on their behalf. It is not something that concerns in any embodied way the moral agent himself.

This is also the tradition of detective fiction, which is, like the American western, another indigenous American art form. Much of the action of detective fiction is the journey in the dark, both literally and figuratively, of the lone man, able to trust no one fully and accountable, ultimately, only to himself.

There is another literary tradition of embeddedness, of immersion, in the community itself, however. This tradition of community, of particular place and story, emerges from turn-of-the-century immigrant fiction in the work of Anzia Yezierska, Henry Roth, and others.

Whitman, identified by Bellah as typifying the expressive individualist with his poetry of romantic merger with nature, can also be said to represent a counter to the Melvillesque model. Consider his Civil War writings, where the actual work created the details of the actual text. Whitman worked as a nurse. His choice for justice and moral action was rooted in his own family, in his neighborliness. The language of justice in American social policy and in American bioethics reflects this dialectic. Rawls and Nozick, twentieth-century theorists coming from opposite sides of the spectrum in terms of their solutions to the problem of justice, were in a deeper sense heirs to this tradition of agency. Both postulated a choice made with consequences that would predominantly affect the life of the individual understood as an individual.

25. Hauerwas has many counterparts in the larger world of Christian ethics. One that I believe is most interesting in this context is the Mennonite John Yoder. For Yoder, the sectarian community was the social ground of ethics itself. The redemptive act of nonviolence and pacifism has its real meaning in creating a resistance community that, by its message and example, will triumph over the power of history by letting go of the will to control everything in history.

Yoder's community is also an elect. A new creature—a human being empty of self, pride, and power—is created by the renunciation of "effectiveness" in history. The community thus created is one where true commitment and recognition of the other are possible. The real work of the religious person of faith is the radical "war of the lamb." Yoder pointed out that this vision of redemption makes sense only if Christ really was/is the master, if the Christ story is true, and if resurrection happened. Of necessity this limits Yoder to believing Christians.

Yoder asserted that the message need not be universal to be true. He believed in progressive redemption—that the "hereafter is later on this road," that the redemption is an act in human history that has already begun and whose manifestation is revealed in the present actions of community, in recognition or responsibility, between friends and companions along the way.

26. Although in "Communitarians and Medical Ethicists" Hauerwas hotly denied the charge that he is a communitarian and a bioethicist, his contributions to the field have been remarkably persistent for two decades and have in part shaped the discourse of ethics in the arena of health, medicine, and healing.

27. In private conversation with the author in the fall of 1992, Hauerwas noted that other believing communities exist with differing tasks but corresponding parameters—for example, the Jewish community.

28. Because Hauerwas is a Christian theologian, the place of Christ is very important. He was careful in his writing to locate Christ at the "center of life," and he cautioned against a generalized sense of "community" without this specific content. Along with Calvin and Edwards, he contended that the character and the journey of the self can be seen only in the evidence of good works in community—that is what wholeness will bring. A real renewal of self is made when one is justified and sanctified by God's grace. Sanctification itself is the subjective change in persons as they make virtuous choices to act in the real and specifically responding, contextual world.

Language is important here. The language of faith enables the moral agent to see the world in a new way and to undertake and act on the premise that the divine acts (the indicative) and what our obligations are (the imperative) can be unified as character-forming events if we understand that the indicative is part of the imperative itself.

29. Hauerwas, *Naming the Silences*, p. 148. Indeed I am not sure if such an America ever existed and, even if it did, whether it was a good thing. The "longing" for community so prevalent in our time, from my perspective, is but the working out of liberal theory and practice. Accordingly I fear all appeals for community as an end in itself. For communities formed by the alienated selves created by liberalism can too quickly become a kind of fascism. No one should want community as an end in and of itself but because the forms of cooperation offered by those communities provide for the achievement of goods otherwise unavailable—such as the worship of God. See Hauerwas, "Communitarians and Medical Ethicists."

30. Hauerwas, "Communitarians and Medical Ethicists," p. 11.

31. "What we are able to discern and do results from our participation in various communities. A variety of social worlds have shaped us, determined our general bearing in life, even engendered our specific responses to issues. We cannot and do not muster moral

insight for ourselves by ourselves apart from our communities, any more than we are or can be human beings apart from others. Everything we know about morality and the moral life, or anything else, for that matter, is finally a community enterprise and achievement" (Birch and Rasmussen, *Bible and Ethics in Christian Life*, p. 18).

Birch and Rasmussen, both Lutherans, talked about the issue of authority as power. Authority is given via Christ in scripture because of God's power: it empowers/authorizes those to whom he spoke. However, they noted that all scripture is directed at communities, at peoples with common vision and common tasks. Jesus spoke to an actual, real group; he made a community in history. The call *to* community is the call of all the prophets.

32. In this Birch and Rasmussen are like Hauerwas, who also saw community as setting context.

33. Birch and Rasmussen continue:

While it is true that individuals are not simply community clones, are unique and may well rise well above the moral level of their communities, it is true with equal force that even the most private decision and achievements are the results of our social experience and could neither exist nor be understood apart from that experience. The word "conscience" nicely illustrates this. While we often depict conscience as the individual's "still small voice" within, the etymological meaning betrays its true source. Com + scire means "knowing in relation" or "knowing together." [*Bible and Ethics in Christian Life*, p. 18]

34. The paradigm of the responsive community is a legacy from the work of H. Richard Niebuhr. Hauerwas, Yoder, and Birch and Rasmussen all owe to Niebuhr in part the understanding of the self as in responsible relationship to the moral whole. Hence, while not analyzing his complete argument, below I note some basic Niebuhrian points that emerge as implied centerpieces in the work of those who follow. Niebuhr's community is broader and less specific than the community described by Hauerwas or Yoder. He believed in the reality of the Christ experience but at critical moments tended to universalize Christian ethics as simply an ethics of response for all people. In most instances, however, Niebuhr claimed the historical, cultural, and religious clarity that led him to understand that his ethical stance came from his life as a Christian in community. The final step in his method of ethical reflection is central in emphasizing the importance of community. He postulated the importance of social solidarity. By this he meant that every ethical act is ultimately judged as good and right (as redemptive-directed) by the constant and durable community of others. For Niebuhr, all actions take place and are judged by this constant community.

Sharing language, sharing outcomes, and sharing worldview are only some of the ways in which acts assume communal life. Niebuhr's responsible self can only exist in society. Every act is understood only because of its relationship to the society, history, and moment in which it arises. Every action is *one* act amidst a world of actions and possible choices.

Finally, the Christian community understands that death has no final dominion over action in the world. Redemption in this community will be understood not only as social solidarity, but also as participation in the paschal mystery of reconciliation.

35. In fact, the individual relationship of self to God is usually the hallmark of Luther, Calvin, and the theologians traditionally associated with Protestantism. For the purpose of this book I am deliberately seeking only the sources that are critical of individualism. I am aware of the weight and measure of the traditional texts.

36. John Mahoney, a Jesuit scholar, wrote post–Vatican II of the necessity to go beyond the specific language of natural law in reflecting on ethics. Natural law, historically the basis for the language of the ethical casuistry and principle in Catholic teaching, is not a sufficient ground on which to base ethics, claimed Mahoney; an understanding of faith, or consciousness, and of new social demands is needed. He wanted us to understand how charity, as a "gift of self," is central to ethics. Mahoney used the word "totality" to express the good understanding that humanness and totality of persons must be considered in ethics. His totality meant that he would use a "wider lens" that would include consequences of acts, the whole Christian church (not just Catholics), and the whole order of nature, as in Aquinas, to define and consider what is the right and good act. He stressed not only totality but diversity and mystery in his proposal for moral theology. Like Hauerwas (and Augustine) his metaphor was of pilgrimage; he made the claim that diversity is the power behind positive change in social ethics. His discussion of diversity led to a consideration of the key part played by *koinonia* in the creation of an ethics of community.

37. Mahoney believed the Paulist idea of *koinonia* was a new contribution of the early church and that these fellowships were not a part of Judaism: "Entirely absent from the Old Testament [*sic*] as a description of men's [*sic*] relationship with God, or with each other in God's purpose" (Mahoney, *The Making of Moral Theology*, p. 343). This, however, is not true. Historically, there were other Jewish sects who lived in community, but let us allow him this.

According to Mahoney,

> The work of revealing God's sons and daughters is summed up in the equally
> Pauline idea of koinonia, or "the fellowship of the Holy spirit" . . . which has come
> into such prominence in recent years as almost a rediscovery made by the
> ecumenical movement about the nature of the Christian community. . . . The term
> koinonia and its variants denote a passive and active sharing of God's gifts by
> individuals and among individuals, characteristic of the earliest disciples and of their
> material help collected for the Jerusalem church, as well as the spiritual blessings in
> which the gentiles "have come to share." It is expressive, further, of a corporate
> solidarity, and a solidarity in something received. [Ibid., p. 143]

38. He invited all humanity who share in Christ's fellowship to participate, because all are created in God's image.

39. The norm of autonomy and the vision of contemplation are clearly not sufficient for any of these religious ethicists. What distinguishes them is the necessity of sociability, the need to do the work of reshaping the world, not alone, not alone with God or Christ, but as essentially linked to your fellow.

40. Sandel, "Justice and the Good," p. 173.

41. Hobbes, *Leviathan*, p. 103.

42. According to Hobbes,

Whensoever a man transfers his right or renounces it, it is in consideration of some other right reciprocally transferred to himself or for some other good he hopes for thereby . . . *Contract*. The mutual transferring of right is that which men call CONTRACT. There is a difference between transferring of right to the thing and transferring—that is, delivery—of the thing itself. For the thing may be delivered together with the translation of the right, as in buying and selling with ready money or exchange of goods or lands, and it may be delivered some time after. [Ibid., p. 106]

43. The assumption creates language that describes the forces of the market as opposed to the language of intimate human relationship.

44. Hirshmann, "Freedom, Recognition, and Obligation," p. 1239.

45. Sumner, *Moral Foundation of Rights*, p. 1.

46. Obligation and duty are linked to the term "entitlement," and it is here that language is key. There is, of course, no entitlement without a corresponding obligation, just as there is no right without a duty. Yet these terms are often split apart.

47. According to MacIntyre, *After Virtue*, p. 250,

[Nozick's] scheme of justice being based exclusively on entitlements can allow no place for desert. . . . It is in any case clear that for both Nozick and Rawls a society is composed of individuals, each with his or her own interest, who then have to come together and formulate common rules of life. In Nozick's case there is the additional negative constraint of a set of basic rights. In Rawls's case the only constraints are those that a prudent rationality would impose. Individuals are thus in both accounts primary and society secondary, and the identification of individual interests is prior to and independent of the construction of any moral or social bond between them.

48. MacIntyre noted a central point about "entitlements" and "needs." "Rawls makes primary what is in effect a principle of equality with respect to needs. His conception of the 'worst-off' sector of the community is a conception of those whose needs are greatest in respect of income, wealth and other goods" (ibid., p. 251). Questions remain that are not answered by this discourse. Are needs self-expressed or defined from the outside? Is an objective assessment of need even possible? What is the rank ordering of human need? Is the language of need "I must have or I will die or become seriously impaired," or can it mean "I must have and desire even if it will not help"? Consider the case where two patients in an ICU need a ventilator to breathe. One can recover from acute respiratory distress; one will die in a week in any case. Both need to breathe. Do we then judge depth of need by outcome of assistance to the need?

49. Ibid., p. 248.

50. Walzer's work is critical to other discussions in this book. As a theorist who writes about political science, as a philosopher associated with communitarianism, and as a political scientist who writes extensively about the Jewish community as a model for praxis and as possessing a language tradition that is critical in shaping ideology, his contributions to the challenges to the language of liberalism have been impressive. Here I focus on a specific language developed by Walzer, that is, the meaning of "membership" in the community itself.

51. Walzer, *Spheres of Justice*, p. 66.

52. Ibid., p. 65.

53. Ibid., p. 78.

54. Only its culture, its character, and its common understandings can define the "wants" that are to be provided for. But culture, character, and common understandings are not givens; they do not operate automatically. At any particular moment, the citizens must argue about the extent of mutual provision. See ibid.

55. Ibid., pp. 205, 210.

56. Walzer continues:

Here then is a more precise account of the social contract: it is an agreement to redistribute the resources of the members in accordance with some shared understanding of their needs, subject to ongoing political determination in detail. The contract is a moral bond. It connects the strong and the weak, the lucky and the unlucky, the rich and the poor, creating a union that transcends all difference of interest, drawing its strength from history, culture, religion, language and so on. Arguments about communal provision are, at the deepest level, interpretations of that union. [Ibid., p. 82]

57. It would seem at first glance as though the rich would, of course, always "provide" for the poor, that taxes and resources are directed in the public sector toward persons most indebted to the public hand. Consider for a moment the societies of the Industrial Revolution, the antebellum American South, or the period from 1980 to 1990 in the United States. These periods actually reflected a shift in real earned income from the least comfortable to the most comfortable. Walzer's point is that the process of deciding distributive justice is not democratic; the results will inevitably result in shifts of this sort.

58. Beiner, *What's the Matter with Liberalism?*

59. Ibid.

60. Hirshmann, "Freedom, Recognition, and Obligation," p. 1233.

61. Personhood is so strongly linked to rationality that its absence, as happens in severe neurological disease or injury, calls into question the entire moral standing of individuals, the weight of their moral appeal for society's help and resource allocation.

62. By the twentieth century this notion was supported by the entire field of psychology.

63. Hume noted the influence of the subjective but understood the rational will as mastering it. It was the dominant tone of liberal philosophy that the choosing will was the ideal and the precondition for social order in any social contract. See Hume, *Treatise of Human Nature*, p. 57.

64. It was a central aspiration of the Enlightenment to provide for debate in the public realm standards and methods of rational justification by which alternative courses of action in every sphere of life could be adjudged just or unjust, rational or irrational, enlightened or unenlightened. So, it was hoped, reason would replace authority and tradition. See MacIntyre, *Whose Justice?*, pp. 6–7, cited in Hauerwas, *Naming the Silences*, p. 53.

65. This section is a condensation and interpretation of Hauerwas, *Naming the Silences*, chap. 2.

66. Hauerwas explores at length what happens when illness is chronic, or when at stake

is not infectious disease but hereditary mental retardation, as with children born with Trisomy 21 (Down's Syndrome). In this work he again explores the problem of the meaning of the difference imposed by the "suffering presence" of the vulnerable and the responsibility of the responding world.

67. Hauerwas, *Suffering Presence*, p. 167.

68. Hauerwas constructs the moral project in the language of the encumbered self, a self aware of and concerned with the effects of injustice, while he remains alert to the capacity of a responding community to address, not eliminate, injustice. His work is about injustice, not distribution, but it is invaluable in the attempt to reclaim the sensibility of the common good as a common project for good.

69. Ibid., p. 132.

70. Flax, *Thinking Fragments*, pp. 3–187.

71. Ibid.

72. Ibid., p. 41.

73. Beiner, *What's the Matter with Liberalism?*, p. 24.

74. Of the many languages that regard the problem of the limits of liberalism to cope adequately with the praxis of distributive justice, the discourse of communicative or discourse ethics clearly directs the project of alternative language for the application of philosophy in the actual world of the clinical. This language most clearly influences the direction of the next section of the work on ethics and language in the problem of the distribution of health care. The application of the insights of the ethics of the discourse as addressed by the tradition of Jewish thought offers the best hope for a new language of ethical reflection.

75. The richness of her language adds yet another dimension to the moral vocabulary of community itself.

76. Dallmayr, introduction to *Communicative Ethics Controversy*, pp. 8–9.

77. "Act only on that maxim through which you can at the same time will that it should become a universal law" (Kant, *Groundwork of the Metaphysics of Morals*, p. 73). (Is this act universalizable? Is it an act I would accept as moral if applied not only to myself, but to all situations?)

78. Benhabib, "Communicative Ethics," p. 331.

79. Since communicative ethics is usually constructed in opposition to the neo-Aristotelian and neo-Hegelian communitarian thinkers just described as being the source of much of the language of community that I find central to a new discourse of ethics (Taylor, MacIntyre, Sandel, and Walzer), I want to isolate the features of Benhabib's position that are specifically useful to my argument. At the same time, I am alert to the general frame of her argument that the modern split between Kantian- and Aristotelian-inspired traditions may no longer be useful.

80. Ibid., p. 336.

81. Ibid., p. 339.

82. Ibid., p. 352.

83. Ibid.

84. Banking! State Security! Health Care Policy!

85. Ibid., p. 359.

86. Benhabib, *Situating the Self.*

87. Ibid., p. 12.

88. Benhabib contrasted her position from the regretful yearning of the communitarians for the loss of the common moral tradition, for particular community of meaning.

89. The school of philosophy that is charted by postmodernism draws from the varied sources noted in this chapter.

90. One might even say "a parallel universe."

Chapter 6

1. Childress and Macquarrie consider this a "misleading term" in *Westminster Dictionary of Christian Ethics*, s.v. "middle axioms." Perhaps a better description would be a coined term: "middle processes."

2. For this phrasing I wish to thank Peter Ochs in a virtual conversation on the Post-Modern Jewish Philosophy Group Internet Discussion, March 1995.

3. The term "social location" was developed extensively in a course in ethics methodology at the Graduate Theological Union in Berkeley, Calif., in the spring of 1988. Professor Charles McCoy stressed that this term, linked to the word "loyalties," as used later, was a primary tool in the examination of method. Unless we understand and appreciate the social location of the text and our own social location as we evaluate it, we are in danger of misreading the intent of the theory itself. My thanks to Dr. McCoy for his insistence on this point.

4. Robb, "Framework for Feminist Ethics." The terms used were presented at a seminar on feminist ethical method at the Graduate Theological Union in the spring of 1988. They are discussed in several places in Robb's work on feminist ethics.

5. Levinas, "The Face."

6. Herb Basser, as noted on the Post-Modern Jewish Philosophy Network (see n. 2 above).

7. John Puddefoot, from a discussion on the Post-Modern Jewish Philosophy Network (see n. 2 above). In this posting, Puddefoot reminds us that authoritative texts ought to be regarded as living texts carried along by a tradition that simultaneously qualifies them and is itself qualified by them.

8. Plaskow, *Standing Again at Sinai.*

9. Plaskow's work itself is not the only text that urges the reclamation of this voice. Many do. For an excellent and personally detailed reflection on the entrance of women into the world of rabbinics and Torah study, Vanessa Ochs, *Words on Fire*, is important reading. Ochs's point is that the traditional exclusion of women is not inherent to all texts. A careful reclamation is possible if women are taught to study seriously and if men equally regard the task of examining the troubling texts and traditions as fundamental. My thanks to Dr. Elliot Dorff who suggested this resource to me.

10. Buber, *Israel and the World*, p. 33.

11. Plaskow, *Standing Again at Sinai*, pp. 1–10. As Plaskow pointed out, this focus had been used by apologists for the exclusion of women at the deepest level from the language

of the dialogue itself, to which Buber's quotation, cited above, testified. Plaskow's point here is that the realm of the family is important but it is no real substitute for an actual role in the polis. She is correct. My point is a much narrower one, that given the limited terrain assigned to women in the tradition, it is of some significance that the terrain is at least highly valued. It was not simply the exclusivity of the gender-exclusive language. Buber stressed that the details of the daily circumstances were holy yet at the same time reified their place in the hierarchal order.

12. Levinas, "The Pact," p. 202. Daniel Boyarin, in his reading of this paragraph, reminded me that painfully little of this ideal is realized in modern Jewish reality. This is true, but the fact that it is embedded in the texts means that every Jew who reads and prays from them seriously at least has to reflect on them again and again during the course of every day.

13. The exceptions, notably but not exclusively the Muslim world before 1492 in Spain, are noted elsewhere in this chapter, in the discussion of Biale's work.

14. The terms of Greek analysis do not precisely fit the Jewish system.

15. This mode applies for all other norms as well.

16. In fact it is essential to remember that much of the case law turns on elaborate constructs that never happened, or could never be expected to happen. Much of the law concerning the role of the court in judging a murderer can be seen in this way (which, by the way, needs to be understood wherever the text is used to interpret actual historical circumstances; this is one of the major sources of confusion in some traditional interpretations of Jewish tradition by Christians, especially relative to the Christian understanding of the "trial of Jesus").

17. When confronted with a contemporary problem—for example, how to behave in the face of the AIDS crisis—halakhists go first to the text and commentary to seek solutions.

18. The Oral Law or the Oral Tradition is, of course, predominantly written. "In the Talmud, technical discussions dealing with complex legal issues are often juxtaposed with ethical teachings or sayings. The legal and ethical are often fused, as in the tractate Baba Batra where charity and compassion for the poor are defined as religious obligations" (Wineburg and Zoloth-Dorfman, "Jewish Ethics").

19. In other words, "The question stands [until the Messiah comes to resolve it]." Such disputes are among the things that will be resolved once the Messiah comes.

20. It is this vagueness that Peter Ochs claims is another name for multivocity, his term. See Internet posting, Post-Modern Jewish Philosophy Network, 18 May 1995. Baruch Brody has alluded to this in a similar analysis of rabbinic method.

21. There are actually more than 613 in the corpus of halakhah. Six hundred thirteen corresponds to the number of limbs of the body, in rabbinic reckoning 248, added to the number of days of the year.

22. How this works, in fact, reads even more clearly than in principle. It is often the daily blessings and the daily disciplines that bring the entire sacred world into the simplest home setting. Note how this acts as a feminist corrective to a religion that is, of course, patriarchal by historical definition.

23. During the last 150 years, four branches of Judaism have developed. All acknowledge the role of halakhah, but each gives it different weight in the setting of normative standards

for its tradition. For the Orthodox Jew, halakhah is interpreted by his or her rabbi, who then consults leading scholars if the issue is difficult, and that decision is considered halakhically binding. For the Conservative Jew, halakhah has a strong voice in the determination of *din* by the rabbinic community. The Conservative *minhag* is determined by the community. Jewish law is then integrated with insights from the social sciences and Western philosophic norms to facilitate decision making. For Reform Jews, the individual is autonomously responsible for his or her own choices, in light of the tradition and the primary ethical stance of the tradition. For the purposes of this book, the traditional or halakhically grounded position will be described, although the reader should remember that among Jews there is considerable variance. My contention is that, even for Jews not bound by its restraint, halakhah wields a strong methodological influence.

24. Leibowitz, "Commandments."

25. Hartman, "Halakhah." It is instructive to read both chapters as cited to get a full view of the differences between these two highly respected theorists. I could have chosen many other examples. Both Hartman and Leibowitz are Modern Orthodox and are Israeli. Thus, even within the same and very restricted intellectual communities, variances will emerge.

26. This position was taken in the twelfth century by Maimonides, and in the twentieth by one of his major commentators, contemporary Israeli philosopher David Hartman. See Hartman, *Maimonides*.

27. Heschel, *Between God and Man*, p. 161.

28. Jacobs, "Relationship between Religion and Ethics," p. 42.

29. Eruvin 100b, cited in Lichtenstein, "Does Jewish Tradition Recognize an Ethics Independent of *Halakhah*?," p. 62.

30. Ibid., pp. 62–65.

31. Avot 3:17, as cited in ibid., p. 62.

32. Ibid., p. 65.

33. Ibid., p. 63.

34. Ibid., p. 66.

35. Ibid., p. 67.

36. Jeremiah 9:23, cited in ibid., p. 67.

37. This three-part phrase is evocative of the quote in Micah that tells the people what God wants of them: to live justly, to love *hesed*, and to walk humbly with God. See Micah 6:8.

38. Babylonian Talmud, Bava Metzia 6:6. Cited in Lichtenstein, "Does Jewish Tradition Recognize an Ethics Independent of *Halakhah*?," p. 74.

39. Ibid.

40. Ibid., p. 75.

41. As Levinas said, "And what are we to make of circumcision? Can we explain that away with a little psychoanalysis?" See "The Pact."

42. Dorff, "Training Rabbis."

43. "Fundamentalism" is Fox's word. "One of the greatest dangers to Jewish faith and Jewish thought is the fundamentalist tendency that occasionally manifests (in our own time, as in others) and that seeks to freeze doctrine at a particular point." See Fox, "Judaism, Secularism, and Textual Interpretation," p. 24.

44. Ibid.

45. *Shemot Rabbah*, vol. 9. Cf. *Mekhilta, Bahodesh* 9, ed. Horowitz-Rabin, p. 235, as cited in Fox, *Jewish Ethics*, p. 18.

46. This is especially important in bioethics, when much turns on the most technical medical data.

47. According to Daniel Boyarin, in a comment on this passage in the first draft of this chapter, Soloveitchik described this position as Kantian.

48. One can see a stream and note its beauty, its physical properties, or its ritual use, for example. All are "real" views of the same phenomena. Soloveitchik explains that the religious person would first see the ritual use.

49. Soloveitchik, *Halachic Mind*. The entire book is a argument for the summary I have presented here. See especially the last chapter.

50. Established by, finally, the willingness of Abraham to sacrifice Isaac.

51. *Sifre Deuteronomy, Piska* 33, midrash to Deuteronomy 32:10. Professor Herbert Basser, while a visiting professor at the University of California at Berkeley, 1984–85, studied this passage with me and explained this insight. It is also found in his book, *Midrashic Interpretations of the Song of Moses*, p. 140.

52. For a full account of several alternate readings, the best source is Ilana Pardes's book on the uses of such variant readings for feminist scholars. See Pardes, "Creation According to Eve."

53. Unless the death was witnessed, Jewish law considered the woman abandoned and therefore still married. In modern warfare, whole divisions of men can be blown up and their bodies never found. Halakhah had to consider this new circumstance.

54. Hartman, "Halakhah," p. 310.

55. Case law is the most important but not the only way that new data is admitted. It is also admitted via midrash. Philo adds Platonic physics as well. My thanks to Elliot Dorff for this insight.

56. Montefiore and Loewe, *Rabbinic Anthology*, pp. 340–41.

57. Boyarin, *Intertextuality and the Reading of Midrash*, pp. 34–36.

58. David Hartman was a visiting professor of Jewish thought (Taubman professorship) in the fall of 1986. This insight was taken from notes from a seminar on Maimonides taught at the University of California at Berkeley.

59. Ibid.

60. This insight is found in Hartman, *Maimonides*, p. 26.

61. The aspect of God that is alluded to in this context is the *shekhinah* aspect, identified in later Jewish thought as the feminine aspect. In earlier texts, the *shekhinah* refers to the indwelling, immanent presence of God.

62. There have been two earlier interpretations of this phrase. The first place that it occurs is in the *Alenu* prayer, read at the conclusion of the prayer service, in which the Jew asks for a world order in which all the brokenness of the world will be healed under the sovereignty of God (*l'taken olam b'malchut Shadai*). The prayer has nothing to do with human action. The second usage is the way that the Lurianic mysticism of the Kabbalah describes the brokenness at the heart of the world. In the original creation, according to this tradition, God's primordial light was collected and contained in great vessels. These vessels

cracked, releasing sparks into the world. It is the task of the individual Jew to "reclaim the sparks" in all things and through *tikkun olam*, mediation, and study, restore them to their rightful place.

63. Judges in the Talmud are God's partners in the world.

64. Walzer, *Exodus and Revolution*, introduction and conclusion.

65. David Elazar offered a historical sociological theory of a tripartite *edah* that is helpful in understanding both Biale and Walzer. His sociological observation—that the Jewish community is always organized in three parts, Kingship, Torah, and Priests—was useful in shaping Biale's historical interpretation and provided an account of the specifics of power relationships within the community.

66. For Liberation Theology in the Roman Catholic tradition it is one of the single most important features of the method.

67. Ernst Simon and Harold Fisch, in Fox, *Jewish Ethics*, chap. 2, pts. 1 and 2.

68. Walzer, *Exodus and Revolution*.

69. Hartman, "Halakhah," p. 312.

70. This term is from the teaching of Joseph Soloveitchik, the major rabbinic commentator of our time.

71. Hartman, *Joy and Responsibility*, p. 150.

72. Levinas, *Ethics and Infinity*, pp. 1–12, 86–89.

73. Levinas, *Nine Talmudic Readings*, p. 108.

74. See Genesis 2:7.

75. Levinas, *Nine Talmudic Readings*, p. 85.

76. For further detail on this, see the section on the *rodef* in Chapter 7.

77. Levinas, *Nine Talmudic Readings*, p. 108.

78. Note how this is similar to the notion, found in the work of Seyla Benhabib and others in the discipline of communicative ethics, that the key ethical moment was "reversibility."

79. Levinas, *Nine Talmudic Readings*, p. 168.

80. Ibid., p. 171.

81. See Levinas, "Toward the Other," and *Ethics and Infinity*, pp. 93–103.

82. Levinas, *Nine Talmudic Readings*, p. 176.

83. Ibid., p. 39.

84. Ibid., p. 99.

85. Ibid., p. 47.

86. Ibid., p. 48.

87. Ibid.

88. Ibid., p. 21.

89. Ibid.

90. Ibid., pp. 97–98.

91. Ibid., p. 193.

92. Taken alone, the radical encounter of the other is an isolated gesture of martyrdom. It is still essential but then has no historical resonance. Taken outside the context, the gesture of encounter is lost.

93. See Levinas, "The Pact."

94. Ibid., p. 215.

95. This is a very complicated problem in Levinas. He does not comment on the text's assumption that the real people were men and that the women, children, and *gerim* were remarkably included. This text continued the assumption that "women" ought to be in a category other than "person," and their inclusion was generous but surprising in the text.

96. Ibid., p. 225.

97. The practice of the halakhic method itself reinforced the belief in and practice of argument as a teaching process. A good debate and passion in intellect were valued and expected, because the moral agent was supposed to be in dialogue with another in a discursive community. As an example, virtually every quotation in this book could be paired with reliable commentary to the absolute contrary. A good shouting match among theorists was reliably expected; this very disagreement enabled the halakhic method to function over time and circumstance. "Community" in this tradition did not mean consensus; it meant discourse. In traditional teaching academies (*yeshivot*) every person learning has a study partner, and textual studies are done *b'hevrutah*, face-to-face, with this partner. Furthermore, even conducting an argument with diametrically opposed views was seen as serving the cause of the search for divine truth, a concept called in Hebrew *makhloket l'shem shamayim*.

98. Ibid., p. 221.

99. This, of course, is the issue at the heart of the feminist challenge to the tradition. If this is to be true, then girls have to be taught to learn in the same way that boys are taught. See Ochs, *Words on Fire*, for this discussion.

100. Dorff, "Training Rabbis," p. 14.

101. This creation of community is true even for the secular Jew who lives entirely outside the tradition. In a way, the existence of the Orthodox community creates a world that others count on to exist, a Jerusalem of the spirit to which it is possible to return.

102. Hartman, *Joy and Responsibility*, p. 183.

103. In ethicist Larry Churchill's remarkable book about medical triage and justice in the allocation of health care, he calls on ethicists to create a communal alternative to the language of the Good Samaritan story. This discussion of the "Rutharian" choice is such an attempt.

104. Plaskow, *Standing Again at Sinai*, pp. 2–10.

105. Boyarin, in comments on an earlier draft of this book, made this important remark.

106. There is a growing and important literature on this topic. See Pardes, *Countertraditions in the Bible*, for the single best source on how this works in the Jewish tradition.

107. At the core of ethics in Judaism is Franz Kafka's maxim, "The Messiah will come, not on the day the world is perfect, but the day after." (This is Kafka at his most rabbinic.)

108. Buber's work has had strong and consistent appeal among Christian theologians, notably H. R. Niebuhr. In the Jewish context, his work has been more controversial. I am interested in his specific perspective on moral agency, which I argue retains many elements of traditional Jewish thought. Heschel has been regarded as more centrally located in the traditional Jewish textual sources.

109. Dan Zoloth-Dorfman, "Martin Buber."

110. This is a novel formulation for classic Jewish thought, since it does not put the mitzvot at the center of the project of response, but this is one reason why Buber is acceptable to Christians.

111. Ibid., p. 16.

112. There is a danger that self can be consumed by community. Buber called this the political (versus social) principle of collectivity. In collectivity, self is given up and personal responsibility abdicated. The will of the group is substituted for individual will, and I-It relationships for I-Thou relationships.

113. See for example, Buber, "Jew in the World" and "Spirit of Israel and the World Today."

114. For Abraham Joshua Heschel, a contemporary of Buber's and another major theologian of our time, this insight was pivotal, but not sufficient. Heschel, in interpreting moral agency, began with anthropology. He addressed not only human anthropology but "divine anthropology" as well. For Heschel, the Bible was the story of "divine anthropology." But the responding self in relationship to God was shaped by Heschel's view of the human primarily as one who answers God's constant call.

Human anthropology and agency were shaped by three responses to this call: the way of wonder, the way of revelation, and the way of sacred deeds. As adults, Heschel argued, we lost the awe and wonder found in nature that surprised, delighted, and terrified us as children. Heschel believed that this awe, this "radical amazement," was the proper response to God's extraordinary world of nature. It was the beginning of the awareness of the divine that constituted humanity. Despite the human propensity for science, reason, and investigation (which was also central to our nature), we persistently glimpsed the divine behind the world of nature. The true nature of this divine presence was a mystery for us, and it would remain a mystery. But humans were capable of understanding and sensing the ineffable and capturing a sense of the mystery, the absolute meaning of being. Thus, for Heschel, meaning could not be contained by intellectual terms alone; it was intuitive, sensual, preverbal, and ultimately very personal. The compassion and love at the heart of the universe could be sensed and felt even if it could not be expressed. This was the "way of wonder" of which humans were capable. Heschel argued that it must inform our ethical relationships.

As humans, we were also addressed by God in the text of the Bible and in revelation. To be human, for Heschel, was to hear the question of the Other in the world—not to be alone or surrounded by "thick silence." The revelation was mediated by prophecy, but it was the ability to be open to prophecy and to "live with it" (e.g., by reading/hearing and reconstituting the text/call as our own) that constituted the human experience.

Finally, for Heschel, to be fully human was to be capable of the response to the call with sacred deeds. According to Heschel, God's call to us commanded us to be holy. This meant we must *act* to be fully human. Heschel contended that actions in the community are what ultimately make us complete as persons. Simply hearing and responding with passion was neither fully human nor fully moral, until actual deeds were accomplished in the world as a result of this understanding.

For Heschel, the community actions, the mitzvot in their fullest meaning (internal intention in connection with external acts), were the most human response to God's call as encountered in the Bible. Heschel's moral agent must act in the tangible, accountable world. Heschel believed that mitzvot of compassion and justice extended to political and social action (such as joining the fight for civil rights or working against the war in Vietnam). The struggle to be alive to mitzvot, to live them fully and not perfunctorily, was a constant challenge. However, as Levinas noted, for Heschel it was this very challenge, this hard act of listening, that characterized his anthropology.

115. The well-known figures of Buber and Heschel were not the only ones to address the core issue of moral agency, of course. Israel Salanter, the ideological and spiritual leader of the movement known as *musar* (ethics), inspired a program that self-consciously endeavored to construct moral agents through the directed experience of intense study, self-examination, and practical human relationship. It would be impossible to reflect on the system of Jewish ethics without at least a brief mention of the largest, self-conscious, specific, and popular movement for ethical renewal that flourished in recent Jewish history. For some in the tradition, ethics is the equivalent of the "doing of *musar*," meaning a deliberate and separate act of ethical reflection and deliberation. But the term has specific historical roots that make it appropriate to consider when examining the nature of the moral agent and the concept of autonomy in Jewish thought. The *musar* movement flourished from 1841 to 1945 in Eastern Europe, largely in western Russia (the Pale), Lithuania, and Germany. At its height, it attracted thousands of followers, (some) women and men, to an intra-halakhic process of ethical renewal. It was rooted in tradition and text, yet this movement was at all times deeply influenced by its times—a period of tumult and catastrophe in Jewish history.

Halakhic Judaism as a closed and intact system was crumbling under the internal dissolution of rabbinism. The intricate, increasingly demanding system of halakhah was administered in the 1840s by an academic rabbinic leadership that was less interested in the fluid interpretation of halakhah characteristic of earlier periods. Hasidism was one of the social/religious challenges to orthodoxy and control of the Lithuanian rabbinic authorities who led academic Judaism at that time. There were many other challenges. In Germany, the *Haskalah* challenged the source of traditional rabbinic social, political, and magisterial order with new insight derived from the Western intellectual tradition of the Enlightenment. The *Haskalah* was a religious and cultural/social force that asked for the introduction of philosophy, science, sociology, and psychology into the curriculum of Jewish learning. Importantly, it raised the issues of citizenship and participation in the social and political polis of the non-Jewish world. In Western Europe, the movement for Reform Judaism further questioned the very basis of the religious legal structure and authority of Jewish orthodoxy.

In this extraordinary period of tumult in Jewish life, Zionism was another force for change, an option for Jewish self-understanding and a solution to the problem of oppression and powerlessness. Massive emigration, largely to America, suddenly also became possible for Jews, presenting the community with yet another option. Socialism, and the vision of a radically reclaimed world for the Jewish working class, offered another possibility for both social and political transformation.

Meanwhile, while Jewish intellectuals passionately debated these possibilities, and mass movements emerged in support of each idea, the czars tried to cope with the "Jewish

Problem" with options of their own. In various waves of cooptation and repression the czars alternately expelled Jews from cities and opened "Crown schools" to educate Jewish children. The czars enacted the repressive May Laws to establish six years of preliminary cantonment in addition to the twenty-five-year army conscription. This meant that Jewish boys from the age of twelve could be taken into a world where it was impossible to live a commanded life. Families said the *kaddish* (the prayer for the dead) for these children, for they knew they would be lost to them. Plague, pogroms, and revolution were constant realities of this period.

In the midst of this world, Rabbi Israel Salanter, a local spiritual leader, created a movement for ethical renewal, started academies, and instituted a meditative, self-reflective method for personal growth and change. Salanter started with the view that human persons were deeply evil (lustful, sinful, and full of urges/instincts of power and ego), yet deeply mutable as well. Human character, in Salanter's view, was changeable, and persons could strive toward an ideal vision of self. These three characteristics (evil, changeable, and visionary) constituted both his anthropology and his method of ethical reflection.

According to Salanter, men (and women) were capable of daily choices for good or for evil. Presented with this choice, they could respond by "doing *musar*"—that is, rationally controlling impulses toward evil by study, meditation, and action in the world. Doing *musar* meant direct involvement with one's inner life—reflection, meditation, study of the Torah, and study of Musar literature (at least a little each day). This was a kind of cognitive purification. It also meant finding a companion and community with whom to do *musar*. One needed an interpersonal relationship to do this work, along with "worldly wisdom." One had to recruit another person with whom to do *musar*. Together the pair were enjoined to do mutual discernment of faults (criticism and self-criticism) and had to care (including physical acts of care) for each other. A *musar* text on what was needed to do *musar* required an enactment every day of the mitzvah of "loving your neighbor as yourself." Fellowship and caring for the other were critical to personal change.

Finally, exertion—consistent spiritual labor—was required. For Salanter, "despair almost prevails" but might not. Despite brutality, loss, and risk in the world, study, *musar*, intellectual work, reflection, and deeds could lead to serious change. True ideal completion was not possible in exile, but, Salanter believed, the "hereafter can begin right now" for a small community.

God's command required sensitivity, according to Salanter. *Musar* was a process, not a handbook, by which the morality and justice and kindness in the world could be increased with internal work, paradoxically, in social relationship. Salanter's ethics were interpersonal, based on and commanded by psychology. He believed that the ability for human beings to choose this way created the beginning of a more chosen, more sacred world.

116. Dorff, "Training Rabbis," p. 13.

117. Ibid., p. 15.

118. While you can divorce your spouse and choose not to have children, everyone is born into a family of some kind. It is the nature of the primate either to have an other for a prolonged period of dependency or to not become human, capable even of human language.

119. Ibid., p. 14.

120. Talmud Balvi Shabbat 54b. As cited in Dorff, "Training Rabbis," p. 13.

121. Boyarin, *Carnal Israel*. Boyarin, David Biale, and Howard Schwartz, among others, have opened up this entire discourse.

Chapter 7

1. See, for example, Rosner, *Modern Medicine and Jewish Ethics*, p. 348, as a representative source.

2. Bava Metzia 62a, trans. Adin Steinsaltz, in *The Talmud*, p. 29.

3. In other words, the wealthy should keep the resources.

4. Or could it? The encounter in the desert calls the question for the interest discourse. What is at stake, it seems, is the life and death of another. Money is about this, and this interplay between the two texts reminds us sharply that the market metaphor, the rules of business, is actually limited by human life and death.

5. Jewish Publication Society, *Torah Commentary*, p. 175.

6. We might add, What if the radical construct of the "original position," following Rawls, cannot be arranged?

7. For more about this relationship, see Chapter 8.

8. Jewish Publication Society, *Torah Commentary*, p. 178.

9. Sokel, "Allocation of Scarce Medical Resources."

10. Ibid., p. 70.

11. Sokel cited the responsa of the following: Rabbi Moshe Shterbach, *Responsa Teshuvot ve-Hanhahot* (Jerusalem, 1986); *Hoshen Mishpat, Responsa* 858; Rabbi Zadok ha-Cohen of Lublin, *Ozer ha Melekh, Yesodei ha-Torah* 5:5; the Hazon Ish, *Gilyonot le-Hiddusshei R. Hayim ha Levi, Hilkhot Yesodei ha-Torah* (Bnei Brak, 1974); Rabbi Chaim Ozer Grodinski, *Ahi'ezer, Yoreh De'ah* 16 (Vina, 1925), p. 35; Rabbi Eliezer Walenburg, *Responsa Ziz Eliezer*, vol. 9, chap. 28; and Rabbi Shmuel Edels, Bava Metzia 62b, in support of his contention. Of course, even within this response system, as opposed to the first interpretive school, there are dissenters, and Sokel cited two, Rabbi Y. Uterman, in *Shevet Yehuda* (Jerusalem, 1955), p. 18, and Rabbi Moshe S. Shapira, *R. Mshe Shmuel ve Dora* (New York, 1964), p. 236.

12. This quote is taken from Schochet, *Responsum of Surrender*, p. 43; in a footnote the author states that his source is Solomon Pines, from the tenth-century philosopher physician al-Razi.

13. Abraham, "Priorities in Medicine," p. 95. One can only speculate on what happens to the earnest Jewish physician working in the emergency room on this premise.

14. "Horayot," in *Talmud Balvi*, p. 13a.

15. Ibid.

16. Women were seen as being in the same category as the other nonperformers, in this rendering, all handicapped in their discourse with God, unable to speak or hear the language of prayer or to witness reality and testify in court with accuracy.

17. Anal rape was generally considered more physically painful as well as psychologically demeaning in the Greco-Roman world as well. This was noted by Daniel Boyarin in comments on an earlier draft.

18. Bava Metzia, in *Talmud Balvi*, trans. Adin Steinsaltz, p. 71a.

19. Sokel cited the *Tur*, chap. 251, where interfamily hierarchy is worked out. Here we have an example of self, then parents, then older children, then cousins, etc. See Sokel, "Allocation of Scarce Medical Resources," p. 83.

20. Also unclear is the possible application of this text to the allocation of nonmonetary goods. Because health care services in our culture have a commodity value, the text stands as a part of the justice debate rather than as a debate only about loans.

21. Sokel, "Allocation of Scarce Medical Resources," p. 85.

22. Dorff, "Jewish Approach to End-Stage Medical Care," 29. (In my dissertation I was using a draft version of this text.)

23. Schochet, *Responsum of Surrender*, p. 20.

24. Jerusalem Talmud, Tractate Terumot, 7:20.

25. This has enormous resonance in the health care debate: Ought the community to pay for those who are culpable for their illness, who drink and drive, or who smoke?

26. The number quoted is a metaphorical number, the literary equivalent of "a zillion dollars." As we shall see in subsequent texts, the usual ransom amount for a child is 200 (regular) dinars.

27. Schochet, *Responsum of Surrender*.

28. At least if we determine the pressure on the community is the issue (if there are no other captives). It may also be the case for all situations; the text is unclear.

29. My thanks to Rabbi Eliezer Finkelman, Berkeley, Calif., for the translation of these texts, for his explanation of their importance to the siege texts, and for the construction of this last point.

30. Schochet, *Responsum of Surrender*.

31. This exception of course reflected an inherent bias toward the redemption of male captives; females were rarely being groomed to be sages of Israel.

32. Schochet, *Responsum of Surrender*, p. 39.

33. Ibid.

34. Goodman, *Toward a Theory of Justice*, p. 41. Goodman's book deals extensively with the problems of punishment, deserts, and retribution but is useful in this context for his reflection on community.

35. Ibid., p. 40.

36. Schochet, *Responsum of Surrender*, p. 43.

37. The texts are not clear on this point. Perhaps, as Boyarin pointed out in comments on an earlier draft of this book, such a woman is expendable because of differential value or status within the community.

38. Landau's responsum is "cryptic," concluded Schochet. He noted that Landau proposed that certain things may be done to facilitate the conscription of community undesirables rather short of actually handing them over or hiding the chosen.

39. Dorff, "Jewish Approach to End-Stage Medical Care," p. 52, n. 32.

40. Ibid., p. 20.

41. Weisbard, "On the Bioethics of Jewish Law," p. 360. This is a remarkable article. Not only is it enormously detailed, unearthing sources in texts that were new to the field at the time; it is one of the earliest works on the topic. The ideas on the *terefah* are truly

innovative, used in this context. My thanks to the author for his help in getting me a copy and his generous explanation of these passages. (Please note that the spelling difference in the term is a function of our different transliterations of the Hebrew.)

42. Dorff, "Jewish Approach to End-Stage Medical Care," p. 28.

43. Rabbi Shimon Efrati, responsa published in 1961, in Kirschner, *Rabbinic Responsa of the Holocaust Era*, responsa 6, p. 65.

44. Kirschner, *Rabbinic Responsa of the Holocaust Era*, responsa 9.

45. Ibid., p. 119, from the responsa of Rabbi Zvi Hirsch Meisals.

46. Brody has been most obliging in helping me frame my research around the *rodef* text. In personal communication about an earlier draft of this book, he directed me to his related work in this field. In that conversation he most strongly advocated the use of these texts.

47. An extensive and authoritative discussion of the *rodef* defense and its relationship to deserts and justification in Jewish law is presented in the *Wayne Law Review* 33 (Summer 1987); Finkelman, "Self Defense and the Defense of Other in Jewish Law," is particularly useful. See also Baruch Brody, "Economics of the Laws of *Rodef*," and Zohar, Weinrib, Brody, and Levine, "Symposium."

48. *Talmud Balvi*, Sanhedrin 73a.

49. Baruch Brody, "Economics of the Laws of *Rodef*," p. 67.

Paradoxically, you are also saving the *rodef*. The Misnah is clear: The *rodef* must be stopped from violation of the commandment, and you are, in the ultimate Levinasian sense, taking responsibility for his responsibility. You are to go to any expense and to any lengths—even to kill him—to take responsibility for his responsibility. This is not Brody's point, and it does not have a parallel meaning for health care, but it does illustrate further the seriousness with which the rabbis took this problem of communal responsibility, and in which Levinas has found the pattern of community that I addressed in Chapter 5.

50. Ibid., p. 69.

51. Moshe Tendler, "Physician Reimbursement."

52. Ibid.

53. Sanhedrin 17b, Nezikin.

54. Babylonian Talmud, Seder Nezikin, vol. 3, Sanhedrin, author's translation.

55. Women did not count as witnesses in the Great Sanhedrin.

56. All who are defined as witnesses, that is.

57. The "death" involved is different in the two states. Traditionally, women are taught that the end of a menstrual cycle that does not lead to conception is a death of sorts, the loss of the potential child. In childbirth, the traditional texts teach that the *mikvah* acknowledged the risk of death to the woman, and her return to the world of sexuality. The *mikvah* was also used to ritually cleanse the body of a person immediately after death as part of the preparation for burial.

58. One can note that the rabbinic listing is a nearly exact reversal of Maslow's developmental needs scale.

59. Boyarin commented in an earlier draft of this book that it is important to note that the shift in technology has caused the actual role of a surgeon to become unimaginably different from the role of the surgeon listed here.

60. As noted previously, the Talmudic system is constructed so that all commentaries are contemporaneous, so the world that Ruth inhabits does not "influence" the rabbis; it *is* the world of the rabbis, as it is the world of my grandmother, and it is the world that is mine.

Chapter 8

1. The ethics that I am suggesting are meant to apply in all situations of distributive justice.

2. Stout, *Ethics after Babel*. Stout argues that there is no such thing as a "neutral vantage" and "a universal language for ethics" and that each person speaks from the distinctive vantage of his or her own tradition.

3. Recall that in the texts of rescue, which describe how to save a caravan of people under threat of brigands, all men are to be saved before all women, unless the threat is to the sexuality of the travelers. In that case, female virgins take precedence, but since forced male sex is assumed to be more painful than female rape, men take precedence.

4. This insight is not unique to feminists, of course.

5. Levinas's work is richly described in Aronowicz, "Emmanuel Levinas's Talmudic Commentaries."

6. Pardes, *Countertraditions in the Bible*, p. 2.

7. Ibid.

8. Whatever one thinks about preventative health, one must acknowledge its limited link to virtue. Further, the cause of much of what makes us ill is beyond our ability to control or understand.

9. This point was suggested by Daniel Boyarin in a reading of the first draft.

10. Aristotle, *Nicomachean Ethics*, vol. 8, bk. 1, p. 215.

11. Jewish Publication Society, *Torah Commentary*, p. 95. The next lines of the account are as follows: "As he was about to enter Egypt, he said to his wife Sarai, 'I know what a beautiful woman you are. If the Egyptians see you and think "She is his wife" they will kill me and let you live. Please let me say that you are my sister, that it may go well with me because of you, and that I may remain alive thanks to you.' When Abram entered Egypt, the Egyptians saw how beautiful the woman was. Pharaoh's courtier saw her and praised her to Pharaoh, and the woman was taken into Pharaoh's palace."

Even Pharaoh is appalled at this, asking six verses later, "Why did you not tell me that she was your wife!?" What occurs here allows the material enrichment of Abram: he acquires "sheep, oxen, asses, male and female slaves and camels" because Sarai is raped and enslaved by Pharaoh. It is a horrific break in the narrative when Sarai becomes "enthinged" and, for a time, loses even her name ("how beautiful the woman was").

This famine story resonates against the Ruth story, as it deals with similar themes: power, sexuality, the stranger, and a backdrop of desperation.

12. Note that Jacob, son of the blind Isaac, admonishes his sons *not* to look at one another. The Hebrew verb implies reciprocity. Sarna states that it also implies helplessness and the sense of "don't put on a pretense." Note the contrast, of course, with Levinas's conceptualization of Sinai.

13. In an earlier version of this text read at the American Academy of Religion, Hans O. Tiefel asked about my hermeneutical choice of Ruth, which stood so clearly outside the discourse in the traditional texts. I answered that I started with this text in part because I was committed to a feminist reading of the tradition. I am grateful to Dr. Tiefel for asking this question.

14. The Ruth text was dated in a personal communication with Professor Jacob Milgrom, University of California, December 1992.

15. The subtitle of this section is from Pardes, *Countertraditions in the Bible*, p. 99.

16. Rabinowitz, *Midrash Rabbah*, p. 16.

17. I pay particular attention to this commentary, not because it is of such scholarly weight, but precisely because it has been identified as the "woman's text." It is the compilation of the commentary in Yiddish written for the unlearned women of the Eastern European Jewry. It was meant to serve as the guide to the scripture studied in the synagogue. It is through the language of this text that my grandmothers knew Ruth. See *Tz'enah Ur'enah*, p. 848.

18. I cannot resist this interpretation. *Oi Vay!* is not just a Yiddish idiom. It is a Yiddish idiom derived from the Hebrew *oy va-voy*. All quotes are from *Tz'enah Ur'enah*.

19. Sasson, "Ruth," pp. 321–22.

20. Ibid.

21. *Tz'enah Ur'enah*.

22. Rabinowitz, *Midrash Rabbah*, p. 20.

23. "Ruth," in ibid.

24. Rabinowitz, *Midrash Rabbah*, pp. 8, 21.

25. Ozick, "Ruth," p. 369.

26. Sasson, "Ruth," p. 322.

27. Ozick, "Ruth," p. 370.

28. Pardes, *Countertraditions in the Bible*, p. 100.

29. That this was a Republican campaign theme in the 1992 election was no casual choice. The ideology of autonomy is linked to the theme of traditional idealized family values, since to suggest otherwise would be to assert that perhaps a community might have responsibility for the most vulnerable—not a popular election year theme.

30. Ozick, "Ruth," p. 371.

31. There is still no mention of living men in Moab; the midrash explains that their fathers have also died.

32. Rabinowitz, *Midrash Rabbah*, p. 33. Ozick made this point as well: "detritus and ash."

33. Ogletree, *Hospitality to the Stranger*, p. 48.

34. For an interesting commentary on this scene one can examine its treatment in the *Tz'enah Ur'enah*. It contains an explanation of how the life of the women of the household could have been conducted for ten years. The explanation is that while they did not convert to Judaism, they practiced "a little" Jewishly; otherwise what could Naomi have meant by "return"? The conversion of Ruth, explains this commentary further, following the midrash, is done "interlinearly" by Naomi; Naomi does not speak of it and it does not appear in the text of the statement by Ruth of her acceptance of their shared fate.

35. Ozick, "Ruth," p. 372.

36. There is a parallel text. In Jonah, the sailors on the boat act in much the same way. They are like regular religious people; they pray, they offer sacrifice, they know that God acts in the world, and they are reluctant to hurt anybody, but they will do as they are told.

37. Pardes, *Countertraditions in the Bible*, p. 102.

38. Levinas, *Ethics and Infinity*, p. 86.

39. Ogletree, *Hospitality to the Stranger*, pp. 48, 52.

40. Levinas, *Ethics and Infinity*, p. 50.

41. Rabinowitz, *Midrash Rabbah*, p. 38. Also noted in *Tz'enah Ur'enah*, p. 834, as follows: "The Sages learn from the story of Ruth how our forefathers used to conduct themselves with one who approached for conversion. The word 'return' is written three times to show that when a person wished to convert he was first told three times to leave. . . . Ruth said: 'If you will not convert me, I will go to another Jew to convert me, but I wish to become a convert through your hands.' When Naomi heard that she truly desired to convert, she first told her some of the commandments to see if she would heed them."

42. In the spirit of Boyarin, I want to note here that as a mother nursing a child as I write these words, I can scarcely imagine an act more intimate and privileged.

43. Pardes, *Countertraditions in the Bible*, p. 105.

44. This note is inspired by Lebacqz. The text in question, Numbers, Parshah Balak, is read in synagogue each year in connection with a *haftorah*, which is a selection from Micah. The Torah text asks the question, as it were, of how to live in a manner that is holy; here the People are blessed, and next the People are whoring. The answer of the rabbis who placed the two texts together can be found in the conclusion of the passage in Micah. It is the same passage that Lebacqz found to be critical to an understanding of health care ethics. See Lebacqz, "Humility in Health Care," p. 291.

45. Sasson, "Ruth," p. 322.

46. Pardes, *Countertraditions in the Bible*, p. 117.

47. Mieke Bal regards this moment in the text as, in part, an allusion to Boaz's impotence and Ruth's effort to help. Bal, *Lethal Love*.

48. The word in Hebrew has the connotation of maidservant-who-may-be-a-concubine (Hagar was referred to as *amah*). Ruth is saying that she could be considered his concubine, but she is explicitly asking for more than that. She is asking to be his wife.

49. A word which means a woman that can be taken by a freeman either as a wife or as a concubine. See Sasson, "Ruth," p. 323.

50. This is simply a canopy held aloft over the couple, which represents the home they will then make. The *chuppah* is commonly a prayer shawl, thus the connection here to cloak.

51. A period of three months, corresponding to the time that must elapse before a female proselyte is permitted to marry. See Slotki, "Ruth," p. 6.

52. I cannot find reference to this in any of the midrashim. But surely the rabbis can (and did) count! Perhaps this is the female difference in close textual reading.

53. Walzer, *Exodus and Revolution*, pp. 73–98. Walzer, as noted in the previous chapter, insisted on the political meaning of the Exodus metaphor.

Conclusion

1. Robert Pear, "New Approach to Overhauling Health Insurance: Step by Step," *New York Times*, 11 November 1996. The figure of 42.3 million uninsured comes from the Chicago-based Physicians for a National Health Program. The same group reports that California has experienced the largest increase in uninsured individuals since 1996: an increase of 575,000 to a total of 7.1 million uninsured. Other states with substantial increases include Michigan (up 276,000 to 1.1 million), Illinois (up 169,000 to 1.5 million), Alabama (up 108,000 to 660,000), Florida (up 96,000 to 2.8 million), Maryland (up 96,000 to 680,000), and Pennsylvania (up 76,000 to 1.2 million). More than one out of five persons is uninsured in six states: Texas (where 24.5 percent of the population lacks health insurance), Arkansas (24.4 percent), Arizona (23.8 percent), California (21.5 percent), New Mexico (20.2 percent), and Mississippi (20.1 percent). Between 1996 and 1997, the number of states in which fewer than 1 in 10 persons was uninsured fell from eight to five; the lowest rates were found in Hawaii (7.5 percent uninsured) and Wisconsin (7.9 percent).

2. *Webster's New World Dictionary*, s.v. "conscience."

3. Stanley Hauerwas, "Reflections on Suffering, Death, and Medicine," in *Suffering Presence*, p. 31.

4. Cahill, "Can Theology Have a Role in 'Public' Bioethical Discourse?," p. 10.

5. See Laurie Zoloth-Dorfman, "Community and Conscience."

6. This is not to suggest that the language already insisted on is incorrect. The contribution of Charles Dougherty and others who require that the "preferential option for the poor" be central to an evaluative review of the Oregon project, for example, is crucial. By this insistence Catholic moral theologians have constructed a discussion where the introduction of this language is normative. Yet, it is limited unless much more is brought into the discourse as central.

7. Not, however, for procedures that were experimental, in cases where the risk/benefit burden was very poor, or in cases where the outcome of the illness was self-limiting in any case.

8. Martin Benjamin, "Conscience in Bioethics," p. 25. He calls conscience "the exercise and expression of a reflective sense of integrity."

9. Ibid., p. 5. Benjamin's assertion that conscience can be "heard" by a collective entity allows an understanding of the interior world of institutional ethics committees, institutional review boards, and commissions. His work is interesting in the context of this book because the development of a collective conscience that is the work of a reflective community of moral integrity is formed around the first gesture of ethics, the gesture of encounter.

10. Benjamin has noted a point that Cahill made in her earlier article. iBioethics as a discipline of philosophical inquiry has a broader constituency than public policy.

11. My thanks to Dr. Dina Siden for this point. In her doctoral dissertation, ethicist Siden notes that it is in fact the prophetic voice that makes bioethicists, who stand outside the debate at the bedside, unique.

12. The Oregon plan was only one attempt to grapple with the complex problem of the health care crisis. There were parallels in citizen decision movements in several states.

Vermont, Colorado, Minnesota, and California, among others, have vigorous citizens' groups and parliaments similar to Oregon's. West Virginia in particular has attempted deliberately to structure citizen-based organization and small-group discourse as the citizens of that state struggle to shape health care reform. In New York there were grassroots campaigns aimed at resolving the problem by promoting a single-payer plan.

13. I want to be self-conscious here: if you ask an economist, such as Enthoven, who developed the term "managed competition," you get an economic answer. See Enthoven and Kronick, "Consumer-Choice Health Plan for the 1990s." I am trained as an ethicist, so I have suggested an answer rooted in ethical reflection.

14. The citizens of Oregon used such a measure in one phase of their conversation about health care, in the context of other evaluative tools.

15. We can note this by referring to the first case considered by this book, that of the PVS patient in need of renal dialysis. Saying that his QALY is scant does not give any new information.

16. Further, in constructing these QALYs, much use has been made of the telephone survey, in itself a complicated intervention. There is in the United States a phantom community: the world of manufactured desire created by advertising. The generation that is now constructing public policy was raised in the grip of this phantom communal desire. The television and the phone, the machines that substitute for actuality and embodiment, can create the illusion of intimacy and engagement, but the problem of democracy remains despite this substitute. It would be instructive to see if the answers to what "quality of life" means to each person would differ if the able-bodied and the disabled had to sit in the same room together. Finally, QALYs are by nature adjusted, and the tables are constructed, by an expert with his or her own narrative, values, and beliefs.

17. There are no insurance systems for other basic necessities of life, such as police protection, rescue services, libraries, or parks. Housing costs are not based on this system. Creation of the system carries its own cost. (Estimates are in the range of $30 billion a year, according to Golenski, "Justice and Health Care.")

18. It is not at all clear that patients are better cared for in hospitals—where they eat regimented food and have nurses care for them on a twenty-four-hour schedule—than in their own homes. Healing may best be accomplished in home settings with attendants to assist families and where family members are given time to care for their loved ones. The social organization and convenience of care for the staff is best served by the creation of the hospital as workplace.

19. Small-group meetings even created new paradigms of therapy, as evidenced by the increased longevity of breast cancer patients who attend such small groups.

20. For a longer discussion of how this moral community can be established, see Laurie Zoloth-Dorfman, "Methodology," an unpublished paper written in 1988. Parts of this work were reprinted as Laurie Zoloth-Dorfman, "Methodology," in *Forming a Moral Community*.

21. My thanks here again to Martin Benjamin for a generous discussion at the Society of Bioethics Consultation in the fall of 1992 on this topic. His formulation of this problem enabled me to think through the Oregon problem in this way.

22. For those of us who celebrate the value of human community, not all was lost. As a

woman born and bred in Los Angeles, I can tell you that there was a particular thrill in seeing multinational crowds of people rise up from their living rooms, leave their cars, and walk (walk!) onto the freeway with hand-lettered signs cheering on participants during the car chase or at the trial.

23. It became, for ethicists, the replacement for the World Series.

24. Robin Toner, "Pollsters See a Silent Storm That Swept Away Democrats," *New York Times*, 16 November 1994. Twenty-five percent of polled respondents thought that health care should be left alone, and 41 percent thought only incremental changes were needed. The author concluded that this reflects a sense that Americans do not trust their federal government to act effectively on this issue.

25. See also Carter, *Culture of Disbelief*.

26. Witness the horror of the case of Susan Smith, who drowned her two young children and then blamed an unknown assailant for their murder, prompting a nationwide manhunt for a nonexistent perpetrator.

27. Laurie Zoloth-Dorfman, "The Best-Laid Plans: HMOs and the History of Community," *Journal of Medicine and Philosophy*, 1999.

BIBLIOGRAPHY

•

Primary Sources

Aaron, Henry J., and William B. Schwartz. *The Painful Prescription: Rationing Hospital Care.* Washington, D.C.: Brookings Institute, 1984.

Abraham, Abraham. *Medical Halachah for Everyone.* Jerusalem: Feldheim, 1980.

——. "Priorities in Medicine: Whom to Treat First." In *Medicine and Jewish Law*, edited by Fred Rosner, pp. 89–96. Northvale, N.J.: Jason Aronson, 1986.

Aristotle. *Nicomachean Ethics.* Translated with an introduction and notes by Martin Ostwald. New York: Macmillan, 1986.

Bal, Mieke. *Lethal Love: Feminist Literary Interpretations of Biblical Love Stories.* Bloomington: Indiana University Press, 1987.

Barber, Benjamin. "The Role of the Responsible Citizen." *Trends in Health Care,* Spring/Summer 1992, pp. 9–15.

——. "Who Owes What to Whom?" *Harper's Magazine,* February 1991, pp. 17–25.

Basser, Herbert. *Midrashic Interpretations of the Song of Moses.* New York: Peter Lang, 1984.

Beauchamp, Tom L., and James F. Childress. *Principles of Biomedical Ethics.* 2nd ed. New York: Oxford University Press, 1983.

Beiner, Ronald. *What's the Matter with Liberalism?* Berkeley: University of California Press, 1992.

Bellah, Robert N. *Habits of the Heart: Individualism and Commitment in American Life.* Berkeley: University of California Press, 1986.

Bellah, Robert N., Richard Madsen, William Sullivan, Ann Swidler, and Steven Tipton. *The Good Society.* New York: Alfred A. Knopf, 1991.

Benhabib, Seyla. "Communicative Ethics and Current Controversies in Practical Philosophy." In *The Communicative Ethics Controversy*, edited by Seyla Benhabib and Fred Dallmayr, pp. 330–71. Cambridge, Mass.: MIT Press, 1990.

——. *Situating the Self: Gender, Community, and Postmodernism in Contemporary Ethics.* New York: Routledge, 1992.

Benjamin, Martin. "Conscience in Bioethics." Unpublished paper, 1992.

Biale, David. *Power and Powerlessness in Jewish History.* New York: Schocken Books, 1987.

Birch, Bruce C., and Larry L. Rasmussen. *Bible and Ethics in Christian Life.* Minneapolis: Augsburg Fortress, 1989.

"Black-White Differences in Cervical Cancer Mortality: United States, 1980–1987." *Journal of the American Medical Association* 263 (13 June 1990): 3001–2.

Bleich, J. David. *Contemporary Halachic Problems*. Vol. 1. New York: K'tav Publishing, 1977.

———. *Contemporary Halachic Problems*. Vol. 2. New York: K'tav Publishing, 1983.

———. "The Jewish Entitlements of Valuing Life." *Sh'ma*, 16 November 1990, pp. 1–3.

Boyarin, Daniel. *Carnal Israel*. Berkeley: University of California Press, 1993.

———. *Intertextuality and the Reading of Midrash*. Bloomington: Indiana University Press, 1990.

Brody, Baruch. "The Care of the PVS Patient." *Journal of Law, Medicine, and Health Care* 20 (1992): 12–23.

———. "The Economics of the Laws of *Rodef*." *S'vara* 1 (Winter 1990): 67–70.

———. *Life and Death Decisionmaking*. Oxford: Oxford University Press, 1988.

Brody, Jane. "Doctors Admit Ignoring Dying Patients Wishes." *New York Times*, 14 January 1993.

Buber, Martin. *Between Man and Man*. New York: Macmillan, 1965.

———. *Israel and the World*. New York: Schocken Books, 1965.

———. "The Jew in the World." In *Israel and the World*, pp. 167–72. New York: Schocken Books, 1965.

———. "The Spirit of Israel and the World Today." In *Israel and The World*, pp. 183–94. New York: Schocken Books, 1965.

Cahill, Lisa Sowle. "Can Theology Have a Role in 'Public' Bioethical Discourse?" *Hastings Center Report* 20 (July/August 1990): 10–14.

Callahan, Daniel. "Beyond Individualism: Bioethics and the Common Good." *Second Opinion* 9 (November 1988): 53–69.

———. "The Oregon Initiative: Ethics and Priority Setting." Unpublished paper, 1990.

———. *Setting Limits: Medical Goals in an Aging Society*. New York: Simon and Schuster, 1987.

———. *What Kind of Life: The Limits of Medical Progress*. New York: Simon and Schuster, 1990.

Caplan, Arthur. "How Can We Deny Health Care to Poor While Others Get Face Lifts?" *Los Angeles Times*, 25 April 1989.

Capron, Alexander Morgan. "Oregon's Disability: Principles or Politics?" *Hastings Center Report* 22 (November/December 1992): 18–26.

Carlson, James. "Doesn't Single Out the Poor." Letter to the editor. *New York Times*, 1 September 1992.

Childress, James, and John Macquarrie. *The Westminster Dictionary of Christian Ethics*. S.v. "middle axioms." Philadelphia: Westminster Press, 1967.

Churchill, Larry R. *Rationing Health Care in America*. Notre Dame, Ind.: University of Notre Dame Press, 1987.

———. *Rationing Health Care: Perceptions and Principles of Justice*. Notre Dame, Ind.: University of Notre Dame Press, 1987.

Churchill, Larry R., and Marion Danis. "Autonomy and the Common Weal." *Hastings Center Report* 21 (January 1991): 25–31.

Cleveland, William. "Redoing the Health Care Quilt: Patches or the Whole Cloth." In *Caring for the Uninsured and the Underinsured: A Compendium from the Specialty*

Journals of the American Medical Association, pp. 6–12. Chicago: American Medical Association, 1991.

Cohen, Arthur A., and Paul Mendes-Flohr, eds. *Contemporary Jewish Religious Thought*. New York: Charles Scribner's Sons, 1987.

Collins, James, and Richard David. "The Differential Effect of Traditional Risk Factors on Infant Birth Weight among Blacks and Whites in Chicago." *American Journal of Public Health* 80 (June 1990): 679–81.

Crawshaw, Ralph. Letter to the editor. *New England Journal of Medicine* 327 (27 August 1992): 242.

Crawshaw, Ralph, Michael J. Garland, and Brian Hines. "Developing Principles for Prudent Health Care Allocation: The Continuing Oregon Experiment." *Western Journal of Medicine* 152 (April 1990): 141–42.

——. "Oregon Health Decisions: An Experiment with Informed Community Consent." *Journal of the American Medical Association* 254 (13 December 1985): 3213–16.

Dallmayr, Fred. Introduction to *The Communicative Ethics Controversy*, edited by Seyla Benhabib and Fred Dallmayr, pp. 8–9. Cambridge, Mass.: MIT Press, 1990.

Daniels, Norman. *Am I My Parents' Keeper?* Oxford: Oxford University Press, 1988.

——. *Just Health Care*. Cambridge: Cambridge University Press, 1989.

Davis, Rabbi A., trans. *The Metsudah Siddur*. New York: Metsudah Publications, 1982.

de Tocqueville, Alexis. *Democracy in America*. New York: Vintage, 1945.

Dorff, Elliot N. "A Jewish Approach to End-Stage Medical Care." *Journal of Conservative Judaism* 43 (Spring 1991).

——. "Training Rabbis in the Land of the Free." In *The Seminary at 100: Reflections on the Jewish Theological Seminary and the Conservative Movement*, edited by Nina Beth Cardin and David Wolf Silverman, pp. 11–28. New York: Rabbinical Assembly and Jewish Theological Seminary of America, 1987.

Dougherty, Charles. "Ethical Values at Stake in Health Care Reform." *Journal of the American Medical Association* 268 (4 November 1992): 2409–12.

——. "The Proposal Will Deny Services to the Poor." *Health Progress* 21 (November 1990): 28–31.

——. "Setting Health Care Priorities: Oregon's Next Steps." *Hastings Center Report* 21 (May/June 1991): 1–5.

Dussel, Enrique. *Ethics and Community*. Maryknoll, N.Y: Orbis Books, 1988.

Eddy, David M. "Cost-Effective Analysis: A Conversation with My Father." *Journal of the American Medical Association* 267 (25 March 1992): 1669–74.

——. "Oregon's Plan: Should It Be Approved?" *Journal of the American Medical Association* 266 (6 January 1991): 2439–45.

Edwards, Paul, ed. *Encyclopedia of Philosophy*. Vols. 1, 3–4. New York: Macmillan, 1987.

Egan, Timothy. "Oregon Cut in Transplants Aid Spurs Victims to Turn Actor to Avert Death." *New York Times*, 30 April 1988.

Elazar, Daniel J. *American Federalism*. 3rd ed. New York: Harper and Row, 1984.

Englehardt, H. Tristan, ed. "Rights to Health Care." *Journal of Medicine and Philosophy* 4 (June 1979): 45–57.

Enthoven, Alain, and Richard Kronick. "A Consumer-Choice Health Plan for the 1990s:

Universal Health Insurance in a System Designed to Promote Quality and Economy." *New England Journal of Medicine* 320 (5, 12 January 1989): 29–37, 94–101.

Finkelman, Marilyn. "Self Defense and the Defense of Other in Jewish Law: The Rodef Defense." *Wayne Law Review* 33 (Summer 1987): 5–17.

Flax, Jane. *Thinking Fragments: Psychoanalysis, Feminism, and Postmodernism in the Contemporary West*. Berkeley: University of California Press, 1990.

Fox, Daniel M., and Howard M. Leichter. "Rationing Care in Oregon: The New Accountability." *Health Affairs* 10 (Summer 1991): 7–27.

Fox, Marvin. "Judaism, Secularism, and Textual Interpretation." In *Modern Jewish Ethics*, edited by Marvin Fox, pp. 4–5. Columbus: Ohio State University Press, 1975.

———, ed. *Modern Jewish Ethics*. Columbus: Ohio State University Press, 1975.

Friedman, Emily. "Rationing Healthcare: Crisis and Courage." *Healthcare Forum* 32 (November/December 1991): 10–12.

Garland, Michael J. "Justice, Politics, and Community: Expanding Access and Rationing Health Services in Oregon." *Journal of Law, Medicine, and Health Care* 20 (Spring/Summer 1992): 67–81.

Garland, Michael J., and Romana Hasnain. "Community Responsibility and the Development of Oregon's Health Care Priorities." *Business and Professional Ethics Journal* 9 (Fall–Winter 1990): 183–200.

Gerbert, Barbara. "Why Fear Persists: Health Care Professionals and AIDS." *Journal of the American Medical Association* 260 (16 December 1988): 3481–84.

Gilligan, Carol. *In a Different Voice: Psychological Theory and Woman's Development*. Cambridge, Mass.: Harvard University Press, 1982.

———. "Remapping the Moral Domain." In *Reconstructing Individualism: Autonomy, Individuality, and the Self in Western Thought*, edited by Thomas C. Heller, Morton Sosna, and David Wellbery, pp. 237–52. Stanford, Calif.: Stanford University Press, 1986.

Gillon, Raanan. "Basic Ethics." Presentation to the International Conference on Medical Ethics, Jerusalem, October 1991.

Golenski, John. "Grand Rounds: Ethics and Health Care Economics." Speech to the Kaiser Permanente Physician Group, San Francisco, December 1992.

———. "Justice and Health Care." Presentation to the Holy Cross Hospital System, Holy Cross Hospital, Salt Lake City, Utah, 18 February 1993.

———. "The Oregon Prioritization Experience." Speech to the American Association of Hospital Executives, Berkeley, May 1990.

Golenski, John, and Stephen Thompson. "The Impossible Solution: Expanding Access to Health Care and Reducing Costs." *Stanford Law and Policy Review*, Summer 1991, pp. 44–47.

Goodman, L. E. *Toward a Theory of Justice*. New Haven, Conn.: Yale University Press, 1991.

Government Accounting Office. *Medicaid Expands, Fiscal Problems Mount*. Washington, D.C.: Government Printing Office, 1991.

Hadorn, David. "The Oregon Priority-Setting Exercise: Quality of Life and Public Policy." *Hastings Center Report* 21 (May/June 1991), supplement: 11–16.

———. "The Problem of Discrimination in Health Care Priority Setting." *Journal of the American Medical Association* 268 (16 September 1992): 1439–54.

——. "Setting Health Care Priorities in Oregon: Cost Effectiveness Meets the Rule of Rescue." *Journal of the American Medical Association* 265 (1 May 1991): 2218–25.

Hardwig, John. "What about the Family?" *Hastings Center Report* 20 (March/April 1990): 5–10.

Harrison, Beverly Wildung. "Our Right to Choose: The Morality of Procreative Choice." In *Women's Consciousness, Women's Conscience,* edited by Barbara Andolsen, Christine Gudorf, and Mary Pellauer, pp. 101–21. Minneapolis: Winston Press, 1985.

Hartman, David. "Halakhah." In *Contemporary Jewish Religious Thought,* edited by Arthur A. Cohen and Paul Mendes-Flohr, pp. 309–17. New York: Charles Scribner's Sons, 1987.

——. *Joy and Responsibility.* Jerusalem: Ben-Zvi-Posner, 1978.

——. *Maimonides: Torah and Philosophic Quest.* Philadelphia: Jewish Publication Society, 1976.

Hauerwas, Stanley. "Communitarians and Medical Ethicists: or 'Why I Am None of the Above.' " Speech presented at the Birth of Bioethics Conference, Seattle, Wash., Fall 1992.

——. *Naming the Silences.* Grand Rapids, Mich.: William B. Erdmans, 1990.

——. *Suffering Presence: Theological Reflections on Medicine, the Mentally Handicapped, and the Church.* Notre Dame, Ind.: University of Notre Dame Press, 1986.

Heschel, Abraham Joshua. *Between God and Man.* Edited by Fritz A. Rothchild. New York: Free Press, 1959.

Hilps, Philip J. "Public Hospital Wait for Bed Can Be Days, U.S. Study Says." *New York Times,* 29 January 1992.

Hines, Brian. "Health Policy on the Town Meeting Agenda." *Hastings Center Report* 16 (April 1986): 5–8.

——. *Quality of Life in Allocating Health Care Resources: Principles Adopted by the Citizens Health Care Parliament, September 23–24, 1988.* Portland: Oregon Health Decisions, 1988.

Hirshmann, Nancy J. "Freedom, Recognition, and Obligation: A Feminist Approach to Political Theory." *American Political Science Review* 83 (December 1989).

Hobbes, Thomas. *Leviathan.* Selected and with an introduction by Richard S. Peters. Edited by Michael Oakeshott. London: Collier Books, 1962.

Hume, David. "Justice as Utility." In *Inquiry Concerning the Principles of Morals.* Indianapolis: Bobbs-Merrill, 1957.

——. *A Treatise of Human Nature.* Edited by L. A. Selby-Bigge. Oxford: Oxford University Press, 1978.

Jacobs, Louis. "The Relationship between Religion and Ethics in Jewish Thought." In *Contemporary Jewish Ethics,* edited by Menachem Marc Kellner, pp. 41–57. New York: Sanhedrin Press, 1974.

Jakobovits, Immanuel. *Jewish Medical Ethics.* New York: Bloch Publishing, 1959.

Jennings, Bruce. "A Grassroots Movement in Bioethics." *Hastings Center Report,* special supplement (June/July 1988).

Jewish Publication Society. *The Jewish Publication Society Torah Commentary.* Philadelphia: Jewish Publication Society, 1989.

Jonsen, Albert. "Bentham in a Box: Technology Assessment and Health Care Allocation." *Journal of Law, Medicine, and Health Care* 14 (1986): 172–74.

Kant, Immanuel. *Groundwork of the Metaphysics of Morals.* Translated by H. J. Paton. New York: Harper and Row, 1953.

Kellner, Menachem Marc, ed. *Contemporary Jewish Ethics.* New York: Sanhedrin Press, 1974.

Kirshner, Robert, trans. *Rabbinic Responsa of the Holocaust Era.* New York: Schocken Books, 1985.

Kitzhaber, John. "The Oregon Experience." Speech at the Bioethics Intensive Session, Oakland, Calif., 1988.

Lebacqz, Karen. "Humility in Health Care." *Journal of Medicine and Philosophy* 17 (1992).

——. *Six Theories of Justice.* Minneapolis: Augsburg Publishing House, 1986.

Leibowitz, Yeshayahu. "Commandments." In *Contemporary Jewish Religious Thought,* edited by Arthur A. Cohen and Paul Mendes-Flohr, pp. 67–81. New York: Charles Scribner's Sons, 1987.

Levinas, Emmanuel. *Ethics and Infinity.* Translated by Richard A. Cohen. Pittsburgh: Duquesne University Press, 1985.

——. "The Face." In *Ethics and Infinity,* translated by Richard A. Cohen, pp. 83–93. Pittsburgh: Duquesne University Press, 1985.

——. *Nine Talmudic Readings.* Translated and with an introduction by Annette Aronowicz. Bloomington: Indiana University Press, 1990.

——. "The Pact." In *The Levinas Reader,* edited by Sean Hand, pp. 211–26. Cambridge, Mass.: Basil Blackwell, 1986.

——. "Toward the Other." In *Nine Talmudic Readings,* translated and with an introduction by Annette Aronowicz, pp. 12–29. Bloomington: Indiana University Press, 1990.

Lewin, Tamar. "Health Care System Is Issue in Jailing of Uninsured Patient." *New York Times,* 8 January 1993.

Lichtenstein, Aaron. "Does Jewish Tradition Recognize an Ethics Independent of *Halakhah?*" In *Modern Jewish Ethics,* edited by Marvin Fox, pp. 62–88. Columbus: Ohio State University Press, 1975.

"Life Expectancy Differences Widen." *New York Times,* 16 March 1989.

Locke, John. *The Second Treatise of Government.* Indianapolis: Bobbs-Merrill, 1952.

Lumberg, George. "National Health Care Reform: An Aura of Inevitability Is upon Us." Editorial. *Journal of the American Medical Association* 265 (15 May 1991): 2566.

MacIntyre, Alasdair. *After Virtue.* Notre Dame, Ind.: University of Notre Dame Press, 1984.

——. *Whose Justice? Which Rationality?* Notre Dame, Ind.: University of Notre Dame Press, 1988.

Mahoney, John. *The Making of Moral Theology: A Study of the Roman Catholic Tradition.* Oxford: Clarendon Press, 1987.

Maimonides. *The Guide of the Perplexed.* Translated by Shlomo Pines. Chicago: University of Chicago Press, 1963.

——. *Mishnah Torah.* Translated by Isaac Klein. New Haven, Conn.: Yale University Press, 1972.

Matthiessen, Constance. "Code Blue." *Mother Jones*, November/December 1992, pp. 26–33, 62.

Menzel, Paul T. "Oregon's Denial: Disabilities and the Quality of Life." *Hastings Center Report* 22 (November/December 1992): 21–25.

———. "Some Ethical Costs of Rationing." *Journal of Law, Medicine, and Health Care* 20 (Spring/Summer 1992).

Meyer, Harris, and Brian McCormick. "Disability Law Fear: What Price Equal Access?" *American Medical News*, 9 November 1992.

Mill, John Stuart. *Utilitarianism*. Indianapolis: Bobbs-Merrill, 1971.

Montefiore, C. C., and H. Loewe. *A Rabbinic Anthology*. New York: Schocken Books, 1974.

Nozick, Robert. *Anarchy, State, and Utopia*. New York: Basic Books, 1974.

Ochs, Vanessa. *Words on Fire*. San Diego: Harcourt Brace Jovanovich, 1990.

Ogletree, Thomas W. *Hospitality to the Stranger*. Philadelphia: Fortress Press, 1985.

O'Neill, Patrick. "Profiles: Oregonians Awaiting Transplants." *Oregonian*, 24 November 1987.

———. "State Denies Funds for Two Transplants." *Oregonian*, 3 November 1987.

Oregon Health Services Commission. *Prioritization of Health Services: A Report to the Governor and the Legislature*. Salem, Ore.: Health Services Commission, 1991.

Oregon Legislative Assembly. Sixty-Fifth Regular Session, 1989. Senate Bills 27, 534, and 935.

Ozick, Cynthia. "Ruth." In *Congregation*, edited by David Rosenberg, pp. 361–82. San Diego: Harcourt Brace Jovanovich, 1987.

Pardes, Ilana. *Countertraditions in the Bible*. Cambridge, Mass.: Harvard University Press, 1992.

———. "Creation According to Eve." In *Countertraditions in the Bible*, pp. 13–37. Cambridge, Mass.: Harvard University Press, 1992.

Pinkerson, Mary Enid. "The Oregon Health Plan: A Story of an Experiment in Governance." Ph.D. dissertation, University of Southern California, 1992.

Plaskow, Judith. *Standing Again at Sinai*. San Francisco: Harper and Row, 1990.

Rabinowitz, L., trans. *Midrash Rabbah*. New York: Soncino Press, 1983.

Ramsey, Paul. *The Patient as Person*. New Haven, Conn.: Yale University Press, 1970.

Rawls, John. *A Theory of Justice*. Cambridge, Mass.: Harvard University Press, 1971.

Relman, Arnold. "The Trouble with Rationing." *New England Journal of Medicine* 323 (27 September 1990): 911–13.

Relman, Arnold, and Norman Levinsky. "Is Rationing Inevitable?" *New England Journal of Medicine* 322 (21 June 1990): 1808–16.

Robb, Carol S. "A Framework for Feminist Ethics." In *Women's Consciousness, Women's Conscience*, edited by Barbara Andolsen, Christine Gudorf, and Mary Pellauer, pp. 211–34. Minneapolis: Winston Press, 1985.

Roberts, Barbara. "Bush Blows It on Health Care." Letter to the editor. *New York Times*, 11 August 1992.

Rosenberg, David, ed. *Congregation*. San Diego: Harcourt Brace Jovanovich, 1987.

Rosner, Fred. *Medicine in the Bible and the Talmud*. New York: K'tav Publishing, 1989.

——. *Modern Medicine and Jewish Ethics*. New York: Yeshiva University Press, 1986.

Rosner, Fred, and J. David Bleich. *Jewish Bioethics*. New York: Sanhedrin Press, 1979.

Rothman, David J. "Rationing Life." *New York Review of Books*, 5 March 1992, pp. 32–37.

Sandel, Michael. "Justice and the Good." In *Liberalism and Its Critics*, edited by Michael Sandel, pp. 159–78. New York: New York University Press, 1984.

——. *Liberalism and the Limits of Justice*. Cambridge: Cambridge University Press, 1982.

Sasson, Jack M. "Ruth." In *The Literary Guide to the Hebrew Bible*, edited by Robert Alter and Frank Kermode, pp. 320–28. Harvard, Mass.: Belknap Press, 1987.

Schochet, Elijah Judah, trans. and interpreter. *A Responsum of Surrender*. Los Angeles: University of Judaism Press, 1973.

Slotki, Judah J. "Ruth: Introduction and Commentary." In *The Five Megilloth*, edited by A. Cohen, pp. 35–40. London: Soncino Press, 1975.

Sokel, Moshe. "Allocation of Scarce Medical Resources: A Philosophic Analysis of the Halakhic Sources." Paper presented at the Association of Jewish Studies, Boston, 1990.

Solomon, Robert C., and Mark C. Murphy, eds. *What Is Justice?* New York: Oxford University Press, 1990.

Soloveitchik, Joseph. *The Halachic Mind*. New York: Free Press, 1986.

Sontag, Susan. *AIDS as Metaphor*. New York: Farrar, Straus and Giroux, 1988.

Spicker, Stuart, and H. Tristan Englehardt Jr., eds. *Philosophical Medical Ethics: Its Nature and Significance*. N.p.: D. Reidel, 1977.

Spiegel, Claire, and Irene Wielawaski. "Care Rationed at Overcrowded County-USC." *Los Angeles Times*, 16 December 1991.

Steinberg, Abraham, ed. *Jewish Medical Law: Compiled from the "Tzitz Eliezer."* Translated by David Simas. Israel: Gefen Press, 1980.

Steinbrook, Robert, and Bernard Lo. "The Oregon Medicaid Demonstration Project: Will It Provide Adequate Medical Care?" *New England Journal of Medicine* 326 (30 January 1992): 340–44.

Stevens, William K. "Racial Difference Found in the Kind of Medical Care Americans Get." *New York Times*, 13 January 1989.

Stout, Jeffrey. *Ethics after Babel: The Language of Morals and Their Discontents*. Boston: Beacon Press, 1988.

Sullivan, Louis. "Oregon Health Plan Is Unfair to the Disabled." Letter to the editor. *New York Times*, 1 September 1992.

Sumner, L. W. *The Moral Foundation of Rights*. Oxford: Clarendon Press, 1989.

Swartz, William, and Henry Aaron. "The Achilles Heel of Health Care Rationing." *New York Times*, 9 July 1990.

The Talmud. Translated by Adin Steinsaltz. New York: Random House, 1991.

Talmud Balvi. Selections. New York: Soncino Press, 1964.

Taylor, Charles. "Atomism." In *Powers, Possessions, and Freedom*, edited by Alkis Kontos, pp. 75–103. Toronto: University of Toronto Press, 1979.

Tendler, Moshe. "Physician Reimbursement." Paper delivered at the Third International Conference of Medical Ethics, San Francisco, 1991.

Tz'enah Ur'enah. Translated by Miriam Stark Aakon. Vol. 3, *Devarim*. Jerusalem: Mesorah Publications, 1984.

Urbach, Ephraim. *The Sages*. Cambridge, Mass.: Harvard University Press, 1975.

Veatch, Robert M. *The Foundations of Justice*. New York: Oxford University Press, 1986.

———. *A Theory of Medical Ethics*. New York: Basic Books, 1979.

Walzer, Michael. *Exodus and Revolution*. New York: Basic Books, 1985.

———. *Spheres of Justice*. New York: Basic Books, 1983.

"Wasted Health Care Dollars." *Consumer Reports*, July 1992, pp. 435–50.

Webster's New World Dictionary of the American Language. S.v. "conscience." Cleveland, Ohio: World Publishing, 1966.

Weisbard, Alan J. "On the Bioethics of Jewish Law: The Case of Karen Quinlan." *Israel Law Review* 14 (July 1970): 337–68.

Wineburg, Samuel, and Laurie Zoloth-Dorfman. "Jewish Ethics." In *A Bibliographic Guide to the Comparative Study of Ethics*, edited by Mark Juergensmeyer and John Carmen, pp. 309–37. Cambridge: Cambridge University Press, 1991.

Winslow, Gerald R. *Triage and Justice*. Berkeley: University of California Press, 1982.

———. "Watching Coby Howard Die: Ethics, Economics, and Politics in the Allocation of Medical Care." *Bioethics News* 8 (July 1989): 2–3.

Wise, Paul H. "Infant Mortality as a Social Mirror." *New England Journal of Medicine* 326 (4 June 1992): 1558–59.

Zohar, Noam, Ernest Weinrib, Baruch Brody, and Baruch Levine. "Symposium: After the Rodef." *S'vara* 1 (Winter 1990): 51–73.

Zoloth-Dorfman, Dan. "Martin Buber: Religion, Community, and the Life of Dialogue." Unpublished paper, 1972.

Zoloth-Dorfman, Laurie. "Community and Conscience." Ph.D. dissertation, Graduate Theological Union, 1993.

———. "Methodology." In *Forming a Moral Community*, pp. 30–64. Berkeley: Bioethics Consultation Group, 1992.

Secondary Sources

Alford, Robert R. *Health Care Politics*. Chicago: University of Chicago Press, 1975.

Annas, George. "Adam Smith in the Emergency Room." *Hastings Center Report* 15 (August 1985): 6–8.

———. *The Rights of Patients*. 2nd ed. Carbondale: Southern Illinois University Press, 1989.

Arato, Andrew, and Eike Genhardt. *The Essential Frankfurt School Reader*. New York: Continuum Publishing, 1985.

Aronowicz, Annette. "Emmanuel Levinas's Talmudic Commentaries: The Relation of the Jewish Tradition to the Non-Jewish World." In *Contemporary Jewish Ethics and Morality: A Reader*, edited by Louis E. Newman and Elliot N. Dorff, pp. 212–18. New York: Oxford University Press, 1995.

Arras, John, and Andrew Jameton. "Medical Individualism and the Right to Health Care." In *Intervention and Reflection: Basic Issues in Medical Ethics*, edited by Ronold Munson. Belmont, Calif.: Wadsworth, 1979.

Arras, John, and Nancy Rhoden, eds. *Ethical Issues in Modern Medicine*. 3rd ed. Pt. 6,

"Allocation, Social Justice, Health Policy." Mountain View, Calif.: Mayfield Publishing, 1989.

Barry, Brian. *Theories of Justice*. Berkeley: University of California Press, 1989.

Bayer, Ronald, Arthur Caplan, and Norman Daniels, eds. *In Search of Equity: Health Need and the Health Care System*. New York: Plenum Press, 1983.

Beauchamp, Dan E. "Community: The Neglected Tradition of Public Health." *Hastings Center Report* 15 (December 1985): 4–6.

——. "Public Health as Social Justice." *Inquiry*, March 1976, pp. 9–17.

Bellah, Robert N. *The Broken Covenant*. New York: Seabury Press, 1975.

Berger, Peter L. *The Sacred Canopy*. New York: Anchor, 1969.

Blank, Robert H. *Life, Death, and Public Policy*. Dekalb: Northern Illinois University Press, 1988.

Bleich, J. David. *Judaism and Healing*. New York: K'tav Publishing, 1987.

Blendon, Robert J., and Drew E. Altman. "Public Attitudes about Health Care: A Lesson in National Schizophrenia." *New England Journal of Medicine* 311 (30 August 1984): 643–47.

Byrne, Peter, ed. *Health, Rights, and Resources*. Kings College Studies, 1987–88. London: King Edward's Hospital Fund for London, 1988.

Califano, Joseph A. *America's Health Care Revolution: Who Lives? Who Dies? Who Pays?* New York: Random House, 1986.

Callahan, Daniel. "Minimalist Ethics." *Hastings Center Report* 11 (October 1981): 19–25.

Carter, Stephen. *The Culture of Disbelief*. New York: Anchor, 1994.

Churchill, Larry R. "Reviving a Distinctive Medical Ethics." *Hastings Center Report* 19 (May/June 1989): 28–34.

Code, Lorraine. *Epistemic Responsibility*. Hanover, N.H.: University of New England Press, 1987.

——, ed. *Philosophic Essays in Method and Morals*. Toronto: University of Toronto Press, 1988.

Cohen, Alfred. "Halachic Aspects of Organ Transplants." *Journal of Halacha and Contemporary Society*, no. 5 (1983): 8–13.

Curran, Charles E. *Directions in Fundamental Moral Theology*. Notre Dame, Ind.: University of Notre Dame Press, 1985.

Dan, Joseph. *Jewish Mysticism and Jewish Ethics*. Philadelphia: Jewish Publication Society of America, 1986.

deKerrasdaude, Jean, John Kimberly, Victor G. Rodurn. *The End of an Illusion*. Berkeley: University of California Press, 1989.

Dorff, Elliot N. *Choose Life: A Jewish Approach to Medical Ethics*. Los Angeles: University Papers, University of Judaism, 1987.

Dorff, Elliot N., and Arthur Rosett. *A Living Tree: The Roots and Growth of Jewish Law*. Albany: State University of New York Press, 1986.

Dworkin, Gerald. *The Theory and Practice of Autonomy*. Cambridge: Cambridge University Press, 1988.

Dworkin, Ronald. "The Right to Death." *New York Review of Books*, 31 January 1991, pp. 2–7.

——. *Taking Rights Seriously*. Cambridge, Mass.: Harvard University Press, 1977.

Easton, Lloyd D., and Kurt H. Guddat, eds. *Writings of the Young Marx on Philosophy and Society*. Garden City, N.Y.: Anchor, 1967.

Elazar, Daniel J. *Community and Polity*. Philadelphia: Jewish Publication Society, 1980.

Elazar, Daniel J., and Stuart Cohen. *The Jewish Polity*. Bloomington: Indiana University Press, 1985.

Englehardt, H. T., ed. "Rights to Health Care." *Journal of Medicine and Philosophy* 4 (June 1979).

Fein, Rashi. "On Achieving Access and Equity in Health Care." *Milbank Quarterly* 50 (1972): 53–70.

Feldman, David M. *Health and Medicine in the Jewish Tradition*. New York: Crossroad Publishing, 1986.

——. *Marital Relations, Birth Control, and Abortion in Jewish Law*. New York: Schocken Books, 1974.

Feldman, David M., and Fred Rosner. *Compendium on Medical Ethics*. 6th ed. New York: Federation of Jewish Philanthropies of New York, 1989.

Fisher, Sue. *In the Patient's Best Interest: Women and the Politics of Medical Decisions*. New Brunswick, N.J.: Rutgers University Press, 1988.

Fox, Renee C., Linda H. Aiken, and Carla M. Messikomer. "The Culture of Caring: AIDS and the Nursing Profession." *Milbank Quarterly* 68, supp. 2 (1990): 12–23.

Frankena, William K. *Ethics*. 2nd ed. Englewood Cliffs, N.J.: Prentice Hall, 1973.

Gilligan, Carol, Jamie Victoria Ward, and Jill McLean Taylor, eds. *Mapping the Moral Domain*. Cambridge, Mass.: Harvard University Press, 1988.

Gillon, Raanan. *Philosophical Medical Ethics*. Chichester, England: John Wiley and Sons, 1985.

Ginsburg, Eli. *American Medicine*. Totowa, N.J.: Rowner and Allanheld, 1985.

Glendon, Mary Ann. *Rights Talk: The Impoverishment of Political Discourse*. Boston: Free Press, 1991.

Golenski, John. "Executive Summary." Oregon Basic Health Service Act, Summary of Bill 27, 31 March 1989.

——. "A Report on the Oregon Medical Priority Setting Project." Unpublished manuscript, 1990.

Green, Ronald. "Contemporary Jewish Bioethics: A Cultural Assessment." In *Theology and Bioethics*, edited by Earl Shelp, pp. 245–67. Dordreek, Netherlands: D. Reidel Publishing, 1985.

——. "Health Care and Justice in Contract Theory Perspective." In *Ethics and Health Policy*, edited by Robert Veatch and Roy Branson, pp. 113–20. Cambridge, Mass.: Ballinger, 1976.

Greenspahn, Frederick E. *Contemporary Ethical Issues in the Jewish and Christian Traditions*. Hoboken, N.J.: K'tav Publishing, 1986.

Gusfield, Joseph R. *Community: A Critical Response*. New York: Harper and Row, 1975.

Hardin, Garrett. "The Tragedy of the Commons." *Science*, 13 December 1968, pp. 1243–48.

Harrison, Beverly Wildung. "The Dream of a Common Language: Towards a Normative

Theory of Justice in Christian Ethics." In *The Annual of the Society of Christian Ethics*, 1983. Dallas, Tex.: Society of Christian Ethics, Perkins School of Theology, Southern Methodist University, 1983.

Hauerwas, Stanley. *A Community of Character: Toward a Constructive Christian Social Ethic*. Notre Dame, Ind.: University of Notre Dame Press, 1981.

——. *Who Is Man?* Stanford, Calif.: Stanford University Press, 1965.

Hiatt, Howard H. "Protecting the Medical Commons: Who Is Responsible?" *New England Journal of Medicine* 293 (31 July 1975): 235–41.

Jacob, Walter. *Contemporary American Reform Responsa*. New York: Central Conference of American Rabbis, 1987.

Jonsen, Albert R. "Responsibility as a Principle in Contemporary Religious Ethics." Ph.D. dissertation, Yale University, 1967.

Jonsen, Albert R., and Stephen Toulmin. *The Abuse of Casuistry*. Berkeley: University of California Press, 1988.

Kilner, John F. *Who Lives, Who Dies? Ethical Criteria in Patient Selection*. New Haven, Conn.: Yale University Press, 1990.

Kittay, Eva Feder, and Diana T. Meyers. *Women and Moral Theory*. Savage, Md.: Rowman and Littlefield, 1987.

Langan, John. "Defining Human Rights: A Revision of the Liberal Tradition." In *Human Rights in the Americas: The Struggle for Consensus*, edited by Alfred Hennely, S.J., and John Langan, S.J., pp. 97–135. Washington, D.C.: Georgetown University Press.

Lebacqz, Karen. *Justice in an Unjust World*. Minneapolis: Augsburg Publishing House, 1987.

——, ed. *Genetics, Ethics, and Parenthood*. New York: Pilgrim Press, 1983.

Levinas, Emmanuel. *Difficult Freedoms: Essays on Judaism*. Baltimore: John Hopkins University Press, 1990.

Lifton, Robert Jay. *The Nazi Doctors*. New York: Basic Books, 1986.

McKinley, John. *Issues in the Political Economy of Health Care*. New York: Tavistock Publications, 1989.

Marty, Micah, ed. *Healthy People 2000: A Role for America's Religious Communities*. Chicago: Park Ridge Center, 1990.

Meir, Levi. *Values in Bioethics*. New York: Human Science Press, 1986.

Meiselman, Moshe. "Ethical Issues in the Treatment of Kidney Failures." In *Sourcebook for Halachic Resources for Contemporary Ethical Dilemmas*, pp. 57–64. Los Angeles: Yeshiva University of Los Angeles.

Melhade, Evan, Walter Feinberg, and Harold Swartz, eds. *Money, Power, and Health Care*. Ann Arbor, Mich.: Health Administration Press, 1988.

Menzel, Paul T. *Medical Costs, Moral Choices*. New Haven, Conn.: Yale University Press, 1983.

——. *Strong Medicine: The Ethical Rationing of Health Care*. New York: Oxford University Press, 1990.

Mill, John Stuart. *On Liberty*. New York: Viking Penguin, 1988.

Moony, Gavin, and Alistair McGuire, eds. *Medical Ethics and Economics in Health Care*. Oxford: Oxford University Press, 1988.

National Leadership Commission on Health Care. *For the Health of a Nation*. Ann Arbor, Mich.: Health Administration Press, 1989.

Niebuhr, H. Richard. *The Responsible Self*. San Francisco: Harper and Row, 1963.

Niebuhr, Reinhold. *Moral Man and Immoral Society*. New York: Charles Scribner's Sons, 1960.

O'Brien, Mary. *Reproducing the World: Essays in Feminist Theory*. Boulder, Colo.: Westview Press, 1989.

O'Neill, Patrick. "Health Panel Seeks Areas for Priority List." *Oregonian*, 20 May 1990.

——. "Health Plan Spawns Epidemic of Doubt." *Oregonian*, 19 May 1990.

——. "Reformers Define Basic Care." *Oregonian*, 21 May 1990.

Oregon Catholic Conference. "Testimony before the Senate Health Insurance and Bioethics Committee on SB 523," 21 February 1989.

Outka, Gene. "Social Justice and Equal Access to Health Care." *Journal of Religious Ethics* 2 (1974): 54–70.

Plato. *Plato's Republic*. Translated by G. M. A. Grube. Indianapolis: Hackett Publishing, 1974.

Ratcliff, Kathryn Strother, ed. *Healing Technology: Feminist Perspectives*. Ann Arbor: University of Michigan Press, 1989.

Rosenberg, Charles B. *Care of Strangers: The Rise of America's Hospital System*. New York: Basic Books, 1987.

Rosner, Fred. *Medicine in the Mishneh Torah of Maimonides*. New York: K'tav Publishing, 1989.

——, ed. *Biblical and Talmudic Medicine*. New York: Sanhedrin Press, 1978.

Rosner, Fred, and Moses Tendler, eds. *Practical Medical Halacha*. Jerusalem: Feldheim Publishers, 1980.

Rotenstreich, Nathan. *Jewish Philosophy in Modern Times*. New York: Holt, Rinehart and Winston, 1968.

Rousseau, Jean-Jacques. *The First and Second Discourses*. Edited and translated by Roger D. Masters. New York: St. Martin's Press, 1964.

Schuller, Bruno. *Wholly Human: Essays on the Theory and Language of Morality*. Washington, D.C.: Georgetown University Press, 1986.

Spero, Shubert. *Morality, Halakha, and the Jewish Tradition*. New York: K'tav Publishing, 1983.

Spohn, William C. *What Are They Saying about Scripture and Ethics?* New York: Paulist Press, 1984.

Tamari, Meir. *With All Your Possessions: Jewish Ethics and Economic Life*. New York: Free Press, 1987.

Tendler, Moses D. *Medical Ethics*. 5th ed. New York: Federation of Jewish Philanthropies, 1975.

Toulmin, Stephen. "The Tyranny of Principles." *Hastings Center Report* 11 (December 1981): 31–39.

U.S. Bipartisan Commission on Comprehensive Health Care. "A Call for Action." Pepper Commission, Final Report. Washington, D.C.: United States Bipartisan Commission on Comprehensive Health Care, 1 September 1990.

Weiss, Raymond, and Charles Butterworth, eds. *Ethical Writings of Maimonides*. New York: Dover Publishing, 1975.

Wolfe, Alan. *Whose Keeper? Social Science and Moral Obligation*. Berkeley: University of California Press, 1989.

Zborowski, Mark. *People in Pain*. San Francisco: Jossey-Bass, 1961; Ann Arbor, Mich.: University Microfilms, 1981.

Computer-based Material

Bar Elan University Responsa Project: Complete and Historical Listing of all Rabbinic Responsa. Bar Elan University, Israel, 1990.

The Computerized Torah Repository: The On-Line Pentateuch, Mishnah, and Gemara. B'nai B'rok, Israel, 1991.

INDEX

●

Abaye, 175
Abraham, Abraham, 167
Ackerman, Bruce, 108–9
Aggadah, 127, 135, 140, 195, 198, 225
Aging, 12, 13, 58
AIDS patients, 13, 24, 254 (n. 2)
Aid to Families with Dependent Children (AFDC), 22, 24–25, 65
Akiba, R., 161, 162, 163–64, 165, 166, 190, 198
Alabama, 23
American Medical Association, 20
Americans with Disabilities Act, 258 (n. 64)
Anderson, John, 45
Apel, Karl-Otto, 112
Arendt, Hannah, 152
Argument: and communicative ethics, 113; and Jewish ethics, 122, 126–27, 129; and halakhah, 127, 133, 150, 160, 170, 281 (n. 97); and midrash, 128
Aristotle: and bioethics, 8; and humans as social, 58; and justice, 74, 75, 125, 260 (n. 10); and communitarianism, 97–98; and moral agency, 102, 104–5; and rationality, 109; and Maimonides, 140–41; and civic friendship, 196–97; and communicative ethics, 275 (n. 79)
Autonomy: and resource allocation, xi; and liberal theory, xii, 153, 157–59; and common good, 8; and bioethics, 14–15, 93, 95, 97, 228–29, 258 (n. 42); and community, 15, 229, 236; and OHD, 28; and rationing, 54–56; and patients, 55, 60, 74, 95, 256–57 (n. 31); and citizen participation, 69; language of, 74, 93, 96; and libertarian theory of justice, 76–77; and deontology, 85–86; and procedural justice, 87–88; and justice,

92; religious perspectives on, 94; and self, 95–97, 114; and rights theory, 97; and communitarianism, 98; and individualism, 99; and moral agency, 101; and Enlightenment, 101, 110, 157, 240; and Hobbes, 105; and germ theory, 110; and scarce resources, 160; and privacy, 241–42; and health care justice, 255 (n. 15); and Hardwig, 256 (n. 31); and religious ethics, 272 (n. 39); and family values, 289 (n. 29)
Avadim, 217

Baraita, 162
Beauchamp, Tom, 56
Begadav, 146–47
Beiner, Ronald, 96–97, 100–101, 108–9, 112
Bellah, Robert, xi, 98–100, 197, 226, 269 (n. 24)
Beneficence: and bioethics, 8, 14, 56; and rationing, 54–56; and physicians, 55–56, 95, 257 (n. 31); and justice theories, 76; and health care justice, 255 (n. 14)
Benhabib, Seyla, 112–15, 225, 238, 275 (n. 79), 276 (n. 88), 280 (n. 78)
Benjamin, Martin, 226, 229–30, 291 (n. 9)
Berlin, Naftali Zvi Yehuda, 164
Bet midrash, 123
Biale, David, 280 (n. 65)
Biblical narrative, 103, 197–98, 288 (nn. 11, 12). *See also* Ruth story; specific books of the Bible
Bioethics: case stories of, 3–8; and beneficence, 8, 56; language of, 8, 75–76, 92–93; and religious ethics, 10; and autonomy, 14–15, 93, 95, 97, 228–29, 258 (n. 42); and OHD, 27, 29; and physician/patient encounter, 54–56, 60, 222;

Relman, Arnold, 63
Resource allocation: and justice, xi, 50,
73, 93, 124; and Jewish textual tradition, xi–xii, 167–71; government's role
in, 36, 37; and social good services, 49–
50; and libertarian theory of justice,
78; and Rawls, 89; and indivisible resources, 167–71; and Ruth story, 211–
13; and language, 219; and needs,
274 (n. 56). *See also* Health care—
allocation
Responsibility: and language of community, xi, 14; and stranger/self encounter,
146–47, 149; and mitzvot, 149–50; and
Buber, 156; and Ruth story, 204–6; and
citizenship, 226
Right act, 124, 126, 151, 159
Rights theory: and common good, 9; and
health care justice, 53–54, 255 (n. 17);
and rationing, 66; language of, 74, 93,
105–6, 108, 111, 273 (n. 43); and Mill,
82–83; and autonomy, 97; and social
contracts, 105–6, 273 (n. 42); and Jewish ethics, 157–58; and deontology, 264
(n. 51)
Robb, Carol, 121, 124, 134, 140, 144, 151,
159, 255 (n. 17)
Roberts, Barbara, 69–70
Rodef, 169, 184, 186–89, 196, 287 (n. 49)
Roosevelt, Franklin D., 268 (n. 18)
Rosner, Fred, 161–62, 167
Roth, Henry, 269 (n. 24)
Rousseau, Jean-Jacques, 261 (n. 20)
Ruth story: and justice, xiii, 198, 201, 209,
212, 216, 217–18; interpretations of,
134; and halakhah, 163; and scarce resources, 198, 200–204, 209, 211, 215, 219;
and marginal as central, 199–217; language of, 200, 207–8, 210, 211, 213, 216–
20; and community, 200–204, 216–18;
and citizenship, 204–6, 216, 218; and
stranger/self encounter, 206–19 pas-
sim; and Ruth's conversion, 209–10,
290 (n. 41); and resource allocation,
211–13; and kinship, 213–14; and ethics of encounter, 223, 226, 245; and
bioethics, 224; and public policy, 225;
and moral community, 230, 237; and

Oregon health care reform plan, 238;
and Jonah, 290 (n. 36)

Saint Augustine, 136
Salanter, Israel, 283 (n. 115)
Sandel, Michael, 98, 104–5, 108, 275
(n. 79)
Sasson, Jack, 201
Scarce resources: and allocation of public goods, xi–xii, 73; and health care allocation, xii; and health care access,
38; and health care justice, 47, 52, 119;
and justice, 49, 52, 54–62, 91, 198, 266
(n. 83); and utilitarian theory of justice, 83; and procedural justice, 88;
and Hume, 92; and needs, 106; and
Jewish ethics, 116, 159, 240; and autonomy, 160; and Jewish textual tradition,
160–67, 197; and halakhah, 194; and
Ruth story, 198, 200–204, 209, 211, 215,
219; and language, 218–19; and health
care reform, 223, 226; and Locke, 260
(n. 16)
*Schlondorff v. The Society of New York
City Hospital*, 55
Schochet, Elijah, 172, 178, 181
Secular ethics, xii, 10, 121, 153
Self: and community, 9, 99, 102, 112, 115,
181, 192, 224, 270 (n. 28), 271 (n. 34);
and citizen participation, 27; and liberal theory, 94, 98; and society, 95,
96, 99; and autonomy, 95–97, 114;
and communitarianism, 98, 104–5;
and social contracts, 105; and rationality, 109, 274 (n. 61); as male and autonomous, 114; and Jewish textual tradition, 116; and Jewish ethics, 122, 158;
and Levinas, 148, 150; and Buber, 156,
282 (n. 112); and conscience, 230; defense of, 241; and justice, 275 (n. 68).
See also Stranger/self encounter
Shamash, 171, 172
Shimon ben Gamiel, Rabbi, 174, 175, 176
Shlomo Abu Zimra, David ben, 177
Shlomo ben Yehiel Luria, Rabbi, 180
Shostack, Daniel, 250 (n. 41)
Simon, Ernst, 143
Simpson, O. J., 239